Molecular Pathology
in Clinical Practice: Infectious Diseases

Molecular Pathology in Clinical Practice: Infectious Diseases

Editor

Debra G.B. Leonard, MD, PhD
Professor and Vice Chair for Laboratory Medicine, Department of Pathology and Laboratory Medicine, Weill Medical College of Cornell University and New York Presbyterian Hospital, New York, New York

Section Editor Infectious Diseases

Angela M. Caliendo, MD, PhD
Vice Chair and Associate Professor, Department of Pathology and Laboratory Medicine, Emory University Hospital, Atlanta, Georgia

Section Editors

Adam Bagg, MD
Director, Hematology, Department of Pathology and Laboratory Medicine, University of Pennsylvania, Philadelphia, Pennsylvania

Karen L. Kaul, MD, PhD
Professor, Northwestern University Feinberg School of Medicine, Evanston, Illinois; Department of Pathology and Laboratory Medicine, Evanston Northwestern Healthcare, Evanston, Illinois

Vivianna M. Van Deerlin, MD, PhD
Director, Molecular Pathology Laboratory, Department of Pathology and Laboratory Medicine, University of Pennsylvania Health System, Philadelphia, Pennsylvania

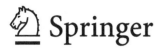
Springer

Editor

Debra G.B. Leonard, MD, PhD
Professor and Vice Chair for Laboratory Medicine, Department of Pathology and Laboratory Medicine, Weill Medical College of Cornell University and New York Presbyterian Hospital, New York, New York

Section Editor Infectious Diseases

Angela M. Caliendo, MD, PhD
Vice Chair and Associate Professor, Department of Pathology and Laboratory Medicine, Emory University Hospital, Atlanta, Georgia

Section Editors

Adam Bagg, MD
Director, Hematology, Department of Pathology and Laboratory Medicine, University of Pennsylvania, Philadelphia, Pennsylvania

Karen L. Kaul, MD, PhD
Professor, Northwestern University Feinberg School of Medicine, Evanston, Illinois; Department of Pathology and Laboratory Medicine, Evanston Northwestern Healthcare, Evanston, Illinois

Vivianna M. Van Deerlin, MD, PhD
Director, Molecular Pathology Laboratory, Department of Pathology and Laboratory Medicine, University of Pennsylvania Health System, Philadelphia, Pennsylvania

ISBN 978-0-387-87367-1   ISBN 978-0-387-87369-5 (eBook)
DOI 10.1007/978-0-387-87369-5

Library of Congress Control Number: 2008934314

Printed on acid-free paper

springer.com

To Greg
With love and thanks

Preface

Molecular pathology is the newest area of pathology subspecialty practice, with the first molecular genetic pathology board examination having been given by the American Board of Pathology and the American Board of Medical Genetics in November 2001. The primary boards in anatomic and clinical pathology given by the American Board of Pathology have an increasing emphasis on molecular pathology knowledge in general pathology practice. The clinical practice of molecular pathology is becoming fundamental to almost every aspect of healthcare delivery, assisting with diagnosis of disease, therapeutic choice, therapeutic outcome monitoring, prognosis, prediction of disease risk, directing preventive strategies, beginning-of-life decisions, patient and specimen identification, and clinical epidemiology. With this growing emphasis on molecular pathology, a textbook focused on the clinical practice of molecular pathology is essential.

While the original textbook *Molecular Pathology in Clinical Practice* addresses all areas of molecular pathology clinical practice in a single textbook, *Molecular Pathology in Clinical Practice: Infectious Diseases* contains only the chapters relevant to infectious disease molecular pathology practice. The purpose of this textbook focused on molecular infectious disease testing is to provide a comprehensive reference for individuals whose practice is more focused on medical microbiology. *Molecular Pathology in Clinical Practice: Infectious Diseases* is not a meant to be a recipe book for molecular tests currently in clinical practice. Instead, the emphasis of this volume is on the molecular variations being detected for clinical use, how test results are used, and clinical and specific laboratory issues that require special attention.

Molecular Pathology in Clinical Practice: Infectious Diseases aims to present the current state of our knowledge about molecular infectious disease testing. Some of the chapters include relatively nascent knowledge that is anticipated to be useful for clinical practice in the future, while other chapters present testing that is better established. My hope, as editor of this textbook, is that many editions will be needed in the future as we continue to apply the fruits of the Human Genome Project to the practice of medicine, resulting in improved outcomes for our patients.

Debra G.B. Leonard, MD, PhD

Contents

Contributors

Angela M. Caliendo, MD, PhD
Vice Chair and Associate Professor, Department of Pathology and Laboratory Medicine, Emory University Hospital, Atlanta, GA 30322, USA

Daniel H. Farkas PhD, HCLD
Director, Molecular Diagnostics, Department of Pathology, The Methodist Hospital, Houston, TX, 77030; Associate Professor, Department of Pathology and Laboratory Medicine, Weill Medical College of Cornell University, New York, NY 10021, USA

Andrea Ferreira-Gonzalez, PhD
Professor, Department of Pathology, Director, Department of Molecular Diagnostics Laboratory, Molecular Diagnostics, Virginia Commonwealth University, Richmond, VA 23298, USA

Betty A. Forbes, PhD
Professor, Department of Pathology and Medicine, Virginia Common University Health Systems; Medical College of Virginia Campus, Richmond, VA 23298, USA

Julie D. Fox, BSc, PhD, MRCPath (UK)
Associate Professor, Microbiology and Infectious Diseases and Provincial Laboratory for Public Health (Microbiology), University of Calgary, Calgary, Alberta T2N 4W4, Canada

Christine C. Ginocchio, PhD, MT (ASCP)
Director, Microbiology/Virology and Molecular Diagnostics, North Shore Long Island Health System Laboratories, Lake Success, NY 11042, USA

Jeanne A. Jordan, PhD
Associate Professor, Department of Pathology, University of Pittsburgh/Magee Women's Hospital, Pittsburgh, PA 15213, USA

Debra G.B. Leonard, MD, PhD
Professor and Vice Chair for Laboratory Medicine, Department of Pathology and Laboratory Medicine, Weill Medical College of Cornell University and New York Presbyterian Hospital, New York, NY 10065, USA

Ruth Ann Luna, MS
Assistant Director, Molecular Microbiology Laboratory, Department of Pathology, Baylor College of Medicine, Houston, TX 77030, USA

Frederick S. Nolte, PhD, D (ABMM), F (AAM)
Professor, Pathology and Laboratory Medicine, Emory University School of Medicine; Director, Clinical Microbiology and Molecular Diagnostic Laboratories, Emory Medical Laboratories, Atlanta, GA 30322, USA

Deborah Ann Payne, PhD, ClSp(MB), CLDir(NCA)D
Associate Professor, Director of Molecular Diagnostics, Department of Pathology, University of Texas Southwestern Medical Center-Veripath, Dallas, TX 75390, USA

Joseph F. Pulliam, MD
Department of Pathology, Baylor College of Medicine, Methodist Hospital, Houston, TX 77030, USA

Hanna Rennert, PhD, FACMG
Director, Molecular Pathology Laboratory, Department of Pathology and Laboratory Medicine, New York Presbyterian Hospital, Weill Medical College of Cornell University, New York, NY 10065, USA

Megan J. Smith-Zagone, MD
Pathologist, St Joseph Hospital, Eureka, CA 95501, USA

Karen Snow-Bailey, PhD, FACMG, FHGSA
Director, Department of Diagnostic Genetics, LabPlus, Auckland District Health Board, Auckland, New Zealand

Peter A. Tilley, MD, FRCPC
Medical Microbiologist, Department of Microbiology and Infectious Diseases and Provincial Laboratory for Public Health (Microbiology), University of Calgary, Calgary, Alberta T2N 4W4, Canada

James Versalovic, MD, PhD
Assistant Professor, Department of Pathology and Molecular Virology and Microbiology, Baylor College of Medicine; Director, Microbiology Laboratories, Texas Children's Hospital, Houston, TX 77030, USA

Chapter 1

Basics of Molecular Biology

Deborah Ann Payne

Introduction

Molecular biology entails the analysis and study of the chemical organization of the cell. Molecules comprise the smallest chemical component capable of performing all the activities (structural or catalytic) of a substance. One or more atoms constitute each molecule. This chapter describes the physical organization of cells, cellular organelles, and molecules important in cell division, inheritance, and protein synthesis.

Organization of the Cell

The cell is a mass of protoplasm surrounded by a semipermeable membrane.[1] Cells constitute the smallest element of living matter capable of functioning independently; however, within complex organisms, cells may require interaction with other cells. To function independently, cells must produce nucleic acids, proteins, lipids, and energy. In complex organisms, these organic processes form and maintain tissues and the organism as a whole.

Genes consist of discrete regions of nucleic acids that encode proteins, and control the function of the cell. Deoxyribonucleic acid (DNA) and ribonucleic acid (RNA) comprise the two types of nucleic acids found in all cells. Chromosomes, made up of double-stranded DNA complexed with proteins, contain all the genes required for the cell to live and function.

Prokaryotic Cells

Prokaryotic cells are simple organisms lacking subcellular compartments, such as bacteria. The majority of prokaryotic nucleic acids form circular strands comprising approximately 1×10^6 base pairs (bp) (Table 1-1). Additional extrachromosomal genetic elements consist of circular plasmids also known as episomes and linear mobile genetic elements called transposons (30–40 bp). Plasmids range in size from 33 bp to 230 bp[2] and first gained notoriety in the 1950s by being associated with antibiotic resistance in bacteria.[3,4] Transposons also may confer antibiotic resistance on the host bacteria. All these genetic elements exist in direct contact with the bacteria's cytoplasm.

Eukaryotic Cells

Cytoplasm

In contrast to prokaryotic cells, eukaryotic cells are complex, highly compartmentalized structures. The cytoplasm contains multiple membrane-bound compartments known as organelles. The cellular membrane separates the cellular cytoplasm from the external environment. The membranes consist of hydrophobic lipid bilayers. The lipid bilayer contains proteins that serve as receptors and channels.

Nucleus and Nucleolus

The nucleus of the cell contains the cell's linear chromosomes and serves as the primary locus of inherited genetic material. Inner- and outer-pore-containing membranes define the nucleus and separate the chromosomes from the surrounding cytoplasm. Further partitioning occurs within the nucleus to generate the nucleolus, which functions as the ribosome-generating factory of the cell. Instead of additional membranes, fibrous protein complexes separate the nucleolus from the rest of the nucleus. In this structure, the nucleolus organizer (a specific part of a chromosome containing the genes that encode ribosomal RNA) interacts with other molecules to form immature large and small ribosomal subunits. Following processing, immature subunits exit the nucleolus and enter the nucleus. Eventually, mature ribosomal subunits and other molecules exit the nucleolus through the nuclear pores and enter the cytoplasm.

Table 1-1. Comparison of DNA Sizes of Various Genetic Elements

Genomic Element	Size in Base Pairs
Human chromosome	$1–3 \times 10^9$
Bacterial chromosome	$1–4 \times 10^6$
Mitochondrial chromosome	16,569
Bacteriophage	39,000
CAM plasmid	230
R388 plasmid	33
Transposons	30–40

Mitochondria

Mitochondria are membrane-bound organelles within the cytoplasm of cells that have several cellular functions. Inheritable genetic material, independent from the nuclear chromosomes, resides in mitochondria. These maternally derived organelles contain their own circular chromosomes (16,569 bp) and replicate independently from the cell and one another. As a result, not all mitochondria in a given cell have the same mitochondrial chromosomal sequence, resulting in genetic diversity of these organelles within and between different cells of the same organism, which is known as heteroplasmy. Mitochondrial genes encode mitochondria-specific transfer RNA molecules (tRNA). In addition, the mitochondrial chromosomes contain genes that encode proteins used in oxidative phosphorylation, including subunits of the cytochrome c oxidase, cytochrome b complex, some of the ATPase complex and various subunits of NAD dehydrogenase. Other components of the oxidative phosphorylation pathway are encoded by nuclear genes. For this reason, not all mitochondrial genetic diseases demonstrate maternal transmission. Analysis of mitochondrial DNA has applications for diagnosis of mitochondrial-inherited genetic diseases as well as for forensic purposes in the identification of severely decomposed bodies.

Other Cellular Organelles

Membranes not only segregate heritable genetic molecules into the nucleus and mitochondria, but also separate various cellular functions into distinct areas of the cell. The compartmentalization of cellular functions, such as molecular synthesis, modification, and catabolism, increases the local concentration of reactive molecules, thus improving the cell's biochemical efficiency. This partitioning also protects inappropriate molecules from becoming substrates for these processes. One example of this segregation is the endoplasmic reticulum (ER), which consists of a complex of membranous compartments where proteins are synthesized. Glycoproteins are synthesized by ribosome-ER complexes known as rough ER (RER), while lipids are produced in the smooth ER. The Golgi apparatus consists of numerous membrane-bound sacs where molecules generated in the ER become modified for transportation out of the cell.

In addition, peroxisomes and lysosomes segregate digestive and reactive molecules from the remainder of the cellular contents to prevent damage to the cell's internal molecules and infrastructure.

Biological Molecules

Carbon can covalently bond to several biologically important atoms (i.e., oxygen, hydrogen, and nitrogen) and forms the scaffold for all biomolecules. Basic subunit biomolecules can combine to form more complex molecules such as carbohydrates, nucleic acids, and amino acids.

Carbohydrates

Carbohydrates serve as energy reservoirs and are a component of nucleic acids. In addition, carbohydrates also attach to lipids and proteins. The basic unit of a carbohydrate consists of the simple sugars or monosaccharides. These molecules have carbon, oxygen, and hydroxyl groups that most commonly form ringed structures. The oxygen can react with the hydroxyl group of another simple sugar to form a chain. As a result, the formula for a simple sugar is $(CH_2O)_n$, where n represents various numbers of these linked building block units.

Two pentose sugars, deoxyribose and ribose, comprise the sugar element of DNA and RNA molecules, respectively. As the name indicates, deoxyribose ("de-," a prefix meaning "off" and "oxy," meaning "oxygen") lacks one hydroxyl (OH) group compared to ribose.

Nucleic Acids

Nucleic acids are composed of chains of nucleotides. Each nucleotide is composed of a sugar (either ribose or deoxyribose), a phosphate ($-PO_4$) group, and a purine or pyrimidine base. The nucleotides are joined into a DNA or RNA strand by a sugar-phosphate-linked backbone with the bases attached to and extending from the first carbon of the sugar group. The purine and pyrimidine bases are weakly basic ring molecules, which form N-glycosidic bonds with ribose or deoxyribose sugar. Purines are comprised of two rings, a six-member ring and a five-member ring ($C_5H_4N_4$), while pyrimidines consist of a single six-member ring ($C_4H_2N_2$). Purines (guanine, G, and adenine, A) pair with pyrimidines (cytosine, C, and thymine, T) via hydrogen bonds between two DNA molecules (Figure 1-1). The additional hydrogen bond that forms between G and C base pairing (i.e., three hydrogen bonds) dramatically enhances the strength of this interaction compared to the two hydrogen bonds present between A and T nucleotides. This hydrogen-bonding capacity between G:C and A:T forms a pivotal molecular interaction for all nucleic acids and assures the passage of genetic information during

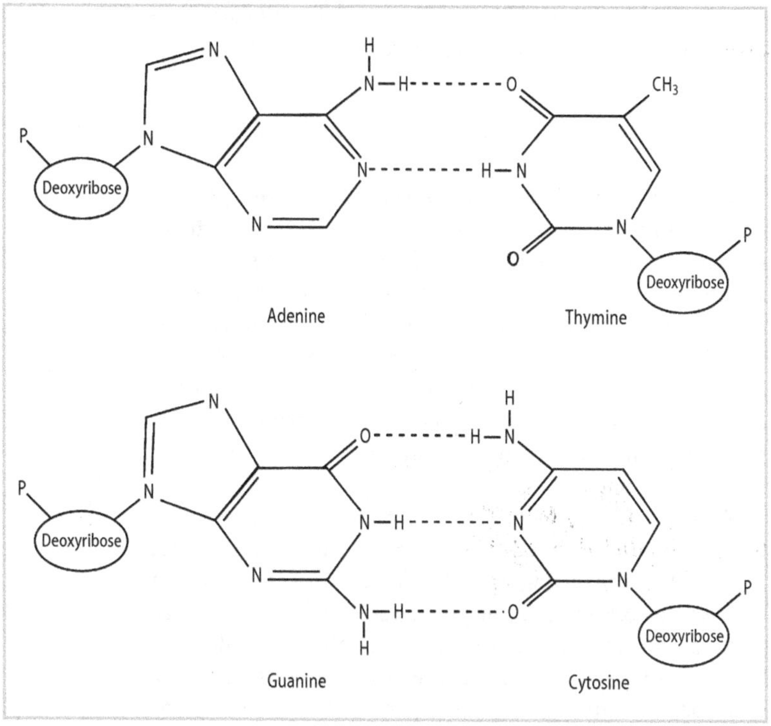

Figure 1-1. DNA base pairing. DNA nucleotides are composed of three moieties (e.g., sugar, base, and phosphate groups). The bases are either purine (adenine and guanine) or pyrimidine (thymine and cytosine). Note the difference in hydrogen bonds between adenine and thymine base pairs, with two hydrogen bonds, compared to cytosine and guanine base pairs, with three hydrogen bonds. (Reprinted from Leonard D. *Diagnostic Molecular Pathology*, copyright 2003, with permission from Elsevier.)

DNA replication, RNA synthesis from DNA (transcription), and the transfer of genetic information from nucleic acids to the amino acids of proteins.

Amino Acids

Amino acids are the building blocks of proteins. Amino acids linked together via peptide bonds form large, complex molecules. Amino acids consist of an amino group (NH_3), a carboxy group (COO−), an R group, and a central carbon atom. The R group can be a simple hydrogen, as found in glycine, or as complex as an imidazole ring, as found in histidine. Twenty different R groups exist; and determine whether an amino acid has a neutral, basic, or acidic charge (Table 1-2). The amino group of the polypeptides is considered the beginning of a protein (N-

Table 1-2. Amino Acids

Amino Acid	Amino Acid Symbols		R Group
	Three Letter	Single Letter	
Alanine	ala	A	$CH_3—CH(NH_2)—COOH$
Arginine	arg	R	$HN=C(NH_2)—NH—(CH_2)_3—CH(NH_2)—COOH$
Asparagine	asn	N	$H_2N—CO—CH_2—CH(NH_2)—COOH$
Aspartic acid	asp	D	$HOOC—CH_2—CH(NH_2)—COOH$
Cysteine	cys	C	$HS—CH_2—CH(NH_2)—COOH$
Glutamine	glu	Q	$H_2N—CO—(CH_2)_2—CH(NH_2)—COOH$
Glutamic acid	gln	E	$HOOC—(CH_2)_2—CH(NH_2)—COOH$
Glycine	gly	G	$NH_2—CH_2—COOH$
Histidine	his	H	$NH—CH=N—CH=C—CH_2—CH(NH_2)—COOH$
Isoleucine	ile	I	$CH_3—CH_2—CH(CH_3)—CH(NH_2)—COOH$
Leucine	leu	L	$(CH_3)_2—CH—CH_2—CH(NH_2)—COOH$
Lysine	lys	K	$H_2N—(CH_2)_4—CH(NH_2)—COOH$
Methionine	met	M	$CH_3—S—(CH_2)_2—CH(NH_2)—COOH$
Phenylalanine	phe	F	$Ph—CH_2—CH(NH_2)—COOH$
Proline*	pro	P	$NH—(CH_2)_3—CH—COOH$
Serine	ser	S	$HO—CH_2—CH(NH_2)—COOH$
Threonine	thr	T	$CH_3—CH(OH)—CH(NH_2)—COOH$
Tryptophan	trp	W	$Ph—NH—CH=C—CH_2—CH(NH_2)—COOH$
Tyrosine	tyr	Y	$HO—p—Ph—CH_2—CH(NH_2)—COOH$
Valine	val	V	$(CH_3)_2—CH—CH(NH_2)—COOH$

*Proline has a ring shape arising from the covalent bond formed between the amino group and the central carbon.

terminus), while the carboxyl group is at the opposite end, providing directionality to the protein.

Genetic Molecules

Nucleic acids encode genetic information but also participate in additional physiological processes ranging from metabolism to energy transfer. Nucleotides constitute the monomeric units of nucleic acids (Figure 1-1). Nucleosides consist of two components (ribose or deoxyribose in RNA and DNA, respectively, and either a purine or pyrimidine base). A nucleotide is produced from a nucleoside by the addition of one to three phosphate groups through a covalent bond with the hydroxyl group of the 5′ carbon of the nucleoside's sugar ring.

Nucleic acids are formed by chains of nucleotides linked by phosphodiester bonds between the 3′ carbon of the first nucleotide's sugar ring and the 5′ carbon of the adjacent nucleotide's sugar ring. The phosphodiester linkages cause nucleic acids to have a 5′ to 3′ directionality. The alternating sugar-phosphate chain forms a continuous molecule with bases extending from the 1′ carbon of each sugar. For this reason, the sugar-phosphate chain is referred to as the backbone of nucleic acids (Figure 1-2). The phosphate groups give nucleic acids a negative charge that imparts important physiochemical properties to nucleic acids. The negative charge of DNA facilitates the binding of mammalian DNA to various proteins and allows separation of nucleic acid molecules by charge and size during gel or capillary electrophoresis.

Structure

In double-stranded DNA, the two DNA strands are held together by exact A:T and G:C hydrogen bonding between the bases of the two strands, in which case the two strands are said to be complementary. The two strands are oriented in opposite 5′ to 3′ directions, such that one strand is oriented 5′ to 3′ (↓) and the complementary strand is oriented 3′ to 5′ (↑) in an antiparallel fashion (see Figure 1-2). In this case, "anti-" refers to the head (or 5′ end) of one DNA strand being adjacent to the tail (or 3′ end) of the opposite strand.

The molecular curves of the two DNA strands form antiparallel helices known as the DNA double helix. This double helix form (the B form) has ten nucleotide pairs (base pairs) per turn, occupying 3.4 nm. Because the bonds between the sugar and the base are not perfectly symmetrical, the strands curve slightly. The slight curve of the offset glycosidic bonds results in major and minor grooves characteristic of the B form of the double helix.[5] Many molecular diagnostic assays target the minor groove of DNA with sequence-specific probes known as minor groove binding (MGB) probes. Two other forms of DNA exist as the Z and A forms. The Z form acquires a zigzag shape, while the A form has a very shallow and very deep groove.

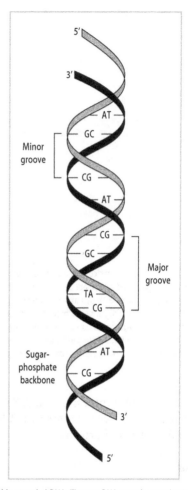

Figure 1-2. Double-stranded DNA. The two DNA strands are oriented in an antiparallel relationship, with asymmetric base pairing of two DNA strands that generates the minor and major grooves of the DNA double helix. (Reprinted from Leonard D. *Diagnostic Molecular Pathology*, copyright 2003, with permission from Elsevier.)

Thermodynamics of Nucleotide Base Pairing

Thermodynamics plays a major role in the structure and stability of nucleic acid molecules. The core mechanism of nucleic acid thermodynamics centers on the hydrogen-bonding capabilities of the nucleotides. The stability of these interactions not only influences the formation and stability of duplex nucleic acids but also impacts the structure and catalytic characteristics of single-stranded nucleic acids through intramolecular base pairing. In addition to these physiological functions, the phenomenon of complementary base pairing profoundly impacts clinical diagnostic assay development. Prior to the advent of clinical molecular diagnostic testing, many diagnostic tests required obtaining an antibody to identify or detect a target protein. The procedures for generating and validating diagnostic antibodies required extensive time and expense. The application of techniques utilizing the capability of two molecules to form a base pair as the basis for detection and characterization of target nucleic acids has greatly facilitated diagnostic test development. The formation of hydrogen bonding between two pieces of nucleic acid is called hybridization, or annealing, and the disruption of the hydrogen bonds holding two nucleic acid molecules together is called denaturation, or melting. The fact that molecular diagnostic tests use hybridization techniques based on A:T and G:C base pairing underscores the necessity for understanding the thermodynamics of hydrogen base pairing of nucleic acids.

Short pieces of DNA or RNA called probes, or primers, that contain a specific sequence complementary to a disease-related region of DNA or RNA from a clinical specimen are frequently used in the molecular pathology laboratory. To achieve hybridization of a DNA or RNA probe to genomic DNA for a diagnostic test, the two genomic DNA strands must be separated, or denatured, prior to probe hybridization. Increasing the temperature of a DNA molecule is one mechanism for disrupting the hydrogen bonds between the DNA base pairs and denaturing double-stranded DNA into single-stranded form. The temperature at which 50% of the double-stranded DNA molecules separate into single-stranded form constitutes the melting temperature (T_m). The shorter the two complementary DNA molecules are, the easier it is to calculate the T_m. This primarily results from the decreased likelihood of nonspecific intramolecular annealing or base pairing compared to inter- and intramolecular base pairing. The simplest and least accurate formula for determining the T_m for short double-stranded DNA multiplies the sum of the G:C base pairs by 4 and multiplies the sum of the A:T base pairs by 2 and then adds these numbers together.

$$T_m = [4(G:C)] + [2(A:T)]$$

Although this is the least accurate method for calculation of the T_m of a double-stranded DNA molecule, it mathematically illustrates that G:C bonds are roughly twice the strength of A:T bonds. This formula works fairly well for short DNA molecules (i.e., ≤18 bp); however, as the length of the DNA molecule increases to 100 bp, the nearest neighbor T_m calculation for DNA and RNA is more accurate.[6,7]

$$T_m = \frac{\Delta H}{\Delta S + R \ln(Ct)} - 273.15$$

where

ΔH = enthalpy of the nucleic acid fragment
ΔS = entropy of the nucleic acid fragment
R = 1.987 cal K^{-1} mol^{-1}
Ct = total strand concentration

For longer sequences (>100 bp), the most accurate formula for calculation of T_m is as follows:[8]

$$T_m = 81.5 + 16.6 \log[NA] + 0.41 [\%G = \%C] - 0.65 (\% \text{ formamide}) - 675/\text{length} - \% \text{ mismatch}$$

Table 1-3 demonstrates the effect of increasing the relative amounts of G:C base pairs on the T_m using these formulas.

Intramolecular base pairing also generates complex three-dimensional forms within single-stranded nucleic

Table 1-3. Melting-Temperature Calculations for Short Oligomers

Total Length	Number of G:C	Number of A:T	T_m*	%G:C†	A:T + G:C‡
30	30	0	106.2	100.0	100.0
30	25	5	101.2	93.2	100.0
30	20	10	89.5	79.5	90.0
30	10	20	83.4	72.7	80.0
30	0	30	71.6	59.0	60.0
20	20	0	90.4	88.8	80.0
20	10	10	72.7	65.1	60.0
20	0	20	55.9	47.8	40.0

*Nearest neighbor calculation of T_m.[6]
†T_m method for sequences over 100 bases.[8]
‡4(G + C) + 2(A + T) formula.

acid molecules. As a result, the single-stranded nature of eukaryotic RNA molecules affords great structural diversity via intramolecular base pairing. These conformations strain the linear RNA molecule and produce chemically reactive RNA forms. Catalytic RNA molecules play pivotal roles in cellular functions and in gene-targeting therapies.

Intra- and intermolecular base pairing can negatively affect hybridizations. Dimers, bulge loops, and hairpin loops exemplify some of these interactions. Hairpins inhibit plasmid replication and attenuate bacterial gene expression.[2] These detrimental effects may also include initiation of spurious nonspecific polymerization, steric hindrance of hybridization of short stretches of nucleic acids (i.e., 10 to 30 base pieces of single-stranded nucleic acids, known as oligomers or primers), and depletion of probes or primers away from the specific target by either primer dimerization or other mechanisms. These interactions can result in poor sensitivity or poor specificity for diagnostic molecular tests.

Topology

The DNA and RNA molecules assume various geometric shapes or topologies that are independent of base pair interactions. Eukaryotic nucleic acids take on linear forms, in contrast to the circular forms of mitochondrial and bacterial chromosomal DNA. Viral genomes occur as different forms, ranging from segmented linear to circular. Although the conformation of RNA molecules can be complex via intramolecular base pairing, the topology of messenger RNA (mRNA) molecules is primarily linear. An organism's genomic topology influences the biochemical mechanisms used during replication and the number of replication cycles a given chromosome can undertake. In contrast to circular genomes, linear genomes limit the total number of possible replication cycles due to progressive shortening of the linear chromosome.

Mammalian Chromosomal Organization

The human genome contains approximately 10^9 base pairs of DNA. The total DNA is contained in 46 double-stranded

DNA pieces complexed with proteins to form chromosomes. The diploid human genome, therefore, is contained in 46 chromosomes: two of each of the 22 autosomal chromosomes, plus either two X chromosomes, in females, or one X and one Y chromosome, in males. Since the length of each helical turn of a double-stranded DNA molecule is 3.4 nm, consisting of ten bases, the length of the total genomic DNA in each cell measures approximately 1 m in length. For each cell to contain this long molecule, the double-stranded DNA must be compressed. A complex of eight basic histones (two copies of histone 2 [H2], H3, H4, and H5) package the DNA.[9] The histone complex contains positively charged amino acids that bind to 146 bases of negatively charged DNA. Histones fold the DNA either partially or tightly, resulting in compression of the DNA strand. Tight folding of the DNA condenses the DNA into heterochromatin. Following packaging and condensation, the nucleic acid strand widens from 2 nm to 1400 nm, with extensive overall shortening of the nucleic acid in the metaphase chromosome. Light microscopy easily permits the visualization of condensed metaphase chromosomes.

Less-condensed DNA binds histone 1 (H1) proteins or other sequence-specific DNA-binding molecules. Some of these DNA-binding molecules regulate gene expression (discussed later in this chapter). In contrast, tightly condensed chromosomes lack the "open spaces" for binding of regulatory proteins and prevent gene expression from tightly condensed DNA regions. These proteins may also prevent access to nucleic acid probes or primers for molecular diagnostic tests. As a result, many DNA extraction protocols include a protein-digestion step to liberate the DNA from these DNA-binding proteins. Removal of these proteins facilitates hybridization with short pieces of nucleic acid, such as primers or probes.

DNA Replication

Eukaryotic DNA Replication

The replication of DNA is a complex process requiring specific physiological temperatures and a host of proteins. As mentioned previously, molecular diagnostic techniques rely on the ability to denature or melt a double-stranded DNA template. Using chemical or physical conditions, separation of DNA strands can be accomplished with alkali or high temperatures (i.e., 95°C). Under physiological conditions, dissociation of DNA strands for replication is accomplished by numerous enzymes, such as helicases and topoisomerases. The region of transition from the double-stranded to separated single-stranded DNA is called the replication fork. The replication fork moves along the double-stranded DNA molecule as replication proceeds. At the replication fork, various primases, initiating proteins, and polymerases bind to the original or parental DNA strands and generate new daughter strands. Known collectively as a replisome, these enzymatic activities gener-

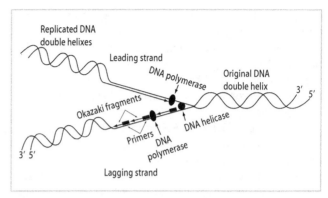

Figure 1-3. DNA replication. Replication fork depicting the leading and lagging strands and the numerous proteins and Okazaki fragments involved with replication. (Reprinted from Leonard D. *Diagnostic Molecular Pathology*, copyright 2003, with permission from Elsevier.)

ate two new nucleic acid strands that are complementary to and base paired with each of the original two template or parent DNA strands. This replication process is known as semiconservative because each resulting double-stranded DNA molecule consists of one new and one old DNA strand (Figure 1-3).

Polymerases function to synthesize new nucleic acid molecules from nucleotide building blocks. The sequence of the new strand is based on the sequence of an existing nucleic acid molecule, and the polymerase adds nucleotides according to the order of the bases of the parent strand, using G:C and A:T pairing. The new strand is antiparallel to the parent strand and is synthesized in a 5′ to 3′ direction. Of the two parent strands of genomic DNA, one strand (called the leading strand) can be read by the polymerase continuously in a 3′ to 5′ direction, with the new strand generated in a continuous 5′ to 3′ direction. In contrast, the opposite strand (known as the lagging strand) cannot be read continuously by the polymerase. The replication fork moves along the lagging strand in a 5′ to 3′ direction, and polymerases synthesize only by reading the parent strand in a 3′ to 5′ direction while synthesizing the new strand in a 5′ to 3′ direction. Therefore, synthesis cannot proceed continuously along the lagging strand, which must be copied in short stretches primed from RNA primers and forming short DNA fragments known as Okazaki fragments. The new strand complementary to the lagging strand is formed by removal of the RNA primer regions and ligation of the short DNA fragments into a continuous daughter strand complementary to the lagging strand. Discontinuous 3′ to 5′ replication results in the progressive loss of ends of the chromosomes known as telomeres in normal cells. Some malignant cells retain telomerase activity that permits the addition of these terminal telomeric sequences to the chromosomes.

While replication requires many proteins, the polymerase determines the speed and accuracy of new strand synthesis. The rate that the four nucleotides are polymerized into a nucleic acid chain defines the processivity of the enzyme. The processivity of most polymerases approximates 1000 bases per minute.

Table 1-4. Fidelity of Various Polymerases

Polymerase	Error Rate
pol β*	8×10^{-4}
pol α*	1×10^{-4}
pol θ*	$1.7–4 \times 10^{-5}$
Pfu†	1.3×10^{-6}
Deep vent†	2.7×10^{-6}
Vent†	2.8×10^{-6}
Taq†	8×10^{-6}
UITma†	55×10^{-6}
Klenow‡	$1–10 \times 10^{-7}$
HIV reverse transcriptase	$6–30 \times 10^{-4}$

*Reference 37.
†Reference 38.
‡Reference 39.

The fidelity of the polymerase refers to the accuracy of the enzyme to incorporate the correct complementary bases in the newly synthesized DNA. Incorporation of incorrect bases or other replication errors can result in cell death or oncogenesis. The error rate of polymerases varies widely from 1 in 1200 to 1 in 1,000,000 bases (Table 1-4). To correct the erroneous incorporation of bases or other replication errors, protein complexes proofread and correct synthesis errors. In normal cells, the cell cycle pauses to facilitate error repair in the G2 phase of the cell cycle (Figure 1-4). Malignant cells may not pause to allow for error correction, resulting in the accumulation of damaged or mutated DNA.

The complexity of the biochemical reactions necessary for replicating eukaryotic nuclear DNA demonstrates a high degree of regulation for generating two strands from one replication fork. In addition to these complexities, replication in eukaryotic cells occurs at multiple origins of

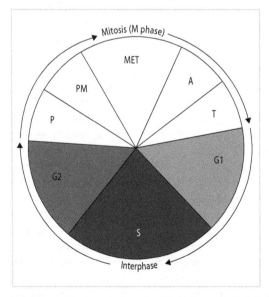

Figure 1-4. Cell cycle. The clear panels are the ordered phases of mitosis (M phase), while the gray and black panels are the ordered stages of interphase. P, prophase; PM, prometaphase; MET, metaphase; A, anaphase; T, telophase; G1, gap 1; S, DNA synthesis; G2, gap 2.

replication (Ori). These multiple sites grow progressively until the newly generated strands join to form complete chromosomal-length DNA.

Bacterial and Mitochondrial Replication

The relatively small chromosomes of bacteria (~10^6 base pairs) utilize a simpler mechanism than eukaryotic replication. A single origin of replication initiates the duplication of the bacterial chromosome, and replication occurs simultaneously on both strands in opposite directions from the origin of replication. This efficient replication process depends on the circular topology of the bacterial genome.

Another unique feature of prokaryotic chromosomal replication is the mechanism bacteria have evolved to protect their chromosomes. The lack of a protective nuclear membrane in bacteria makes the chromosome susceptible to attack by viruses (bacteriophages). As a result, many bacteria produce restriction enzymes that degrade foreign nucleic acids. These restriction enzymes recognize specific short sequences and cleave the DNA at those sites. However, methylation of the recognition sequences in the bacterial chromosomal DNA prevents most restriction enzymes from digesting the chromosomal DNA of the bacteria. In this way, methylating enzymes add methyl groups to the replicated bacterial chromosome, preventing chromosomal degradation by its own restriction enzymes. This methylation and restriction process functions as a primitive immune system by destroying foreign bacteriophage DNA before it can usurp the bacteria's replication system. Bacterial restriction enzymes are used to specifically cleave DNA in molecular diagnostic tests and are useful for identifying genetic variations.

Additional types of replication occur in some viruses and bacteria. The rolling-circle mechanism of replication proceeds with an initial single-strand cut or nick in double-stranded circular genomes, followed by replication proceeding from the nick in a 5′ to 3′ direction. The new strand displaces the old strand. RNA viral genomes use the enzyme transcriptase for replication. In the case of retroviruses, a reverse transcriptase generates an intermediate DNA molecule, which integrates into the host chromosome and then is used for generation of progeny RNA molecules. The high error rate of human immunodeficiency virus (HIV) reverse transcriptase produces numerous mutations in the viral genome.[10,11] Some of these mutations confer resistance to antiretroviral therapies and can be identified by clinical molecular tests.

Cell Division and Cell Cycle

In eukaryotic cells, the cell cycle refers to the entire process of generating two daughter cells from one original cell, with chromosomal replication as one of the steps. The two parts of the cell cycle are called interphase and mitosis.

DNA synthesis occurs during interphase and consists of three stages: gap 1 (G1), synthesis (S), and gap 2 (G2) (Figure 1-4). Regulation of cell division depends on specific cell-cycle-dependent proteins known as cyclins and growth factors. Some of these factors cause the cycle to progress while others stop the cycle at certain stages. Checkpoints, or times when the cycle may be paused, exist at the G1/S and G2/mitosis interfaces and allow the cell time to repair any DNA damage that may be present in the cell before and after replication of the DNA, respectively.

Growth factors initiate the G1 phase via cell surface receptors. Several molecular events such as the dephosphorylation of the retinoblastoma protein and cyclin binding to cyclin-dependent kinases (Cdk) transition the cell toward the G1/S checkpoint. The amount of cellular P53 protein determines whether the cell progresses beyond this checkpoint, with higher levels preventing cell cycle progression. Because various DNA-damaging events, such as ultraviolet light, radiation, carcinogens, and double-stranded DNA breaks, induce production of P53 protein, this molecule serves as a sentinel for mutated DNA. The functional failure of P53 removes this sentinel from the cell cycle process and results in the accumulation of genetic errors. Therefore, inactivation of P53 facilitates oncogenesis.

Once DNA repairs have taken place during G1 prior to replication of the DNA, the cell proceeds to S phase. DNA synthesis occurs in the S phase, followed by the G2 phase. Replication errors occurring during the S phase are corrected in the G2 phase, the G2/M checkpoint. This final checkpoint marks the end of interphase.

Mitosis, the process of physical division of the parent cell into two daughter cells, occurs during the mitosis or M phase of the cell cycle. During mitosis, the duplicated chromosomes are physically separated so that each daughter cell receives the correct number of chromosomes. Mitosis consists of five phases: prophase, prometaphase, metaphase, anaphase, and telophase. The duplicated chromosomes condense during prophase. A structural element known as the mitotic spindle originates from two structures called centrioles, which move to opposite poles of the cell and the spindle forms between the centrioles. The nuclear membrane dissipates, proteins form kinetochores on the chromosmes, and microtubules attach to the kinetochores during prometaphase. The duplicated chromosome pairs attach at central points along the spindles. The arrangement of the highly condensed chromosome pairs along an equatorial cell plane denotes metaphase. As previously discussed, highly condensed chromosomes cannot bind proteins necessary for gene expression. As a result, the cell's internal machinery focuses solely on cell division during metaphase. The centriole-derived spindle guidelines pull the duplicate chromosomes apart and drag them toward each centriole during anaphase. With the separation of the daughter chromosomes (chromatids) into opposite poles of the cell and the reformation of nuclear membranes around the two daughter sets of chromosomes, telophase begins. Cytokinesis, or the division of the cytoplasm, is the last step in cell division. During cytokinesis, the mitochondria are randomly and potentially unevenly distributed in the daughter cells. The cell cycle can then be reinitiated by one or both of the daughter cells to generate additional cells. Alternatively, some cells become quiescent in a G0 phase (between telophase and G1) and either have a prolonged delay before initiating replication again or no longer divide.

Cell division to generate gametes is called meiosis and consists of two divisions, meiosis I and meiosis II. Like mitosis, this process begins with the duplication of chromosomes in prophase I. During metaphase I, the maternal and paternal homologous chromosomes pair (i.e., pairing occurs between each of the pairs of the 22 autosomal chromosomes, the two X chromosomes in females, and the X and Y chromosomes in males). Each pair attaches to the spindle apparatus along the equatorial plane of the cell spindle. DNA may be exchanged between the paired chromosomes by either crossing-over or recombination mechanisms during this pairing stage of meiosis I. During anaphase I, homologous chromosomes separate into daughter cells, resulting in 23 duplicated chromosomes in each daughter cell. A second cell-division cycle, meiosis II, separates the duplicated chromosomes, resulting in haploid cells, egg or sperm, containing only one copy of each of the 22 chromosomes plus an X (egg or sperm) or Y (only sperm) chromosome.

From Gene to Protein

The genomic DNA content is the same in all cells of the same person and encodes all the genetic information for cellular function. Encoded in the DNA are the blueprints for all the RNA and protein molecules present in any type of cell. Different parts of the genetic information are used by different types of cells to accomplish each cell's specific function. DNA is used to produce RNA and protein molecules by processes called transcription and translation, respectively. The regions of DNA that encode RNA and protein molecules are called genes.

Replication requires an increase in building materials for the duplicated daughter cells. Highly condensed metaphase chromatin cannot produce gene products because proteins that initiate gene expression cannot bind to the chromosomes at this phase of replication. In contrast, partially condensed or unfolded chromatin permits the binding of specific proteins (e.g., RNA polymerases) that synthesize mRNA and tRNA. Ultimately, these molecules facilitate the production of gene products, specifically proteins.

RNA molecules function as the mediators between DNA and protein. These molecules essentially speak the same language as DNA because, as nucleic acids, they can base pair with complementary DNA sequences. Like transferring spoken language to a written form, this process of copying information from DNA to RNA is referred to as transcription. The transcription complex of proteins must unwind the double-stranded DNA at the specific gene site to be copied, locate the polymerase binding site on one of the DNA strands, and generate a primary (1°) transcript, which is one component of heterogeneous nuclear RNA (hnRNA) by reading the DNA strand in a 3′ to 5′ direction, with RNA synthesis proceeding in a 5′ to 3′ direction. The 1° RNA transcript is processed into mRNA, and finally the DNA in the region of the gene becomes double-stranded again. Numerous DNA sequences bind proteins that regulate and coordinate gene expression. These sequences can be used to identify the locations of genes within the entire human genome sequence. Since the generation of the first draft of the human genome, the interest in understanding gene structure has increased with the goal of identifying disease-associated genes.[12–14]

Gene Structure

Promoting Transcription

Sequences that bind RNA polymerases in combination with transcription factors drive and regulate the production of 1° RNA transcript (Table 1-5). Proteins and transcription factors bind to sequences located 5′, or upstream, of the gene to be expressed and are collectively called the promoter region of a gene. Negative numbering denotes the location of these sequences upstream of the first protein-encoding base. The promoter sequence initiates (or promotes) transcription of the downstream gene and harbors conserved sequences that are recognized by the transcription complex of enzymes.

The complexity and organization of the transcription regulatory sequences of genes differ between prokaryotic and eukaryotic cells. Prokaryotes contain a simple gene structure with sequences for polymerase binding occurring at −35 and −10 for each gene. The −10 sequence contains a consensus sequence of TATAAT, while the −35 region consists of TTGACA. Variations of these sequences as well as the sequences located adjacent to the gene determine the strength of the promoter's transcriptional activity. For example, small differences such as having a TATATA sequence rather than the consensus sequence at the −10 position will decrease the promoter's ability to bind to the RNA polymerase and result in decreased production of mRNA for that gene. In bacteria, operons regulate expression of multiple genes with related functions from the same promoter.

Table 1-5. Examples of Nucleic Acid Motifs

Name	Sequence
AP1 binding site	TGASTCAG
AP2 binding site	CCCCAGGC
AP3 binding site	GGGTGGGAAAG
AP4 binding site	YCAGCTGYGG
C/EBP	TGTGGAAAG
CCAAT box	CCAAT
CP1 binding site	YN(6)RRCCAATCA
CP2 binding site	YAGYN(3)RRCCAATC
CREB	TGACGTCA
CTF/NF1 binding sites	GCCAAT
GCN4 target site	ATGASTCAT
Glucocorticoid receptor	GGTACAN(3)TGTTCT
Homeobox protein-binding site	TCAATTAAAT
HSTF	CNNGAANNTTCNNG
INF-stimulated response	RGGAANNGAAACT
Lariat consensus sequence	YNYTRAY
MALT box	GGAKGGA
NF-1	TTGGMN(5)GCCAAT
Octamer sequence	ATTTGCAT
Poly A signal	AATAAA
Splice acceptor	Y(11)NYAGG
Splice donor	MAGGTRAGT
TATA box	TATA
Translational initiation sequence	RNNMTGG

R = A/G; Y = C/T; M = C/A; W = A/T; N = A/T/C/G.

In eukaryotic genes, various promoter sequences bind multiple proteins, which catalytically modify and activate other bound proteins. Enhancer sequences increase the production of mRNA but are far removed from the gene. One of the pivotal proximally located sequences comprises a TATA box (TATAAA) located at −25 (Figure 1-5). These bases initiate binding of a TATA-binding protein (TBP) within the transcription factor D complex. Following this binding, transcription factors B, H, and E bind to and open the DNA strands downstream from the promoter. Finally, transcription factor F and RNA polymerase II bind to the transcription complex. The close proximity of these proteins to RNA polymerase II permits phosphorylation of the polymerase and initiation of transcription. In eukaryotic cells, variations in the recognition sequences alter the efficiency of transcription. These variations may be base pair changes or base modifications. For example, promoter sequences that are highly methylated do not bind well to the transcription factors or polymerase. As a result, a gene

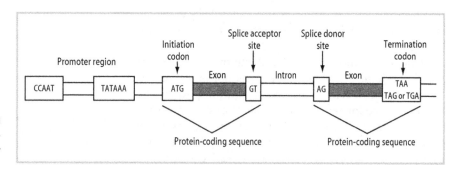

Figure 1-5. Gene structure. Gene structure depicting coding and noncoding regions of the eukaryotic gene. (Reprinted from Leonard D. *Diagnostic Molecular Pathology*, copyright 2003, with permission from Elsevier.)

may appear to be unaltered or intact but may be transcriptionally silent due to methylated bases in the promoter region.

Elongation and Termination of the mRNA

Once the RNA polymerase binds to the promoter, transcription begins at position +1. The polymerase reads the DNA in a 3′ to 5′ direction, while synthesizing the 1° RNA transcript in a 5′ to 3′ direction. In bacteria, the complete transcript serves as the template for translation. Transcription ends with termination. The mRNA must be terminated in bacteria; termination of the transcript can result from attenuation or the formation of hairpin structures. Termination occurs at several sites beyond the polyadenylation signal in eukaryotic cells and is dependent on bases near the stop codon.[15] Because the eukaryotic cell transcripts are polyadenylated, a termination of the transcription process by a process similar to attenuation is not necessary to regulate gene expression. Specifically, transcripts produced after the polyadenylation signal lack a 5′ cap, resulting in rapid degradation.[16,17]

In eukaryotic cells, once the 1° RNA transcript has been produced in the nucleus, this transcript is processed to form an mRNA by splicing to remove the non-protein-coding introns (intervening sequences) and join the protein-coding exons. Introns are located between sequences called exons, which encode the protein sequence and are translated during protein synthesis. Splicing involves a complex of ribonucleoproteins known as a spliceosome, which recognizes consensus sequences at the 5′ and 3′ ends of the intron. Genetic changes to these splice donor (A/C AG G U A/G AGU) and splice acceptor ([U/C]$_{11}$ N C/U AG G/A) consensus sequences may prevent the spliceosome from recognizing and catalyzing the splicing event.[18,19] Autoantibodies directed to or alterations in the steady-state level of the spliceosome may play a role in some diseases.[20-22] Alternate splicing may generate multiple distinct transcripts from a single gene. That is, some exons may be spliced out in one mRNA molecule but retained in another. As a result, alternate splicing generates different proteins from the same gene and 1° RNA transcript.[23-24]

An additional mechanism of generating diversity from 1° RNA transcripts entails trans-splicing (initially identified in *Drosophila* cells). Essentially, two separate, unrelated transcripts form a hybrid molecule by using the splice donor from the first transcripts and the splice acceptor from the second transcripts. Complementary intronic sequences in both transcripts facilitate the generation of the chimeric mRNA. This process has not been demonstrated in other eukaryotic cells. However, when the process is used for gene therapy applications, normal gene function has been restored from defective genes using trans-splicing.[25-26] Other therapeutic applications for catalytic RNA molecules involve innovative treatments for HIV-infected patients. In this application, synthetic ribozymes cleave drug-resistant variants of HIV.[25,27-29]

Additional modifications of the 1° RNA eukaryotic transcript enhance the stability and transport of the mRNA. One such modification occurs immediately on the generation of the 1° transcript and involves addition of a 7-methyl guanosine linked in an unusual 5′ to 5′ linkage to the triphosphate at the 5′ end of the transcript, also known as the 5′ cap. This cap protects the transcript from degradation. Another 1° transcript modification is cleavage at a polyadenylation signal (AAUAA) near the 3′ end of the transcript, followed by the addition of 100 to 200 adenosine residues (poly-A tail) by polyadenylate polymerase. The poly-A tail facilitates transportation of the mature mRNA into the cytoplasm and protection of the transcript from degradation by exonucleases. A given gene may have several polyadenylation signals, providing another level of variation for a single gene.[30-32]

Translation

Translation is the next step in using information from the DNA gene to produce a functional protein. This process changes the genetic information from a nucleic-acid-based language into an amino-acid-based language of polypeptides and proteins. For these reasons, the term "translation" describes this complex cascade of events.

Following transportation of the mRNA into the cytoplasm, translation begins with the mRNA binding to a ribosome and requires additional nucleic acids, specifically protein-associated RNA molecules (Figure 1-6). A ribosome is a complex of about 50 different proteins associated

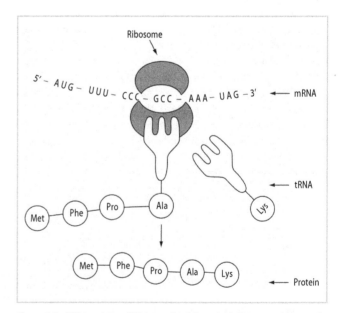

Figure 1-6. RNA translation. RNA is translated through binding events between the mRNA, a ribosome, tRNA, and amino acids, resulting in the production of a protein polypeptide chain. (Reprinted from Leonard D. *Diagnostic Molecular Pathology*, copyright 2003, with permission from Elsevier.)

Table 1-6. The Human Genetic Code

		SECOND BASE OF CODON			
		U	C	A	G
FIRST BASE OF CODON	**U**	**UUU** Phenylalanine (Phe/F)	**UCU** Serine (Ser/S)	**UAU** Tyrosine (Tyr/Y)	**UGU** Cysteine (Cys/C)
		UUA Phenylalanine (Phe/F)	**UCA** Serine (Ser/S)	**UAA** Tyrosine (Tyr/Y)	**UGA** Cysteine (Cys/C)
		UUC Leucine (Leu/L)	**UCC** Serine (Ser/S)	**UAC** **STOP**	**UGC** **STOP**
		UUG Leucine (Leu/L)	**UCG** Serine (Ser/S)	**UAG** **STOP**	**UGG** Tryptophan (Trp/W)
	C	**CUU** Leucine (Leu/L)	**CCU** Proline (Pro/P)	**CAU** Histidine (His/H)	**CGU** Arginine (Arg/R)
		CUA Leucine (Leu/L)	**CCA** Proline (Pro/P)	**CAA** Histidine (His/H)	**CGA** Arginine (Arg/R)
		CUC Leucine (Leu/L)	**CCC** Proline (Pro/P)	**CAC** Glutamine (Gln/Q)	**CGC** Arginine (Arg/R)
		CUG Leucine (Leu/L)	**CCG** Proline (Pro/P)	**CAG** Glutamine (Gln/Q)	**CGG** Arginine (Arg/R)
	A	**AUU** Isoleucine (Ile/I)	**ACU** Threonine (Thr/T)	**AAU** Asparagine (Asn/N)	**AGU** Serine (Ser/S)
		AUA Isoleucine (Ile/I)	**ACA** Threonine (Thr/T)	**AAA** Asparagine (Asn/N)	**AGA** Serine(Ser/S)
		AUC Isoleucine (Ile/I)	**ACC** Threonine (Thr/T)	**AAC** Lysine (Lys/K)	**AGC** Arginine (Arg/R)
		AUG START Methionine (Met/M)	**ACG** Threonine (Thr/T)	**AAG** Lysine (Lys/K)	**AGG** Arginine (Arg/R)
	G	**GUU** Valine (Val/V)	**GCU** Alanine (Ala/A)	**GAU** Aspartic Acid (Asp/D)	**GGU** Glycine (Gly/G)
		GUA Valine (Val/V)	**GCA** Alanine (Ala/A)	**GAA** Aspartic Acid (Asp/D)	**GGA** Glycine (Gly/G)
		GUC Valine (Val/V)	**GCC** Alanine (Ala/A)	**GAC** Glutamic Acid (Glu/E)	**GGC** Glycine (Gly/G)
		GUG Valine (Val/V)	**GCG** Alanine (Ala/A)	**GAG** Glutamic Acid (Glu/E)	**GGG** Glycine (Gly/G)

with several ribosomal RNA (rRNA) molecules. Prokaryotic ribosomes consist of 30S and 50S subunits. Svedberg (S) units are the sedimentation rate of a particle. In eukaryotes, rRNA molecules associate with proteins in the nucleolus to form 40S and 60S subunits. Recognition of the 5′ cap of the eukaryotic mRNA by a ribosome initiates the process of translation.[33]

Each amino acid is encoded by one or more 3-nucleotide sequences, which are collectively known as the genetic code (Table 1-6). Each set of 3 nucleotides of an mRNA that encodes an amino acid is called a codon. As is seen in Table 1-6, the first and second nucleotide positions largely determine which amino acid is encoded by the mRNA codon, while the third base has less effect on which amino acid will be incorporated. In addition to encoding amino acids, certain mRNA codons are used to initiate (START) or terminate (STOP) translation. The genetic code differs slightly between organisms and between mitochon-drial DNA and eukaryotic DNA (Table 1-7). Thus, while one mRNA encodes only one protein sequence, a protein sequence can be encoded by several different mRNA sequences. This is referred to as the degeneracy of the genetic code.

Synthesis of the encoded protein begins at the initiation codon of the mRNA, the first AUG codon after the promoter and encodes a methionine amino acid. This methionine codon establishes the reading frame of the mRNA. The next step in the translation process uses RNA molecules to bridge the information from the sequential mRNA codons to the encoded amino acid in the growing polypeptide chain of the protein. Another set of RNA molecules, tRNA, contain a sequence complementary to each mRNA codon known as the anticodon. The 3′ end of each type of tRNA binds the specific amino acid corresponding to its anticodon sequence. Base pairing of codons with complementary anticodons permits sequential alignment of new amino acids of the polypeptide chain and occurs in the

Table 1-7. Exceptions to the Universal Code in Mammals

Codon	Nuclear Code	Mitochondrial Code
UGA	Stop	Trp
AUA	Ile	Met
AGA	Arg	Stop
AGG	Arg	Stop

small subunit of the ribosome. The large subunit of the ribosome catalyzes the covalent bonds linking each sequential amino acid to the growing polypeptide chain.

Translation ceases when the ribosome encounters a stop codon (UAA, UAG, or UGA). Release factors bound to the stop codon catalyze the addition of a water molecule rather than an amino acid, thus resulting in a COOH terminus to the completed polypeptide chain.[34] Some factors bound to the 3′ untranslated portion of the gene also affect termination.

Structure of Proteins

Just as nucleic acids form various structures via intra- and intermolecular base pairing, proteins also assume various structures depending on the types and locations of amino acids. The primary structure of a protein is the sequence of amino acids from amino terminus (NH) to carboxy terminus (COOH) of the protein. The secondary structure refers to how amino acid groups interact with neighboring amino acids to form structure called an alpha helix or beta sheet. The tertiary structure of a protein is created by amino acids sequentially distant from one another creating intramolecular interactions. The quaternary structure of a protein defines the three-dimensional and functional conformation of the protein. The shape that is ultimately assumed by the protein depends on the arrangement of the different charged, uncharged, polar, and nonpolar amino acids.

Posttranslational Modifications

After generation of the polypeptide chain of amino acids, additional enzymatic changes may diversify its function. These changes are termed posttranslational modifications and can include proteolytic cleavage, glycosylation, phosphorylation, acylation, sulfation, prenylation, and vitamin C– and vitamin K–mediated modifications. In addition, selenium may be added to form selenocysteine. The selencysteinyl-tRNA recognizes the UGA stop codon and adds this unusual amino acid.

Mutations: Genotype Versus Phenotype

Genetic information exists in the form of nucleic acids known as the genotype. In contrast, the encoded proteins function to create a phenotype, an outwardly observable characteristic. Genotypic alterations may or may not cause phenotypic alterations. For instance, missense mutations refer to genetic changes that result in the incorporation of a different amino acid at a specific codon location. These changes may not dramatically alter the protein if the replacement amino acid is similar to the original amino acid (for example, a hydrophobic amino acid replaces another hydrophobic amino acid). However, replacement of an amino acid with a different type of amino acid may significantly change the conformation of the protein and thus change its function. For example, in sickle cell anemia, a valine replaces a glutamic acid at a single position and permits the polymerization of the beta globin molecules to cause stiffening and sickling of the red blood under low oxygen conditions. Different forms of proteins (known as conformers) provide the mechanism for diseases ranging from Creutzfeldt-Jacob disease to Huntington disease. Nonsense mutations describe base changes that replace an amino-acid-encoding codon with a stop codon, which causes premature termination of translation and results in a truncated protein.[35] Truncation may result from the addition or deletion of one or two nucleotide bases, resulting in a shift in the reading frame. Frameshifts often result in premature termination when stop codons are formed downstream from the mutation. Alterations in splice donor or acceptor sites may either erroneously generate or pre-vent appropriate splicing of the 1° transcript, resulting in a frameshift mutation.[36] Genetic changes in the untranslated portions of the gene affecting the promoter, enhancer, or polyadenylation signals may affect the expression of the gene product and result in a phenotypic change. Not all genotypic changes affect the phenotype. Genetic changes affecting the third base of the codon rarely alter the gene code and would therefore be less likely to cause incorporation of a different amino acid.

With the sequencing of the human genome, numerous single nucleotide polymorphisms have been identified, demonstrating the individual nature of human beings. Numerous studies currently target correlating genotype variations to disease phenotypes. These efforts, in combination with improved understanding of gene structure and function, hold the promise of improved diagnosis, treatment, and patient outcomes in the future.

Acknowledgment

I would like to acknowledge Laurie Sower, PhD, for her helpful advice and editorial assistance and our numerous discussions that greatly facilitated the preparation of this chapter.

References

1. Passarge E. *Color Atlas of Genetics*. 2nd ed. Stuttgart: Thieme; 2001.
2. Willets N. Plasmids. In Scaife DLJ, Galizzi A, eds. *Genetics of Bacteria*. London: Academic Press; 1985:165–195.
3. Hewitt WL. Penicillin-historical impact on infection control. *Ann N Y Acad Sci*. 1967;145:212–215.
4. Livermore DM. Antibiotic resistance in staphylococci. *Int J Antimicrob Agents*. 2000;16(suppl 1):S3–S10.
5. Crick JWJF. A structure for deoxyribonucleic acid. *Nature*. 1953;171: 737.
6. Breslauer KJ, Frank R, Blocker H, Marky LA. Predicting DNA duplex stability from the base sequence. *Proc Natl Acad Sci U S A*. 1986; 83:3746–3750.

7. Freier SM, Kierzek R, Jaeger JA, et al. Improved free-energy parameters for predictions of RNA duplex stability. *Proc Natl Acad Sci U S A.* 1986;83:9373–9377.

8. Lewis ME, Arentzen R, Baldino F Jr. Rapid, high-resolution in situ hybridization histochemistry with radioiodinated synthetic oligonucleotides. *J Neurosci Res.* 1986;16:117–124.

9. Felsenfeld G, Groudine M. Controlling the double helix. *Nature.* 2003;421:448–453.

10. Preston BD, Poiesz BJ, Loeb LA. Fidelity of HIV-1 reverse transcriptase. *Science.* 1988;242:1168–1171.

11. Roberts JD, Bebenek K, Kunkel TA. The accuracy of reverse transcriptase from HIV-1. *Science.* 1988;242:1171–1173.

12. Kochetov AV, Ischenko IV, Vorobiev DG, et al. Eukaryotic mRNAs encoding abundant and scarce proteins are statistically dissimilar in many structural features. *FEBS Lett.* 1998;440:351–355.

13. Gotoh O. Homology-based gene structure prediction: simplified matching algorithm using a translated codon (tron) and improved accuracy by allowing for long gaps. *Bioinformatics.* 2000;16:190–202.

14. Olivier M, Aggarwal A, Allen J, et al. A high-resolution radiation hybrid map of the human genome draft sequence. *Science.* 2001;291:1298–1302.

15. McCaughan KK, Brown CM, Dalphin ME, Berry MJ, Tate WP. Translational termination efficiency in mammals is influenced by the base following the stop codon. *Proc Natl Acad Sci U S A.* 1995;92: 5431–5435.

16. Frischmeyer PA, Dietz HC. Nonsense-mediated mRNA decay in health and disease. *Hum Mol Genet.* 1999;8:1893–1900.

17. Wilkinson MF, Shyu AB. Multifunctional regulatory proteins that control gene expression in both the nucleus and the cytoplasm. *Bioessays.* 2001;23:775–787.

18. Bruno C, Lofberg M, Tamburino L, et al. Molecular characterization of McArdle's disease in two large Finnish families. *J Neurol Sci.* 1999;165:121–125.

19. Hou VC, Conboy JG. Regulation of alternative pre-mRNA splicing during erythroid differentiation. *Curr Opin Hematol.* 2001;8:74–79.

20. Lipes J, Skamene E, Newkirk MM. The genotype of mice influences the autoimmune response to spliceosome proteins induced by cytomegalovirus gB immunization. *Clin Exp Immunol.* 2002;129: 19–26.

21. Seidl R, Labudova O, Krapfenbauer K, et al. Deficient brain snRNP70K in patients with Down syndrome. *Electrophoresis.* 2001; 22:43–48.

22. Wehner KA, Ayala L, Kim Y, et al. Survival motor neuron protein in the nucleolus of mammalian neurons. *Brain Res.* 2002;945:160–173.

23. Garzon D, Yu G, Fahnestock M. A new brain-derived neurotrophic factor transcript and decrease in brain-derived neurotrophic factor transcripts 1, 2 and 3 in Alzheimer's disease parietal cortex. *J Neurochem.* 2002;82:1058–1064.

24. Sakata N, Yamazaki K, Kogure T, Mukai T. Alternative splicing of Rh blood group polypeptide mRNA produces a novel transcript containing a short nucleotide insertion on human erythroleukemia K562 cells. *Cell Biol Int.* 2001;25:697–703.

25. Liu X, et al. Partial correction of endogenous DeltaF508 CFTR in human cystic fibrosis airway epithelia by spliceosome-mediated RNA trans-splicing. *Nat Biotechnol.* 2002;20:47–52.

26. Phylactou LA, Darrah C, Wood MJ. Ribozyme-mediated trans-splicing of a trinucleotide repeat. *Nat Genet.* 1998;18:378–381.

27. Phylactou LA, Kilpatrick MW, Wood MJ. Ribozymes as therapeutic tools for genetic disease. *Hum Mol Genet.* 1998;7:1649–1653.

28. Lan N, Howrey RP, Lee SW, Smith CA, Sullenger BA. Ribozyme-mediated repair of sickle beta-globin mRNAs in erythrocyte precursors. *Science.* 1998;280:1593–1596.

29. Mansfield SG, Kole J, Puttaraju M, et al. Repair of CFTR mRNA by spliceosome-mediated RNA trans-splicing. *Gene Ther.* 2000;7:1885–1895.

30. Urano Y, Watanabe K, Sakai M, Tamaoki T. The human albumin gene. Characterization of the 5′ and 3′ flanking regions and the polymorphic gene transcripts. *J Biol Chem.* 1986;261:3244–3251.

31. Lin B, Rommens JM, Graham RK, et al. Differential 3′ polyadenylation of the Huntington disease gene results in two mRNA species with variable tissue expression. *Hum Mol Genet.* 1993;2:1541–1545.

32. Boyd CD, Mariani TJ, Kim Y, Csiszar K. The size heterogeneity of human lysyl oxidase mRNA is due to alternate polyadenylation site and not alternate exon usage. *Mol Biol Rep.* 1995;21:95–103.

33. Gallie DR. Protein-protein interactions required during translation. *Plant Mol Biol.* 2002;50:949–970.

34. Chavatte L, Frolova L, Kisselev L, Favre A. The polypeptide chain release factor eRF1 specifically contacts the s(4)UGA stop codon located in the A site of eukaryotic ribosomes. *Eur J Biochem.* 2001;268:2896–2904.

35. Stratakis CA. Mutations of the gene encoding the protein kinase A type I-alpha regulatory subunit (PRKAR1A) in patients with the "complex of spotty skin pigmentation, myxomas, endocrine overactivity, and schwannomas" (Carney complex). *Ann N Y Acad Sci.* 2002;968:3–21.

36. Valentine CR. The association of nonsense codons with exon skipping. *Mutat Res.* 1998;411:87–117.

37. Cline J, Braman JC, Hogrefe HH. PCR fidelity of pfu DNA polymerase and other thermostable DNA polymerases. *Nucleic Acids Res.* 1996; 24:3546–3551.

38. Maga G, Shevelev I, Ramadan K, Spadari S, Hubscher U. DNA polymerase theta purified from human cells is a high-fidelity enzyme. *J Mol Biol.* 2002;319:359–369.

39. Kuchta RD, Cowart M, Allen D, Benkovic SJ. Kinetic and structural investigations of the replicative fidelity of the Klenow fragment. *Biochem Soc Trans.* 1988;16:947–949.

Chapter 2

Molecular Pathology Methods

Megan J. Smith-Zagone, Joseph F. Pulliam, and Daniel H. Farkas

Introduction

Molecular pathology is based on the principles, techniques, and tools of molecular biology as they are applied to diagnostic medicine in the clinical laboratory. These tools were developed in the research setting and perfected throughout the second half of the 20th century, long before the Human Genome Project was conceived. Molecular biology methods were used to elucidate the genetic and molecular basis of many diseases, and these discoveries ultimately led to the field of molecular diagnostics. Eventually the insights these tools provided for laboratory medicine were so valuable to the armamentarium of the pathologist that they were incorporated into pathology practice. Today, molecular diagnostics continues to grow rapidly as in vitro diagnostic companies develop new kits for the marketplace and as the insights into disease gained by the progress of the Human Genome Project develop into laboratory tests.

Molecular pathology is a natural extension of anatomic and clinical pathology. As molecular research identifies the most fundamental causes and markers of disease, clinical testing is moving to the nucleus and its genetic material. Underlying mutations responsible for genetic diseases, including cancers, are being discovered and used in molecular diagnostic tests. Some have become routine tests in molecular pathology and are described in detail elsewhere in this book.

In this chapter, fundamental and more advanced molecular biology techniques, as practiced in the molecular pathology laboratory, are reviewed. The entire field of molecular pathology is relatively new, having begun in the 1980s and matured through the 1990s. The new century has brought important advances in automated nucleic acid preparation,[1-3] polymerase chain reaction (PCR), real-time PCR, and deoxyribonucleic acid (DNA) sequencing. More and more, the underlying biochemistry occurring in laboratory instruments may be invisible to the user. The goal of this chapter is to describe the principles of these methods so that practitioners have adequate information for instrument troubleshooting and test interpretation.

Obviously, gene products, that is, proteins and polypeptides, are molecules and could technically be classified within "molecular pathology." This chapter focuses on nucleic acid diagnostics, including investigation of deoxyribonucleic acid (DNA) and ribonucleic acid (RNA). The field will eventually move beyond genomics to proteomics. Proteomics is not addressed in this chapter since clinical proteomics is in its most nascent stages and is in extremely limited practice in molecular pathology today.

Basic Science Discoveries: The Foundation

Molecular pathology techniques are rooted in fundamental molecular biology discoveries of the 1940s to 1980s.[4] The clinical laboratory application of molecular biology techniques would not be possible without the discovery by Griffith and Avery that nucleic acid is the genetic material. The foundation of work by Chargaff and Franklin was capitalized on by Watson and Crick, who elucidated the structure of DNA. Understanding DNA structure is seminal to understanding nucleic acid hybridization, which is central to almost all molecular methods used in the clinical molecular laboratory. Additionally, work by Nirenberg (unraveling the genetic code); Wilcox, Smith, Nathans, and others (use of restriction endonucleases for DNA manipulation); Baltimore and Temin (discovery of RNA-dependent DNA polymerase or reverse transcriptase); Britten and Davis (hybridization kinetics); Kornberg and Okazaki (work on DNA polymerases and DNA replication, respectively); Southern (development of solid-phase nucleic acid hybridization, or the Southern blot); Sanger, Maxam, and Gilbert (development of DNA sequencing); Mullis (discovery of PCR for in vitro nucleic acid amplification); and their scientific collaborators and competitors led to a refined understanding of how DNA may be manipulated in vitro for research and ultimately diagnostic purposes.

General Methods

Nucleic Acid Isolation

The first step of most molecular pathology tests is isolation of DNA or RNA from a patient specimen, by either manual or automated methods. Nucleic acid purification begins with lysis of the cells in the sample. Cell lysis liberates cellular macromolecules including proteins, lipids, and nucleic acids. Cell lysis can be accomplished using a detergent solution to break cell membranes and remove lipids. Proteins are enzymatically degraded with protease, usually proteinase K, or selectively precipitated. Protein digestion is performed at about 56°C and will permanently denature many proteins but does not affect nucleic acids. This process is followed by selective extraction that takes advantage of the physical and chemical differences between nucleic acids and other cellular molecules, forming the basis for their isolation. The nucleic acid is then purified from the soluble contaminants produced in the extraction method by precipitation in an ethanol-salt solution. A variation on this theme that combines extraction and purification is the selective adsorption of nucleic acids to silica columns under chaotropic salt conditions. The isolated nucleic acid is then resuspended in a dilute salt buffer, for example, 10 mM Tris/1 or 0.1 mM EDTA pH 7.6 to 8.0 (TE buffer).

The initial lysis step is modified according to the specimen. If the specimen is fresh or frozen solid tissue, it is first homogenized in an appropriate buffer (often TE buffer). If the specimen is formalin-fixed, paraffin-embedded (FFPE) tissue, the paraffin is removed with an organic solvent such as xylenes, followed by rehydration through an alcohol series to a dilute salt buffer before protease digestion. FFPE tissue is also heated during the prolonged protease digestion step to reverse formalin cross-linking between proteins (primarily histones) and nucleic acids. Although this reduces the degree of nucleic acid shearing in subsequent vortexing or centrifugation steps, DNA longer than that packaged into a nucleosome (about 200 base pairs [bp]) is difficult to recover from FFPE tissue. Whole blood specimens may require a centrifugation step to remove erythrocytes prior to recovery of nucleic acids from leukocytes because of the inhibition of PCR by hemoglobin. This cell fractionation step generally is not performed in automated nucleic acid extraction instruments.

Organic (Phenol) Extraction

Nucleic acids have a strong negative charge because of the phosphate groups in the sugar-phosphate backbone, and thus are highly soluble in an aqueous environment. By contrast, proteins, lipids, and carbohydrates contain varying proportions of charged and uncharged domains producing hydrophobic and hydrophilic regions. This difference makes proteins entirely soluble in organic solutions or selective for the interface between the organic and aqueous phases during an organic extraction. This characteristic forms the basis for phenol: chloroform extraction, in which phenol is added to an aqueous solution containing cellular constituents, mixed, and then centrifuged to separate the aqueous and organic phases. If the pH of the extraction is near neutral, both DNA and RNA stay in the aqueous phase, while proteins are in the phenol: chloroform phase or aqueous-phenol interface. If the pH is acidic, the phosphate groups of DNA are preferentially neutralized, driving DNA into the organic phase (or interface) and allowing RNA to be selectively extracted. This method produces high-quality nucleic acids but is relatively labor-intensive, uses hazardous chemicals, and produces liquid organic waste.

Ethanol-Salt Precipitation

Nucleic acids can be precipitated in an aqueous solution by the addition of concentrated ethanol and salt. Ethanol makes the solution hydrophobic, while salt increases the ionic strength of the solution, thereby reducing the repulsion of the negatively charged sugar-phosphate backbone of the nucleic acid. Centrifugation allows the precipitate to be collected and resuspended in a dilute salt buffer (TE buffer).

Chaotropic Salt–Silica Column Extraction

Chaotropic salts such as sodium iodide (NaI) or guanidinium isothyocyanate (GITC) disrupt the structure of water, promoting the solubility of nonpolar substances, such as proteins, in polar solvents, such as water. Saturated chaotropic salts also promote the adsorption of nucleic acids to glass or silica columns. The nucleic acid is purified by a series of washing steps including reducing agents such as sodium azide to further remove contaminants and inhibit remaining enzymes. The nucleic acid is eluted from the column with a dilute, nonchaotropic salt buffer. Since the method is simple, fast, offered in commercial kits by several manufacturers, and adaptable to high-throughput robotic nucleic acid isolation, this method is widely used by clinical molecular laboratories.

RNA Versus DNA Isolation

DNA is the repository of genetic information, which is then transcribed into RNA. RNA forms ribosomes, transfer RNA (tRNA), and messenger RNA (mRNA) for protein translation, and is used for other special functions in the regulation of gene expression that have only recently been discovered. DNA is a hardy molecule present at stable cellular levels, with such well-known exceptions as the amplification and deletion of genes in tumor cells. By contrast, the level of RNA corresponding to a gene can fluctuate dramatically within a very short time in response to changes in the cell's microenvironment and functional needs. This fluctuation results from changes in both the rate of transcription and degradation of an RNA.

DNA is relatively easy to isolate and store because deoxyribonucleases (DNases) are easily denatured by heating or inhibited by sequestration of divalent cations. RNA, by contrast, is rapidly degraded by a variety of ribonuclease (RNase) enzymes that are replete within the cell and on the skin surface. While this is necessary for cellular homeostasis, the ubiquity of RNases leads to a problem for the molecular analysis of RNA. RNases are very stable, active in virtually any aqueous environment, and can regain their activity after denaturation. As a result, RNA is subject to rapid degradation by RNases in most laboratory settings, making RNA a notoriously labile molecule. The rate of degradation varies among RNA species, leading to further analytical complexity.

RNA analysis depends on successful RNA isolation and preservation. The overall techniques are similar to those described above for nucleic acid isolation, but with the mandatory addition of steps to inhibit or degrade cellular RNases and prevent their reintroduction into the isolated RNA. RNA isolation must be performed promptly after specimen collection, particularly if quantitation of RNA is desired. If RNA isolation is delayed, the sample should be stored at −80°C, or at an intermediary isolation point in a stable buffer with RNase inhibitors. Scrupulously clean laboratory technique is required, including careful cleansing of laboratory equipment with bleach, autoclaving of glassware, preparation of reagents with nuclease-free water, and wearing gloves with frequent glove changes. Addition of GITC or beta-mercaptoethanol to the RNA isolation reagents will inhibit or denature RNases present in the sample. The isolated RNA is rehydrated in water or TE buffer that is nuclease free, and stored at −80°C to further inhibit the activity of any residual RNases.

Despite these difficulties, RNA is valuable in the clinical molecular laboratory for several reasons. Many clinically significant viruses such as human immunodeficiency virus (HIV) and hepatitis C virus (HCV) have RNA genomes. Quantitation of RNA provides an important measure of gene expression, which can be used in the diagnosis or monitoring of disease. In addition, mRNA does not contain introns, which is an advantage when analyzing neoplastic translocations with variable intronic breakpoints such as BCR-ABL.[5]

Nucleic Acid Measurement for Quantity and Quality

Nucleic acid quantitation is optional for many protocols that utilize in vitro nucleic acid amplification. Some methods, however, require use of more accurate quantities of nucleic acid, so assessment of the yield and concentration of purified nucleic acids is useful. This is typically done using ultraviolet (UV) spectrophotometry. The absorbance of a nucleic acid solution is measured at several wavelengths. The maximal absorbance for nucleotides is at 260 nm of UV light (A_{260}), while for proteins the maximal absorbance is at 280 nm (A_{280}). Nucleic acids can therefore be quantified by the A_{260} measurement, while the A_{260}/A_{280} ratio provides an estimate of the purity of the sample. Pure DNA has an A_{260} of 1.0 at a concentration of 50 μg/ml and an A_{260}/A_{280} ratio of 1.8, while pure RNA has an A_{260} of 1.0 at a concentration of 40 μg/ml and an A_{260}/A_{280} ratio of 2.0. Lower A_{260}/A_{280} ratios indicate the presence of protein in the solution. Other contaminants can be detected by their absorbance at other wavelengths, such as phenol at A_{270} and guanidinium at A_{230}.

Ethidium bromide (EtBr) intercalates into DNA strands, causing DNA to fluoresce upon illumination with UV light. The fluorescence of EtBr correlates with the number of base pairs of DNA in which the EtBr is intercalated, which is a result of both the size and quantity of the DNA fragment. Therefore, by staining sample DNA with EtBr in an electrophoresis gel and comparing the brightness to mass standards in adjacent lanes, the quantity of DNA can be estimated. This provides a convenient system for quantification of post-PCR DNA prior to sequencing, since the UV spectrophotometer is usually kept in the pre-PCR area (see below for PCR, sequencing, and amplicon carryover contamination). More important, the image of the EtBr-stained sample DNA can be used to assess DNA quality. High-quality, substantially intact DNA forms a single band close to the well serving as the origin of electrophoresis. In contrast, DNA degradation is apparent as a smear of EtBr-stained DNA extending downward from the well. Ethidium bromide is mutagenic and produces light background staining and is therefore being replaced by other intercalating dyes such as SYBR Green.

Electrophoresis

Electrophoresis uses an electric field to separate charged molecules by differential mobility in a sieving matrix that can be either liquid or solid (gel). The differential mobility is determined by the size of the molecule and its conformation, the net charge of the molecule (as modified by pH), temperature, and the pore size of the matrix. DNA, being negatively charged, migrates towards the anode (+) when an electric field is applied to an electrolyte solution. The size of DNA can be modified by restriction endonuclease digestion (see below), rendering DNA fragments small enough to be mobile in the matrix. Conformation can be modified with denaturing conditions prior to or during electrophoresis. Nucleic acids are usually electrophoresed at a slightly alkaline pH to ionize all phosphate groups in the backbone of the molecule.

The pore size of the matrix is determined by the composition and concentration of the polymer. For any given pore size, the mobility of a molecule through the matrix is inversely proportional to the log of its size. Therefore, for a given size difference between two molecules, the difference in the rate of migration will be substantially less if both molecules are large. The limiting mobility is defined as the rate of migration through the gel at which large molecules can no longer be separated for any given pore size. This may be related to the tendency of sections of long DNA fragments to "snake" through different pores in the gel, retarding the mobility of the fragment. The limiting mobility of gels can be overcome by using pulsed field gel electrophoresis (PFGE), in which the voltage gradient is periodically reoriented.

Polyacrylamide Gels

In clinical molecular laboratories, the matrices used most commonly are acrylamide and agarose. Polyacrylamide gels are formed by cross-linking acrylamide monomers with bisacrylamide in the same salt buffer used for electrophoresis and pouring the solution in a thin space between two glass plates. A comb is inserted at one edge between the plates to form wells for sample insertion. After the gel has formed, the plates are mounted in a vertical electrophoresis unit such that the gel forms a bridge between two buffer chambers. Samples, controls, and sizing standards are loaded into the wells, usually in association with a dye to track the progress of electrophoresis, and glycerol to make the samples sink to the bottom of the wells. Electrodes are attached to the buffer chambers and connected to a power supply providing constant voltage. After electrophoresis, the glass plates are separated and the gel is soaked in EtBr solution. DNA is visualized by EtBr staining under UV light. Polyacrylamide forms very small pores and is useful for high resolution of DNA fragments from 100 to 1000 bp. Single base pair resolution can be achieved, allowing polyacrylamide gels to be used for sequencing under denaturing conditions (see below). However, polyacrylamide gels are thin and fragile, the glass plates are cumbersome to work with, and nonpolymerized acrylamide is a lung irritant and neurotoxin; therefore, alternatives to polyacrylamide gel electrophoresis are desirable in the clinical laboratory. Although more costly, precast acrylamide gels are commerically available to circumvent the biohazards of nonpolymerized acrylamide.

Agarose Gels

Agarose gels are formed by boiling an agarose gel powder until the agarose has completely dissolved in the same buffer used for electrophoresis, optionally adding EtBr, then pouring the solution into a horizontal casting tray. Multiple gel combs can be used to form rows of wells. After cooling and polymerization, the gel is loaded in a horizontal electrophoresis apparatus and covered with buffer in a single chamber. Wells are loaded and electrophoresis performed as described above. Agarose gels have a large pore size. Agarose gels with a concentration of 1% are used to separate DNA fragments of 1 to 20 kilobases (kb), while higher-concentration gels are useful to separate smaller DNA fragments. Agarose gels are thicker and more stable than polyacrylamide gels but do not provide the same degree of resolution. Agarose is safer than acrylamide but still must be handled and disposed of with care if the gel contains EtBr. Other modified agarose compounds are available that can be mixed in various ratios with standard agarose to increase the resolution of agarose gels. Like acrylamide gels, precast agarose gels are commerically available.

Capillary Electrophoresis

Capillary electrophoresis (CE) is a widely used separation technology for analysis of proteins, peptides, chemicals, natural products, pharmaceuticals, and DNA. Capillary electrophoresis systems are commercially available and generally provide more consistent and standardized results with less time and effort than gel electrophoresis. Using CE, DNA fragments are rapidly separated with a high-voltage gradient, because the capillary dissipates heat quickly. Therefore, one CE run takes approximately 0.5 hour or less, and if eight or 16 capillaries are run simultaneously, the process reduces the time from standard electrophoresis, which requires 3 to 4 hours. This is a significant time saving in the clinical laboratory for applications such as sequencing. CE enables more standardized results, maximization of workforce efficiency, increased productivity and throughput, and the potential for error reduction. CE also uses smaller sample volumes.

In CE, electrophoretic separation takes place in a capillary tube ranging in length from 25 to 100 cm and approximately 50 to 75 μm in diameter. Most capillary tubes are made of glass (silica) walls that often are covered with an external polyimide coating. Acid silanol groups impart a negative charge on the internal wall of the capillary. A low-viscosity acrylamide-based flowable polymer acts as the electrolyte solution and sieving matrix within the silica capillary and is responsible for the conductivity of current through the capillary. Polymer concentration affects the pore size and movement characteristics of the DNA.

A small section of the capillary coating is removed at one end of the capillary to create a detection window. The detection window is optically aligned with the detection system of the instrument. The detection system often includes either a diode or argon laser combined with a charge-coupled device (CCD) camera or filter wheel and photomultiplier tube. The opposite end of the capillary and electrode is used for the injection of the sample. Sample injection in CE is frequently performed by electrokinetic injection. In electrokinetic injection, the capillary and electrode are moved into the sample well. The sample enters the capillary when a voltage of 2 to 5 kV is applied for approximately 5 to 15 seconds. The voltage causes sample ions including DNA to migrate electrophoretically into the capillary in a flat flow profile. Electrokinetic injection produces increased resolution compared to hydrodynamic injection, which produces a laminar (curved) flow profile. After the injection, the capillary and electrode are returned to a buffer reservoir for the separation. The DNA fragments separate by size during migration through the capillary and are detected through the window at the far end of the capillary.

In the clinical molecular laboratory, DNA sequencing and DNA fragment sizing or quantitation are the most common applications performed on CE instruments. One negative aspect of CE as opposed to older polyacrylamide gel technology is that CE is more sensitive to contaminants and DNA concentration. DNA, being negatively charged, migrates into the capillary when voltage is applied. If there are any other charged particles in the sample, they also are injected into the capillary. For example, salt is an ionic competitor. If salt is present, the fluorescent signal intensity of the sample will be greatly reduced because of ionic competition during the brief injection. Proper sample preparation is therefore a key to successful CE.

After a postreaction purification step, if needed for the specific CE application, DNA samples are resuspended in a sample loading solution. High-quality deionized formamide often is used as the sample loading solution. If DNA is denatured prior to CE, the formamide maintains the denatured state of DNA and provides a very stable environment for fluorescent dyes. Following the postreaction purification and resuspension of products, the samples are ready for analysis on the CE instrument. The fragments are injected into the capillary and detected by laser-induced florescence, and data are generated for analysis using software supplied by the manufacturer for different CE applications.

Restriction Endonucleases

Restriction endonucleases (REs) cleave DNA at specific nucleotide recognition sequences. Restriction endonucleases are naturally occurring proteins found in and purified from bacteria. Each bacterial species contains one or more REs, each recognizing a unique sequence of base pairs in double-stranded DNA, called recognition sites (most commonly 4 to 8 bp long). Bacteria use REs to digest and inactivate foreign DNA (such as bacteriophage DNA). The frequency of recognition sites in target DNA for any given RE is inversely proportional to the size of the recognition site. Some REs do not cleave DNA when their recognition sites are methylated; this can be useful in certain clinical laboratory applications such as detection of imprinted genes in genetic diseases or promoter hypermethylation in tumors. Some mutations occur at RE recognition sites and can be detected by a change in the RE digestion pattern of a PCR product or genomic DNA. Unique DNA restriction

fragment patterns are generated by digestion with different REs, creating a range of DNA restriction fragment sizes. Fractionated using agarose gel electrophoresis. Restriction endonuclease digestion is commonly used as a component of clinical molecular tests.

Specific Methods

DNA Sequencing

Prior to the performance of a sequencing reaction, the DNA template to be sequenced must be properly purified and quantitated. A sequence-specific complementary primer must be synthesized for use in the sequencing reaction. Sequencing primers must also be high-performance liquid chromatography (HPLC) purified or, at the very least, desalted. Samples must be purified following the sequencing reaction to rid the sample of salts, excess dyes, and excess primers that would compete for injection into the capillary. There are numerous protocols and commercial kits available for the postreaction purification. Ethanol precipitation is the least expensive purification method, but numerous gel-filtration and spin-column methods also can be used.

The ability to sequence DNA has been essential to the field of molecular pathology because sequence information is a prerequisite for PCR, PCR alternatives, and hybridization with probes necessary for successful Southern blot analysis. The method for DNA sequencing developed by Sanger, Nicklen, and Coulson[6] is the basis for most DNA sequencing performed both in clinical laboratories and for the Human Genome Project.

The Sanger sequencing reaction uses a single DNA primer and DNA polymerase with linear amplification rather than the exponential amplification of PCR (see below). Components essential to the Sanger sequencing reaction include (1) an electrophoresis technique capable of clearly distinguishing single nucleotide length differences in DNA strands dozens or hundreds of nucleotides in length, (2) sequence-specific complementary primers, with one primer used in the forward reaction and the other used in the reverse reaction for each DNA template strand, and (3) the addition of small proportions of dideoxynucleoside triphosphates (ddNTPs) in addition to the conventional deoxyribonucleoside triphosphates (dNTPs) used in the polymerase reaction. Dideoxynucleotides differ from deoxynucleotides by having a hydrogen atom attached to the 3′ carbon rather than an OH group, which is present on the deoxynucleotide. Because the ddNTPs lack a 3′-hydroxyl group, elongation of the newly polymerized DNA chain cannot occur once a ddNTP has been incorporated (arabinonucleosides can also be used as inhibitors of elongation). The end result is a set of newly synthesized DNA chains that are complementary to the template DNA but that vary in length, with the length determined by the point at which the ddNTP was incorporated into the 3′ end of the chain.

In the original paper, for each template four reactions were performed with the addition of a single inhibitor to each, either ddGTP, ddATP, ddTTP or araCTP.[6] The DNA chains were separated by polyacrylamide gel electrophoresis under denaturing conditions and visualized using $(\alpha\text{-}^{32}P)$-dATP on a radio-autograph. These reactions were run in consecutive lanes of the gel, and the complementary DNA sequence was determined by manual inspection based on the size of each chain, and the specific ddNTP in the reaction.

Today, sequencing is very similar except that radioactive labeling has largely been replaced by fluorescent labeling. Two major categories of fluorescent labeling exist. In dye-primer labeling, the sequencing primer is labeled, and the sequencing reaction requires 4 tubes differing only in the incorporation of the specific ddNTP. In dye-terminator labeling, the sequencing primer is unlabeled and instead each ddNTP is labeled with a different fluorophore. This enables the entire sequencing reaction to be performed in a single tube. Dye-terminator labeling has therefore taken precedence in sequencing. Dye-primer labeling is frequently used in fragment analysis for detection of microsatellite instability, loss of heterozygosity, forensic identification, or allogeneic bone marrow transplantation monitoring using short tandem repeat polymorphisms. Automated sequencers recognize both the size of the DNA chain and the fluorescent color of the chain to assign the nucleotide sequence, and also function as precise detectors for fragment analysis.[7]

Conventional DNA sequencing with polyacrylamide gel electrophoresis (whether using manual or automated sequence detection) is time-consuming and labor-intensive. Therefore, the introduction of CE was a welcome change that facilitated the incorporation of sequencing and fragment analysis into the clinical laboratory.[8] The sequencing reaction products must be purified before injection into the CE unit to remove excess salts, dyes, and unincorporated primers that would compete for injection into the capillary. Purification is accomplished by ethanol precipitation or a chaotropic salt–silica column technique. After the postreaction purification step, samples are then resuspended in a sample loading solution containing high-quality deionized formamide to denature the DNA. Formamide also provides a very stable environment for fluorescent dyes. The fragments are injected into the capillary, detected by laser-induced florescence, and rendered into sequence by the analysis software. An electropherogram of the DNA sequence is generated by the detection software by correlating the fluorescent intensity of each dye wavelength corresponding to a specific ddNTP as a function of migration time.

Examples of Applications of DNA Sequencing

1. Congenital adrenal hyperplasia mutation analysis
2. Retinoblastoma mutation analysis
3. *BRCA1* mutation analysis
4. HIV genotyping to monitor drug resistance and sensitivity
5. High-resolution human leukocyte antigen (HLA) typing for allogeneic bone marrow transplantation

Southern Blot

The Southern blot was developed by E.M. Southern in 1975 and was the first molecular biology tool to have a major impact on clinical molecular pathology. The Southern blot is still used today, though it is being replaced by amplification methods. The implementation of Southern blot was based on prior knowledge of nucleic acid isolation, gel electrophoresis, RE digestion, and nucleic acid probe labeling for detection of DNA sequences of interest.

The Southern blot is a relatively labor-intensive, time-consuming clinical laboratory method.[9] High-quality DNA is isolated from a patient specimen, subjected to RE digestion, and then fractionated by gel electrophoresis. "Blotting" is the transfer of fractionated DNA from the gel to a solid support such as a nylon membrane. The DNA is then hybridized to a small piece of complementary DNA labeled in a variety of ways and called a probe. This detection step allows the gene of interest to stand out from the vast background of DNA present in the sample. If the pattern of banding visualized on the membrane is different from the normal pattern, this may be indicative of a mutation.

Because no amplification of target DNA occurs, Southern blot analysis requires a large mass of DNA. The DNA must also be intact and of high molecular weight. Therefore, electrophoresis of the isolated DNA prior to analysis is important for assessing the integrity of the DNA, since only a small degree of DNA degradation is tolerable. Degraded DNA may produce false-negative results if a signal from high-molecular-weight DNA is expected, while false-positive results may occur if partially degraded DNA results in unusually sized bands. Fortunately, most tests in the molecular pathology laboratory today are based on PCR, which is less affected by DNA degradation. Polymorphisms within RE recognition sites also change banding patterns, a principle used to advantage in other molecular tests.

The physical movement of the DNA in the gel to the membrane may be accomplished by manual capillary transfer, automated vacuum transfer, or electrotransfer. DNA in the gel must first be "conditioned": depurination with dilute HCl and subsequent denaturation with NaOH. Dilute and brief acid treatment causes hydrolysis of the DNA phosphodiester backbone to occur spontaneously at the sites of depurination. This acid induced fragmentation facilitates efficient transfer of the highest-molecular-weight DNA species from the gel to the membrane. Alkali treatment denatures double-stranded DNA (dsDNA) to single-stranded DNA (ssDNA), essential for subsequent nucleic acid hybridization with a labeled ssDNA probe.

The DNA is permanently fixed to the membrane by thoroughly drying the blot in an oven or by exposing the blot to a precise amount of UV irradiation.

The blot is immersed in prehybridization buffer to prepare the DNA on the blot for hybridization with a probe. Prehybridization buffers contain blocking agents included to minimize unwanted nonspecific DNA probe binding that would otherwise contribute to high background on the final image of the Southern blot used to view the results and make diagnostic conclusions. The prehybridization step equilibrates the membrane and blocks sites on the nylon membrane without DNA to prevent the probe from binding nonspecifically and increasing background. A large volume of blocking agent is therefore advantageous. Addition of the labeled probe to the blot begins the hybridization phase of the Southern blot process. A small volume of buffer is used to facilitate probe and target specifically finding each other, thereby promoting hybridization. Hybridization takes several hours to overnight at an appropriate temperature determined by multiple variables: concentrations of the two species; time permitted for hybridization; complexities of the nucleic acids involved; length of the probe and its target and their complementarity to each other (degree of mismatch); pH; temperature; and ionic strength of the buffer used.

DNA probes are labeled before use in hybridization assays to permit visualization of probe-target binding (in reverse hybridization assays, described below, unlabeled probes are immobilized and the target is labeled during the amplification step that precedes hybridization). Such labeling may be accomplished isotopically or nonisotopically. High-specific-activity DNA probes may be generated by in vitro biochemical reactions that synthesize new stretches of DNA from dNTPs, using the probe as a template. One of these dNTPs is labeled with a reporter molecule such as ^{32}P, biotin, or digoxigenin. When incorporated into the newly synthesized DNA, the labeled dNTP, even though it is only one of the 4 dNTPs in the DNA probe, is sufficient to label the entire probe for detection. The probe is then used in vast molar excess relative to target DNA in nucleic acid hybridization to drive the hybridization reaction as quickly as possible.

After hybridization, the blot is washed with buffers containing sodium chloride and detergent to remove excess probe and reduce background. Sodium chloride concentration and stringency are inversely related: the lower the sodium chloride concentration, the more stringent the wash. Increasingly stringent washes remove more nonspecifically bound probe. The temperature of the wash buffer and stringency are directly related: high-temperature washes are more stringent than lower-temperature washes and further contribute to hybridization specificity. When appropriately stringent washing of the blot is complete, only the specific hybrids of interest should remain. Visualization of these specific hybrids, which appear as bands, is achieved by autoradiography for radioactive probes or by luminography for chemiluminescent probes. Hybridization with biotinylated probes is followed by chemical reactions, resulting in insoluble colored precipitates at the site of hybridization on the blot itself that serve as the endpoint (this is also the detection scheme used in the line probe assay; see below). Simple visual inspection is then applied for both isotopic and nonisotopic Southern blots to determine the position where the labeled probe hybridized to its target patient DNA. That position, relative to detection of appropriate controls, allows interpretation.

Northern blotting is an extension of Southern blotting that uses RNA instead of DNA as the target of investigation. Northern blotting is as labor-intensive as Southern blotting but even more problematic due to the highly labile nature of RNA. While northern blotting has been very useful in the research setting to demonstrate the selective expression of genes in various organs, tissues, or cells, it has not become a routine tool in the clinical molecular pathology laboratory.

Examples of Applications of Southern Blotting

1. B- and T-cell antigen receptor gene rearrangement for leukemia and lymphoma[10]
2. Fragile X syndrome diagnosis
3. Myotonic dystrophy diagnosis

Polymerase Chain Reaction

In the mid-1980s in California, Mullis and coworkers developed a method, the polymerase chain reaction (PCR), to amplify exponentially target sequences of DNA.[11] As the name suggests, the method is a DNA polymerase–mediated chain reaction of nucleic acid amplification. Arguably, it is the single most important "invention" that has led to development of a new discipline in clinical laboratory medicine, that is, molecular pathology. Both PCR and Southern blotting are techniques used to investigate specific genomic targets. However, PCR is orders of magnitude more sensitive and much faster, permitting turnaround time of 24 hours or less. PCR lends itself to much higher test volumes than Southern blotting, a crucial point in its acceptance in the clinical laboratory setting. Opportunity for high test volumes, excellent specificity and sensitivity, and the rapid turnaround times of PCR are the principal reasons this technology has spread so quickly in clinical molecular laboratories.

In PCR, a unique sequence of the target nucleic acid of interest is chosen for amplification, for example, oncogene, invading pathogen DNA, genetic mutation. The inherent specificity of the ensuing reaction is provided by two short oligonucleotides, called PCR primers (see Figure 2-1). These short oligonucleotides serve as primers for DNA polymerase–mediated DNA synthesis using denatured target DNA as a template. The two primers are complementary to opposite strands and opposite ends of the targeted DNA template region. Usually the primers bracket

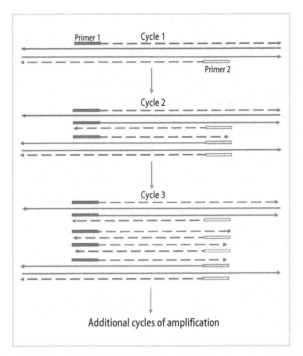

Figure 2-1. The polymerase chain reaction. (Reprinted with permission from Tsongalis GJ, Coleman WB. *Molecular Diagnostics—A Training and Study Guide.* Washington, DC: AACC Press, 2002.)

the area of interest, but one type of PCR (allele-specific PCR; see below) uses primers that overlap the area of interest. Successful PCR depends on temperature cycling, and in the first step of PCR the reaction temperature is raised to 95°C to 98°C to denature the target DNA. After 10 to 60 seconds at this temperature, the temperature is reduced to about 50°C to 70°C, depending on the specific protocol, and held there for usually 10 to 60 seconds. This facilitates hybridization (annealing) between the now-denatured target and the PCR primers, and is thus called the annealing step. This hybridization event is favored over target reannealing because the PCR primers are small and present in vast molar excess, and move more rapidly in solution than larger DNA molecules.

The hybridized PCR primers form local areas of double strandedness with the template DNA, thereby serving as primers for DNA polymerase to bind and synthesize a new strand of DNA, using the target DNA as a template. Subsequent to the initial discovery of PCR, the opportunity for automating the cyclical nature of PCR was realized by using DNA polymerase from hot-spring living bacteria, *Thermophilus aquaticus* (hence the term "*Taq* polymerase"). *T. aquaticus* thrives at very high temperatures, and so its proteins do not denature at the high temperatures needed to denature DNA in the first step of PCR. Catalysis by *Taq* polymerase of a new strand of DNA proceeds at a temperature intermediate to the near-boiling temperature used for denaturation and the relatively lower temperature used for annealing. DNA polymerization occurs during this extension step, typically at 65°C to 75°C. Taken together, these three steps (denaturation, annealing, and extension) define one PCR cycle.

Temperature cycling is automated through the use of an instrument called a thermal cycler. Thermal cyclers hold small capped tubes containing the reagents needed for PCR and cycle between the temperatures needed for the different steps of the PCR.[12] A single PCR tube contains template DNA (<1 ng to 1 μg), *Taq* DNA polymerase, two PCR primers (~15 to 30 nucleotides long), all four dNTPs, Mg^{2+}, and buffer to maintain an elevated pH (~8.4) optimal for *Taq*.

The repetition of the cycles generates exponential amplification of the target DNA because each double-stranded target DNA molecule, theoretically even if there is only one, is replicated after one PCR cycle. Both the original and replicated DNA molecules are then available to function as templates for cycle 2, in true "chain reaction" style, generating another doubling, or four copies of the original target. Cycle 3 ends with eight molecules, and doubling continues with completion of each new cycle. This doubling plateaus in later cycles since reagents, usually dNTPs, become limiting. Additionally, the enzyme may not function at 100% efficiency, and so true exponential amplification is theoretical, although there is a true exponential phase of amplification.

Greater than one billion identical copies of the original target DNA region are generated after 32 cycles of PCR: 2^{32} or more than four billion, the difference owing to the fact that unit-length amplicons are not generated until the end of the second cycle of PCR. Amplicons (PCR products) are defined as replicated target molecules created by PCR. Unit-length amplicons are those whose ends are defined by the primers. During the first cycle, the primers are extended by *Taq* polymerase using template DNA. The termination of this extension is undefined and a function of how far the polymerase moves down the template during the time allotted. The enzyme, therefore, moves beyond the ends of the primer-binding site on the complementary strand. After completion of the first cycle, therefore, the newly synthesized DNA molecules are greater in length than the sequence bracketed on each strand by the primers. In the second cycle, DNA molecules are synthesized from the products of the first cycle whose ends are defined by the two primers. These are so-called unit-length amplicons. While all of the above is true, the practical clinical laboratory difference between one- and four-billion-fold amplification is irrelevant because either number is sufficient for detection of the target, often by electrophoresis with EtBr visualization.

Several factors affect the specificity and sensitivity of PCR. The production of specific PCR amplicons is a function of both the complementarity of the primers to the target DNA and the annealing temperature of the PCR cycle. Heating will denature the primer from its target DNA. The temperature at which the primer melts from the target DNA varies directly with the length of the primer and the guanosine-cytosine (GC) content of the primer, and inversely with the degree of mismatch between the primer and the target DNA. The melting temperature (T_m) of the primer is the temperature at which 50% of the primer is denatured from the target DNA. If the thermal cycler is programmed to reach an annealing temperature higher than the primer T_m, the efficiency of PCR is compromised and sensitivity decreased. In contrast, if the annealing temperature is substantially less than the primer T_m, the primer can bind to both complementary and noncomplementary DNA, resulting in reduced PCR specificity as nontarget DNA is amplified (and potentially decreased sensitivity as reaction components are used nonspecifically). Therefore, the ideal annealing temperature is slightly less than the T_m of both primers, and the primers should be designed to have a very similar T_m. The annealing temperature can be decreased with subsequent cycles during PCR in a process called "touchdown" PCR. This allows the initial cycles to produce specific products at high annealing temperatures, while later cycles amplify previously generated amplicons more efficiently using lower annealing temperatures, thereby increasing sensitivity (see also the use of touchdown PCR in multiplex PCR, below).

Taq polymerase is very sensitive to mismatches between the primer and the target DNA at the 3′ end of the primer but can withstand considerable noncomplementarity at the 5′ end of the primer. Numerous PCR variations have been designed to take advantage of both these facts. *Taq* polymerase also requires Mg^{2+} as a cofactor for stabilization of primer annealing. Insufficient Mg^{2+} decreases PCR efficiency, while too much Mg^{2+} stabilizes nonspecific primer annealing. Primers with a high GC content may show a narrow range of tolerance for variation from ideal PCR conditions, leading to decreased amplification or nonspecific products. This may be alleviated by using PCR additives such as dimethyl sulfoxide (DMSO) or glycerol, but the success of these additives may need to be determined empirically for different primer pairs. Another strategy to improve specificity is the use of "hot-start" PCR, in which a crucial PCR reactant such as *Taq* is either physically or chemically sequestered from other PCR reagents until denaturation begins. This prevents the generation of nonspecific amplification products by inhibiting the activity of *Taq* until after the initial PCR denaturation step.

PCR is more sensitive than Southern blot hybridization because of the amplification of the target sequence. However, the specificity of the amplified PCR product must be verified. Simple agarose gel electrophoresis coupled with EtBr staining may be used to observe the PCR product(s). When a clinical PCR protocol is established, such gels may be subjected the first time to blot hybridization with a specific probe complementary to the internal, non-primer sequence of the amplicon(s). This exercise proves that the PCR-generated band not only is the correct size and highly likely therefore to be the correct target, but also is a DNA fragment that has high or perfect homology with a known probe. For example, hybridization of a particular 302 bp PCR product band detectable on an agarose gel with a defined cytomegalovirus (CMV) DNA probe confirms that the oligonucleotide primers synthesized based on the CMV sequence and used in the PCR are recognizing CMV-specific DNA and that the PCR is indeed specific for detection of CMV. An alternative method to validate the specificity of the PCR product is to sequence the PCR product. Following this one-time validation analysis, electrophoresis alone, as opposed to blot hybridization or sequencing, may be the assay endpoint.

There have been significant commercial endeavors to automate or semiautomate high-volume PCR-based clinical tests. For example, denatured aliquots of completed PCRs can be added to microtiter plates with wells to which specific DNA probes are bound. In the presence of amplicon, for example, if the patient is infected with the pathogen of interest or a specific mutation is present, the amplicons hybridize to the bound probe and are retained in the well during washing. Subsequent biochemical reactions are used to detect labeled moieties in the amplicons ("built in" to the PCR components), facilitating colorimetric detection of a positive patient reaction by an automated plate reader. Absence of colored product in a well indicates a negative result for that patient specimen, provided that all positive and negative controls are within tolerance limits. This scheme has gained US Food and Drug Administration (FDA) approval for clinical PCR-based detection kits for *Chlamydia trachomatis*, *Neisseria gonorrhoeae*, HCV (qualitative) and HIV.[13] (For a complete list of FDA-approved tests, go to the Resources section at http://www.amp.org/, the home page for the Association for Molecular Pathology). Subsequent generations of automated PCR instrumentation are now available that completely automate the amplification and detection process.[14] The field is moving toward real-time PCR detection (described below).

Another aspect of PCR that is attractive for the clincal molecular laboratory is the ability to use relatively crude extractions of patient specimens rather than highly purified DNA. Cell lysis and subsequent DNA liberation accomplished by boiling or treatment with detergent may be sufficient to process a specimen in preparation for PCR.[15] Conventional PCR-based tests may be completed with turnaround times of as short as 2 to 4 hours, while real-time PCR can be completed in 30 minutes, making this technique attractive for stat testing.

Examples of Applications of PCR

1. Detection of the diagnostic *BCL2/IGH* gene rearrangement in follicular lymphoma
2. Detection of *Chlamydia trachomatis* in urine

PCR Variations

PCR-Restriction Fragment Length Polymorphism Analysis

Polymorphisms are inherited differences found among the individuals in a population. The term "polymorphism" is not synonymous with the term "mutation" in that mutations are variations found less frequently in a population or occur as nongermline changes usually in a tumor cell (somatic mutations). In the case of restriction fragment length polymorphisms (RFLP), DNA sequence differences alter RE recognition sites, manifested either as obliteration or creation of a restriction site. With obliteration of an RE site, the DNA of individuals with an RFLP exhibits a larger restriction fragment of DNA than those without the polymorphism. With creation of a new RE site, RE digestion results in two smaller fragments relative to the unaffected individual. In either case, the polymorphism is detectable by creation of a new restriction fragment pattern, that is, a restriction fragment length polymorphism. In PCR-RFLP, the PCR products are digested by one or a combination of REs and electrophoresed to detect polymorphisms or mutations which are seen as changes in the DNA fragment sizes reflected by changes in the band pattern on the gel.

Examples of Applications of PCR-RFLP Analysis

1. Detection of sickle-cell hemoglobin (HbS)
2. Detection of the *Mnl* I restriction enzyme polymorphism created by the Factor V_{Leiden} mutation[16]

Restriction-Site Generating PCR

Some mutations create or abolish RE recognition sites and can easily be detected by PCR-RFLP. Unfortunately, most polymorphisms or mutations do not alter an RE recognition site. In restriction-site generating PCR (RG-PCR) (and a related research technique called PCR-mediated site-directed mutagenesis [PSDM]), an artificial RE recognition site is generated during PCR using a specially designed PCR primer.[17,18] The primer contains a base mismatch to the template DNA adjacent to the variable base of the mutation that creates an RE recognition site in the PCR product. The mismatched base in the primer is located near or at the 3′ end of the primer, which is near or adjacent to the variable base of the mutation, and together they create a novel restriction site within either the mutant or wild-type amplicon. The presence or absence of the RE recognition site is determined from the pattern of digested fragments by gel electrophoresis. Not all sequences are amenable to the generation of a restriction site, and the amplification efficiency is often decreased due to destabilization of the primer with the mismatch.

Examples of Applications of RG-PCR

1. Identification of *KRAS* codon 12 mutations in colon cancer[19]
2. Identification of mutations in the *CTFR* gene in cystic fibrosis
3. Identification of mutations in the *ATM* gene in ataxia-telangectasis

Multiplex PCR

Multiplex PCR (M-PCR) is a demanding technique used for amplification of several discrete genetic loci with multiple PCR primer pairs in a single reaction. Multiplex PCR simultaneously answers several related questions about a specimen without the need for multiple individual PCR reactions. Multiplex PCR is commonly used for verification that amplifiable nucleic acid is present in the sample, for example, amplification of a housekeeping gene in addition to the gene sequence of interest, and to check for the presence of PCR inhibitors that can prevent amplification of target nucleic acid, for example, coamplification of an exogenously added internal control. Multiplex PCR often requires painstaking optimization of PCR conditions and careful design of the multiple primer pairs to prevent the generation of primer-dimers and other nonspecific PCR products that may interfere with the amplification of specific products. Touchdown PCR can be used with multiplex PCR if the primer pairs have different annealing temperatures. Concentrations of individual primer pairs may need to be optimized to account for different amplification efficiencies and competition between the primer pairs.

Examples of Applications of Multiplex PCR

1. Detection of enterovirus and herpes simplex virus (HSV) nucleic acids in cerebrospinal fluid (CSF)
2. Detection of pathogenic enteric bacteria in stool
3. Analysis of multiple *BRCA1* loci in a breast cancer patient[19]
4. Identification of different bacteria in a respiratory infection[20]
5. Amplification of multide microsatellite loci for bone marrow engraftment analysis

Nested PCR

In nested PCR, two pairs of PCR primers with one set internal to the other (nested) are used to sequentially amplify a single locus. The first pair is used to amplify the locus as in any PCR assay. A dilution of the first PCR reaction then is amplified with the nested primers. Alternatively, semi-nested PCR is performed using one of the original PCR primers and one new internal primer in a second round of amplification. Both nested and semi-nested PCR generate a second PCR product that is shorter than the first one.[21] The logic behind this strategy is that if the wrong locus was amplified incorrectly or nonspecifically, the probability is very low that it would be amplified a second time by a second pair of primers. Thus, nested PCR enhances specificity while also increasing sensitivity. The problem with nested PCR is the high risk of amplicon contamination when the first-round PCR products are used to set up the second round of PCR with the nested primers (see section below on amplicon contamination control). For this reason, many clinical laboratories do not use nested PCR procedures.

Allele-Specific PCR

Allele-specific PCR (AS-PCR) also is referred to as amplification refractory mutation system (ARMS), PCR amplification of specific alleles (PASA) and PCR amplification with sequence-specific primers (PCR-SSP). AS-PCR is based on the principle that a 3′ mismatch between a PCR primer and the template DNA prevents PCR amplification.[22] AS-PCR is especially useful for detection of single nucleotide polymorphisms (SNPs) or mutations. For AS-PCR, target DNA is amplified in two separate and simultaneous reactions. Each reaction contains an allele-specific primer (either normal or mutant) and a second primer common to both reactions. PCR is performed under stringent conditions, to prevent PCR amplification if a mismatch is present. Genotype is based on amplification in either one of the reactions alone (homozygous normal or mutant) or both reactions (heterozygous). Detection of the amplicon is by either gel electrophoresis or real-time PCR technology (see below). A disadvantage of AS-PCR is that unsuspected nucleotide polymorphisms or mutations located in the DNA template at or adjacent to the 3′ binding site of the primer would prevent amplification, leading to incorrect genotyping.

AS-PCR can detect one mutant allele in the presence of 40 copies of the normal allele. AS-PCR can be combined with M-PCR using multiple allele-specific primers in the same reaction tube. This technique is known as multiplex ARMS, a useful method when a single disease is caused by different mutations in one or more genes. Multiplex PCR-SSP also is commonly used in low-resolution HLA typing, in which multiple primer pairs for HLA loci are used along with control primers that amplify a housekeeping gene to verify that amplifiable DNA is present in each reaction tube.

Examples of Applications of AS-PCR

1. Detection of multiple cystic fibrosis CFTR mutations
2. Detection of alpha-1 antitrypsin deficiency mutations
3. Defection of phenylketonuria mutations

Allele-Specific Oligonucleotide Hybridization

Allele-specific oligonucleotide hybridization (ASOH), also known as dot-blot analysis, is used for genotyping of highly polymorphic regions of DNA. ASOH can be thought of as a variation of the Southern blot, in that patient DNA amplified by PCR is bound to a membrane and hybridized with labeled allele-specific oligonucleotide probes.[23] Reverse dot-blot analysis differs from ASOH in that unlabeled allele-specific oligonucleotide probes are spotted onto different membrane locations and hybridized with labeled PCR amplicons.

For ASOH, the PCR products are denatured and a small amount of denatured (single stranded) amplicon is spotted onto a nylon or nitrocellulose membrane. The amplicon is permanently bound to the membrane by baking under vacuum or UV cross-linking. Amplicons from different specimens can be spotted at different locations to interrogate the genotype of multiple specimens simultaneously. Duplicate membranes are made for each probe type. Each membrane is hybridized with two different labeled oligonucleotide probes (one complementary to the mutant sequence and another to the normal sequence of the same DNA region). The membranes are washed to remove nonspecifically bound probe. Samples that hybridize strongly to only one probe indicate homozygosity for the normal or mutant allele; those that hybridize with both probes are heterozygous. The oligonucleotide probes are labeled and detected by radioactivity (often avoided in clinical molecular laboratories), fluorescence, colorimetry, chemiluminescence, or mass spectrometry. One criticism of ASOH is the potentially ambiguous discrimination of a positive signal. Optimization of the assay and the use of both positive and negative controls help to define and score ASOH results.

Example of Application of ASOH

1. Low-resolution HLA typing

Oligonucleotide Ligation Assay

Oligonucleotide ligation assay (OLA) is a highly specific method for detecting well-defined alleles that differ by a single base.[24,25] The target sequence is initially amplified using PCR and then denatured. A pair of allele-specific oligonucleotide (ASO) probes (one specific for the wild-type allele and the other specific for the mutant allele), a common reporter probe (complementary to a sequence common to both alleles), and DNA ligase are added to the denatured PCR products. The ASO probes are designed to differ from one another only at the terminal 3′ base. The common reporter probe is positioned immediately adjacent to the 3′ terminal end of the ASO probes. If the ASO is complementary to the amplicon, DNA ligase can covalently join the ASO and the reporter probe. If the ASO is not a perfect match to the amplicon, the 3′ base does not anneal with the amplicon, and DNA ligase cannot join the ASO and reporter probes. The ligation products are analyzed by electrophoresis. Alternatively, one of the probes can be biotinylated at the 5′ end and the other probe tagged at the 3′ end with a reporter molecule such as fluorescein or digoxigenin. If ligation occurs, the ligation product is biotinylated at one end, facilitating capture onto a streptavidin-coated microtiter plate. The opposite end contains the reporter label. Washing removes unbound label and the reporter molecule is detected.

Dynamic Allele-Specific Hybridization

Dynamic allele-specific hybridization (DASH) is a temperature-dependent, real-time variation of ASOH.[26] Dynamic allele-specific hybridization begins with amplification of polymorphic DNA regions by PCR in which one primer is biotinylated. The biotinylated product strand is bound to a streptavidin-coated microtiter plate well, and the non-biotinylated strand is washed away. An oligonucleotide probe complementary to one allele is annealed to a bound PCR product strand, forming a DNA duplex that interacts with a double-strand-specific intercalation dye. On excitation, the dye emits fluorescence proportional to the amount of double-stranded DNA (probe-target duplex) present. The duplex is heated through a temperature range while the fluorescent signal is continually monitored. A rapid fall in fluorescent signal indicates denaturation of the DNA duplex. DNA duplexes with nonhomologous regions denature at a lower temperature than completely homologous DNA. The melting-temperature profile distinguishes homozygosity for either allele alone or a heterozygous mixture of the two.

Reverse Transcription–Polymerase Chain Reaction

Reverse transcription–polymerase chain reaction (RT-PCR) may be thought of as RNA-based PCR. RT-PCR was made possible by the discovery in the early 1970s of retroviral reverse transcriptase (RT), an RNA-dependent DNA polymerase, by David Baltimore and Howard Temin,[27] for which they shared the Nobel Prize in 1975. Reverse transcriptase catalyzes DNA synthesis using RNA as the template, producing a DNA strand complementary to the RNA template, called complementary DNA (cDNA). Because cDNA is not subject to RNase degradation, it is far more stable than the corresponding RNA. Complementary DNA can be treated like any other DNA target in subsequent PCR. Logistically, RT-PCR is trivially more time-consuming than PCR due to the extra enzymatic step of reverse transcription, but there are enzymes that combine reverse transcription and DNA polymerase activities, making RT-PCR more efficient. With the introduction of techniques to successfully isolate and protect RNA from ubiquitous RNases, and to synthesize cDNA by reverse transcription and the discovery of PCR, RNA analysis is now virtually as rapid and sensitive as PCR-based DNA investigation. RT-PCR is a high-volume test method for the clinical molecular laboratory due to its use in the diagnosis and quantitation of RNA virus infections, principally HIV and HCV.

Examples of Applications of RT-PCR

1. HIV and HCV viral load determinations
2. Detection of *BCR*/*ABL* translocation diagnostic of chronic myelogenous leukemia

Real-Time PCR

Real-time PCR is based on the generation of a fluorescent signal by the PCR process, which is detected during PCR cycling (i.e., in real time) and reflects the amount of PCR product synthesized.[28–30] Different real-time PCR methods use alternative ways to generate a fluorescent signal during PCR. These include an intercalating dye such as SYBR Green that binds the minor groove of DNA, or an oligonucleotide used as a primer or probe and labeled with a fluorogenic dye. Instruments that combine in vitro nucleic acid amplification and real-time detection of the PCR product are dramatically increasing test menus for oncology, infectious diseases, and genetics in clinical molecular laboratories because of the wide range of readily available amplification primers and detection schemes, rapid turnaround time, the potential to eliminate the time and costs associated with electrophoresis, and the reduction in PCR contamination risk.

Real-time PCR is different from conventional PCR in several ways.

- Amplicon generation, temperature profiles, and melt curves are monitored in real time, reducing the time required for post-PCR analysis. In most cases, there is no need for postamplification processing of the PCR products. This eliminates the need for gel electrophoresis and, because the reaction tubes remain closed after PCR starts, there is decreased risk of amplicon carryover contamination within the laboratory.
- Results are more reproducible between runs since quantitation of target is based on amplification cycle threshold in the log-linear phase of amplification rather than traditional endpoint analysis in the PCR plateau phase.
- Real-time PCR methods have a wide dynamic range, up to 10 logs.
- Real-time PCR systems with intercalating dye or fluorogenic probes can be used to perform melting-curve analysis. This adds a check for specificity or potentially the detection of unknown sequence variants (see below).

The simplest real-time PCR method uses intercalating dyes that insert into the stacked bases of DNA PCR products, allowing detection of amplification in real time. These dyes, for example, SYBR Green and EtBr, are nonsequence-specific dyes that increase in fluorescence when bound to double-stranded DNA. Intercalating dyes are often used for melting-curve analysis, qualitative and semiquantitative PCR, product discrimination and purity, and determination of primer and probe melting T_m. Intercalating dyes can be used for quantitative PCR. Results, however, are more specific and accurate with a sequence-specific probe since fluorescence is directly proportional to the amount of specific amplicon produced and reduces the background contributed by primer-dimers or nonspecific PCR products. Intercalating dye fluorescence represents all double-stranded DNA, including primer-dimers and other non-specific product that can be visualized with an endpoint melting-curve analysis.

Most fluorogenic oligonucleotide techniques take advantage of the principle of fluorescent resonance energy transfer (FRET), in which the energy from one dye molecule (the donor) is transferred without the emission of a photon to an acceptor dye molecule when the two are in close proximity. If the acceptor is a fluorophore, a photon is emitted at a characteristic wavelength. However, if the acceptor does not emit a photon, the energy is dissipated and fluorescence from the donor is quenched. The reporter dye can be either the donor (if no FRET takes place) or the acceptor (if FRET does take place) and is defined as the one whose fluorescence correlates with the quantity of desired PCR amplicon. Several fluorogenic techniques are described below.

TaqMan

TaqMan uses a short probe complementary to a non-primer internal sequence of the PCR product. The probe is labeled at the 5′ end with a reporter donor dye and at the 3′ end with an acceptor dye that quenches the reporter when the probe is intact. During the extension phase of PCR, probe bound to an amplicon is cleaved by the 5′ endonuclease activity of *Taq* polymerase, freeing the reporter dye from the quencher and resulting in fluorescence. The fluorescent signal increases proportionally to the number of amplicons generated during the log-linear phase of amplification. To ensure that hydrolysis of the probe occurs, a two-step PCR can be used with annealing and extension taking place at the same temperature (~60°C). Ideally, the TaqMan probe binding site is located near one primer and the size of the amplicon is no longer than 200 to 300 bases. One negative aspect of this format is that once the probe is hydrolyzed, it is unavailable for subsequent reactions or melting-curve analysis, thus requiring an excess amount of probe in the reaction mix with the potential to decrease the PCR efficiency.

Molecular Beacon

A molecular beacon is a longer probe with a 5′ reporter dye and 3′ quencher dye. The probe forms a hairpin loop structure when not bound to target DNA, thereby juxtaposing the dyes with quenching of fluorescence. The loop sequence is complementary to the non-primer amplicon sequence. When the loop of the molecular beacon probe hybridizes to the amplicon during the annealing step of real-time PCR, the reporter dye is separated from the quencher, resulting in fluorescence. For the molecular beacon probe to anneal to the amplicon, the amplicon-probe hybrid must be more stable than the internal base-pairing hairpin so that a fluorescent signal is generated. Generally, DABCYL is the nonfluorescent universal quencher and the other dye is a reporter fluorophore such as FAM, Cy3, TET, TAMRA, Texas Red, ROX, or Cy5.

Hybridization

Hybridization is a two-probe system in which one probe contains a donor dye and the other contains the reporter acceptor dye. The probes are designed to anneal to one strand of the PCR product adjacent to one another and internal to the primers. This juxtaposes the dyes, allowing FRET to occur. This probe format works well with the traditional three-step PCR with annealing at ~55°C (primer specific) and extension at 72°C, the optimal temperature for *Taq* polymerase activity. When DNA polymerase encounters the probes, they are displaced from the target strand rather than hydrolyzed and thus available for the next round of amplification as well as endpoint melting-curve analysis.

Uniprimer (Amplifluor, Sunrise)

Like molecular beacon probes, the uniprimer system uses a hairpin structure in the oligonucleotide to quench fluorescence. The 3′ region of the fluorogenic oligonucleotide is identical to a nonbinding region at the 5′ end of the reverse PCR primer. This allows the fluorogenic oligonucleotide to become a primer for the newly formed amplicon by the third round of PCR. The probe is then opened in the fourth and subsequent rounds of PCR by the polymerase action of *Taq*, allowing fluorescence to occur. The advantage of this system is that the same fluorogenic oligonucleotide can be used in any PCR reaction (universal fluorogenic primer).

Scorpion

Scorpion also uses a hairpin structure in the oligonucleotide to quench fluorescence. The fluorogenic oligonucleotide is part of the reverse primer, and the nucleotides in the hairpin are complementary to the PCR amplicon sequence between the primers. The Scorpion primer unfolds and anneals to the PCR amplicon, allowing fluorescence to take place beginning in the first round of PCR.

Lux

Lux is a variation of real-time PCR that uses a single fluorophore in a primer with a hairpin loop structure. The fluorophore is quenched by the complementary structure of nucleotides in the stem of the hairpin loop. When the primer is incorporated into double-stranded DNA, thus opening the hairpin loop, fluorescence is maximal. The advantage of this system is lower production costs with the use of only one fluorophore.

Real-Time PCR Method

The following concepts are important for understanding the use of real-time PCR in a clinical diagnostic laboratory. When optimizing real-time PCR, the growth curve of the fluorescent signal versus the number of PCR cycles should be monitored to determine when optimal conditions have been achieved (Figure 2-2). The growth curve should be sigmoidal (S shaped) with three phases: baseline (background signal or lag phase), log-linear (exponential amplification phase), and plateau. For each phase, several characteristics should be assessed. The baseline phase of the curve represents initial cycles of amplification in which accumulation of the specific signal has not yet exceeded the background signal. The fluorescent signal in this phase is from unbound probe or autofluorescing components in the reaction. The log-linear phase of the curve represents exponential amplification of the target (see Figure 2-1) and provides useful information about the reaction. The curve can be described by the following equation: $T_n = T_0(E)^n$, where T_n is the amount of target sequence at cycle n, T_0 is the initial amount of target sequence at cycle 0, and E is the amplification efficiency of the target sequence. The crossing point represents the number of PCR cycles at which the growth curve enters the log-linear phase. There is an inverse linear relationship between the crossing-point cycle number and the number of template copies present in a reaction.

The slope of the log-linear phase is a reflection of amplification efficiency, and the efficiency of the reaction can be determined by identifying the crossing points of known standards and plotting a line of linear regression (see Figure 2-3). The efficiency can then be determined using the following equation: $E = 10^{-1/slope}$, where E is efficiency and slope is the slope of the standard curve. Using this equation, the slope should be between -3 and -4, with -3.3 indicative of efficiency close to or at 2. The

inflection point is the point at which the log-linear amplification curve goes from positive to negative and begins to enter the plateau phase. If there is no inflection point, the curve may represent not amplification of DNA, but rather signal drift. Drift is characterized by gradual increase or decrease in fluorescence without amplification of product.

Plateau is defined as the phase of growth when critical components become rate limiting and amplicon accumulation is minimized or stops. The plateau is also the point at which incremental increase in fluorescent signal stops. As the rate of accumulation slows and enters the plateau phase, the curve levels. Since endpoint measurements are often made in conventional PCR when reaction components are limited, minor sample variations can have a relatively major effect on endpoint product. Real-time PCR focuses on the rate of amplicon accumulation (log-linear phase and cycle threshold or crossing point), not on endpoint signal. The plateau phase can be shortened by decreasing the number of cycles for a product of greater purity. Several factors contribute to the plateau phase: PCR product reannealing versus primer annealing, enzyme or dNTPs becoming limiting, and amplicon buildup with resultant reaction inhibition.

Real-time PCR utilizes the log-linear phase of the amplification curve for data analysis. This method provides a more accurate measurement than endpoint analysis. The cycle at which the curve crosses a specified threshold is called the cycle threshold (Ct), or crossing point (Cp). The Ct value can be used for qualitative or quantitative analysis. A qualitative analysis uses the defined Ct as a pass/fail measurement. A quantitative assay uses the Ct of defined standards of known template concentration to generate a standard curve. Then the Ct values for unknown samples are used to extrapolate the concentration(s) in the unknown samples from the standard curve. Some real-time instrumentation software allows determination of the Ct by a mathematical analysis of the amplification curve, rather than crossing at a set fluorescent signal threshold. Plotting the second derivative of the growth curve generates a peak that corresponds to a point near the baseline of the growth

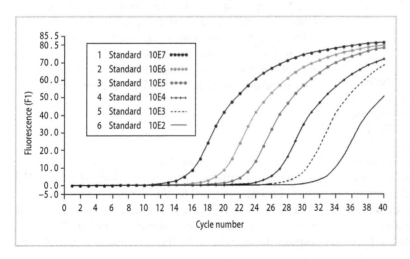

Figure 2-2. Real-time PCR curves for a 10-fold dilution series of a known standard. Data provided by Roche Molecular Diagnostics. (Used by permission. Data © 2003 Roche Diagnostics Corporation, all rights reserved.)

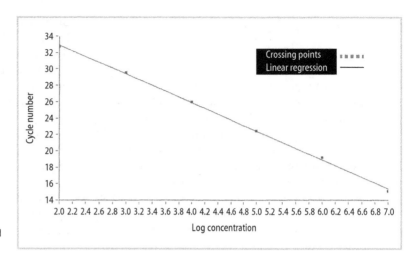

Figure 2-3. Standard curve generated by real-time PCR of a 10-fold dilution series of a known standard.

curve (see Figure 2-4). The cycle at which this peak occurs is designated as the Ct or Cp. This analysis method can provide better run-to-run reproducibility than manually setting the Ct using the primary signal.

DNA Methylation and Methylation-Specific PCR

DNA methylation is a mechanism by which the cell regulates gene expression. Methylation is an enzyme-mediated modification that adds a methyl ($-CH_3$) group at a selected site on DNA or RNA. In humans, methylation occurs only at cytosine (C) bases followed by a guanosine (G), known as CpG dinucleotides. The CpG dinucleotides are prone to spontaneous mutations and have been selectively depleted from the mammalian genome. However, some regions of DNA have retained CpG dinucleotides and are referred to as CpG islands. The CpG islands are found primarily in the 5′ region of expressed genes, often in association with promoters. When the promoter CpG island is methylated, the corresponding gene is silenced and transcription does not occur. This is one method of silencing imprinted genes, as the transcription repression is passed on through cell division. Aberrant CpG island methylation of tumor-suppressor genes is frequent in cancer and appears to be an important mechanism of neoplastic transformation.

Methylated DNA can be distinguished from unmethylated DNA using sodium bisulfite treatment of DNA, which converts unmethylated C to uracil (U) but leaves methylated C intact.[31] This in vitro treatment can then be followed by one of several methods to distinguish C from U, including restriction endonuclease digestion with methylation-sensitive enzymes, sequencing, or methylation-specific PCR (MSP).[32] MSP of bisulfite-treated DNA uses primer pairs that specifically identify either methylated or unmethylated DNA. The primers are designed to hybridize to regions containing one to three CpG sites concentrated in the 3′ region of the primer to increase the specificity of amplification, and enough non-CpG cytosines to ensure that unmodified DNA is not amplified. Gel electrophoresis is used to detect the presence or absence of the amplicon in each of the two reactions, indicating the presence of unmethylated or methylated alleles or both. A novel modification is the use of quantitative MSP, which combines MSP with real-time PCR to distinguish the high-level CpG methylation in neoplasia from low-level methylation that can occur with aging or in nonneoplastic conditions such as metaplasia.[33]

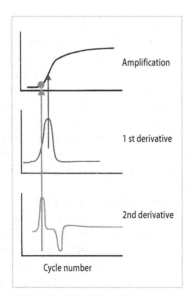

Figure 2-4. Graphical depiction of the second derivative maximum method used to identify the crossing point (Y axis is fluorescence value).

Examples of Applications of Methylation-Specific PCR

1. Analysis of imprinted genes
2. Clonality assessment based on X chromosome inactivation
3. Abnormal methylation in neoplasia

PCR Variations for Unknown Sequence Variants

Most of the techniques discussed above are used to screen for sequence variants (both mutations and polymorphisms) based on previous knowledge of the variant; i.e., the sequence of the variant is either known or defined by the experimental conditions. By contrast, there is an evolving interest in both research and clinical molecular pathology to identify sequence variants by scanning without prior knowledge of their existence; i.e., the sequence of the variant is unknown. Sequencing is the ultimate screening technique, but is costly and labor-intensive. The goal of the scanning techniques described below (denaturing gradient gel electrophoresis [DDGE], and temperature gradient gel electrophoresis [TGGE], heteroduplex analysis [HA], single-strand conformation polymorphism [SSCP], denaturing high-performance liquid chromatography [DHPLC], and protein truncation test [PTT]) is to identify specimens with possible variant sequences, thereby reducing costs relative to sequencing. Should an unknown variant be detected, for example by a shift in the mobility of the PCR product on a gel or capillary, the PCR product with altered mobility is isolated and sequenced. Melting-temperature analysis in real-time PCR also can be used to identify unknown sequence variants.

Denaturing Gradient Gel Electrophoresis and Temperature Gradient Gel Electrophoresis

Denaturing gradient gel electrophoresis (DGGE)[34,35] and temperature gradient gel electrophoresis (TGGE)[36,37] are similar methods for separating DNA fragments with similar lengths but with different sequences according to their mobilities under a linear gradient of increasingly denaturing conditions. The gradient is created in DGGE with a mixture of urea and formamide, and in TGGE with a combination of water baths and a cooling plate under the gel. Both DGGE and TGGE take advantage of the markedly decreased mobility of partially melted dsDNA compared to either fully annealed dsDNA or ssDNA. Melting within a dsDNA fragment occurs within stretches of base pairs called melting domains. The point at which a domain begins to denature is referred to as the melting temperature (T_m), whether melting was induced by temperature or denaturing chemicals. In general, GC-rich sequences are more resistant to denaturation because of the three hydrogen bonds holding G and C together, as opposed to the two hydrogen bonds between A and T. During electrophoresis, once a dsDNA fragment reaches the point at which the melting domain with the lowest T_m begins to denature, mobility of the fragment through the gel nearly ceases. Fragments that melt early in the gel can therefore be separated from those that melt later. Complete denaturation of the dsDNA can be prevented by adding a GC-rich region to the 5′ end of one of the primers (GC clamp), increasing the sensitivity for detection of sequence variants.

In DGGE and TGGE, the denaturing conditions and the time of electrophoresis should be optimized such that normal sequences migrate to an intermediate position in the gel by the end of electrophoresis. This allows sequence variants creating either a higher or lower T_m to be identified. The denaturing gradient may be perpendicular or parallel to the electric field. Perpendicular gradient gels covering a broad range of denaturing conditions are loaded with normal sequence in all lanes to find the optimal, narrower denaturing gradient (chemical or temperature) for later use in parallel gradient gels. Parallel gradients are then used to run samples but also to optimize the time of electrophoresis by loading the normal sequence to different lanes at different times. Double-gradient DGGE adds a sieving gradient, for example, 6% to 12% polyacrylamide, colinear with the denaturing gradient in the gel matrix, further improving band resolution.

Both DGGE and TGGE work best with DNA fragments less than 500 bp in length. When GC-clamped fragments are analyzed, the sensitivity of detecting a SNP is close to 99%. Following electrophoresis, specific bands can be isolated from the gel and sequenced. DNA fragments with a high GC content are not easily analyzed by DGGE, since all fragments are harder to melt.

Examples of Applications of DGGE or TGGE

1. *APC* gene mutation analysis in familial adenomatous polyposis[38]
2. *CTFR* gene mutation analysis in cystic fibrosis[39]
3. *TCRG* gene rearrangements in lymphoma[40]

Heteroduplex Analysis

Heteroduplex formation results when wild-type and mutant alleles are coamplified, denatured, and allowed to reanneal in a post-PCR annealing step, usually heating and cooling.[41] Some of the strands pair with the complementary strand from the same allele and form homoduplexes. However, some strands pair with a strand from the other allele and form heteroduplexes. Because the heteroduplexes have mismatched base pairs between strands, they form a partially open dsDNA sequence that migrates more slowly in electrophoresis than the fully annealed homoduplexes.

Two types of heteroduplex structures can be formed.[42] When the mismatch consists of one or more single-base mutations, small open areas of dsDNA called "bubble-type" heteroduplexes are formed. When the mismatch is formed by insertions or deletions between the two alleles, a pronounced bending of the dsDNA is produced and referred to as a "bulge-type" heteroduplex. Bulge-type heteroduplexes markedly affect the mobility of the dsDNA, whereas bubble-type heteroduplexes may be difficult to detect in polyacrylamide gels. Detection of single base-pair mismatches can be enhanced in two ways. Electrophoresis can be performed with mutation detection enhancement (MDE) gels, an altered form of polyacrylamide that enhances separation of heteroduplexes. The post-PCR introduction of a known sequence with a short deletion to form a bulge-type heteroduplex enhances the separation of sequences with base-pair mismatches in a process known as universal heteroduplex generation (UHG).

Examples of Applications of Heteroduplex Analysis

1. *HIV* subtyping
2. *CFTR* gene mutation analysis in cystic fibrosis
3. *NF1* gene mutation analysis in neurofibromatosis type 1

Single-Strand Conformation Polymorphism

The principle of single-strand conformation polymorphism (SSCP) is the differential gel separation of ssDNA that folds into a specific secondary structure based on its sequence.[43–45] For SSCP, the region of interest is amplified and the resulting amplicons are denatured using heat or a denaturation buffer, or both, prior to gel or capillary electrophoresis. Amplicons with different sequences will assume different folding conformations upon denaturation. Conformational differences reflecting sequence changes are detected as differences in electrophoretic mobility of the ssDNA in a nondenaturing polyacrylamide matrix. In general, a wild-type sample generates two bands, one for each of the two strands of the dsDNA product. Bands of mutant ssDNA migrate to positions different from those of the wild-type ssDNA. A homozygous mutant sample generates two bands, but with different migration patterns from the two wild-type bands. If a heterozygous mutant is present, four bands are generated: two with wild-type mobility and two with mutant mobility. Three also can be observed bands in heterozygous specimens if the mutation changes the conformation of only one strand but not the other. The bands with altered mobility can be isolated from wild-type bands in the gel, allowing even rare somatic mutations in tumors to be sequenced.

Temperature, ionic environment, and pH affect the conformation and therefore must be held constant throughout the SSCP run. Accurate temperature control during SSCP increases reliability and is an easily modifiable parameter in repeatable, nonisotopic experiments that may increase sensitivity. SSCP is adversely affected if unincorporated primers are allowed to bind to the ssDNA during denaturing and cooling prior to electrophoresis, or if nonspecific bands are produced by low-fidelity PCR. In SSCP, electrophoretic mobility patterns of variant alleles can be difficult to distinguish from wild type. Another disadvantage is that multiple experimental conditions are required for 100% sensitivity for detection of all sequence variants.

SSCP is most sensitive when the DNA amplicon is less than 200 bp in length. Sensitivity decreases as fragment length increases. This can be overcome by multiplexing differently sized fragments onto a single gel lane and by restriction enzyme digestion prior to electrophoresis. When restriction endonucleases are used, the procedure is referred to as restriction endonuclease fingerprinting–single-strand conformation polymorphism (REF-SSCP). Additionally, SSCP is relatively less sensitive for detecting G to C mutations. The addition of glycerol enhances mutation detection in this circumstance.

Variations of SSCP include RNA-SSCP (rSSCP), dideoxy fingerprinting (ddF), bidirectional ddF (bi-ddF), and SSCP detection of virtually all mutations (DOVAM-SSCP). RNA is more stable and adopts more conformational structures than does ssDNA, allowing enhanced detection using rSSCP. RNA-SSCP is not widely used because of the relative difficulty in producing RNA for analysis. Dideoxy fingerprinting involves a dideoxy Sanger single-primer termination reaction (cycle-sequencing reaction; for additional information on the Sanger reaction, see the section on sequencing, above) followed by nondenaturing electrophoresis. A fingerprint bandshift is indicative of sequence changes. Bidirectional ddF is an advancement of ddF whereby the dideoxy Sanger termination reaction is performed with two opposing primers in the same tube. SSCP detection of virtually all mutations is a recently described modification in which SSCP is performed under different conditions with different buffers and gel matrices that result in overall increased sensitivity for mutation identification.

The detection of an altered SSCP pattern does not identify the exact sequence variation present in the analyzed DNA. Therefore, positive SSCP results require DNA sequence analysis to confirm and identify sequence variation.

Examples of Applications of SSCP

1. Screening for mutations in the adenomatous polyposis coli (*APC*) gene
2. Mutation analysis of the *ATP7B* gene in Wilson disease
3. Mutation analysis in *BRCA1* (in familial breast cancer)
4. Pathogen identification[46]

Denaturing High-Performance Liquid Chromatography

Denaturing high-performance liquid chromatography (DHPLC) is an ion-paired, reversed-phase, liquid chromatography method used to identify mutations, including SNPs and small insertions or deletions, through its ability to separate heteroduplex DNA from homoduplex DNA[47]. DHPLC is conceptually similar to heteroduplex analysis (HA; see above). Conventional HA makes use of a gel matrix to separate homo- and heteroduplex species in a nondenaturing environment, whereas DHPLC uses partially denaturing conditions in a liquid chromatography column to exaggerate the separation between the two species.

The gene to be studied is first amplified using PCR. High-fidelity PCR is used to prevent the production of PCR artifacts (pseudoalleles) that could produce false-positive results. Optimal amplicon length is between 100 and 500 bp. Purifying the PCR product is usually not necessary, as unincorporated primers, nucleotides, and genomic DNA do not interfere with the analysis. DHPLC requires heteroduplex formation, accomplished by heating and slow cooling. Therefore, for conditions in which only one variant allele type may be present (such as recessive diseases, X-linked conditions in males, or small tumor samples with loss of heterozygosity in all cells), PCR products from normal and patient samples are mixed in equal proportions before heating and cooling to produce heteroduplex DNA and distinguish from homozygous wild-type alleles. The addition of normal PCR amplicons is not required when using DHPLC to test PCR products from heterozygous individuals, which naturally form heteroduplexes when denatured and slowly cooled.

The duplexes are injected into a DHPLC column, and the DNA binds to the stationary matrix. Binding is aided by triethylammonium acetate (TEAA). Because the stability of the binding depends on the temperature, the column is optimally held at the melting temperature of the PCR fragment. The melting temperature can be calculated using a variety of proprietary or free software programs. The DNA is next eluted using acetonitrile, an organic solution that facilitates the subsequent separation of the DNA from the column matrix, and DNA absorbancy is measured at 260 μm. The linear gradient of acetonitrile established in the column allows separation of DNA fragments based on size or the presence of heteroduplexes, or both. All DNA fragments impart a characteristic profile when the absorbance is plotted against elution time. The peak of maximum absorbance is the retention time of that DNA sample at a given acetonitrile concentration. Heteroduplexes are less stable and thus have a lower affinity for the column. The concentration of acetonitrile required to separate heteroduplexes from the column is therefore lower, so heteroduplexes elute from the column earlier than homoduplexes.

The column temperature and gradient conditions can be optimized for the separation of any heteroduplex-homoduplex mixture. Some DNA fragments have more than one melting domain and the analysis may be carried out at more than one temperature. One advantage of DHPLC is that reinjection of the same sample at different temperatures is possible. Other advantages include high detection rates of mutations, rapid separation times per sample, a high degree of automation, and the ability to collect elution fractions and sequence each eluted fragment. Disadvantages of DHPLC include the need for expensive equipment and columns, high-fidelity PCR, and optimization of each reaction required to achieve the highest sensitivity of mutation detection.

Examples of Applications of DHPLC

1. *RET* and *CFTR* mutation detection[48]
2. *BRCA1* and *BRCA2* mutation analysis[49]

Protein Truncation Test

The protein truncation test (PTT) is used to identify mutations that result in premature termination of protein translation. PTT detects mutations at the protein rather than the genomic DNA or RNA levels. Initially developed for Duchenne muscular dystrophy (DMD) testing, PTT now is used more widely,[50] since protein-truncating mutations are associated with multiple types of hereditary cancer syndromes, including breast, ovarian, and colon.

For PTT, the gene segment of interest is amplified by PCR. The amplicons are used for in vitro transcription and translation in a coupled reaction. The resulting proteins are separated using sodium dodecyl sulfate (SDS) polyacrylamide gel electrophoresis. The presence of a premature termination codon is indicated by the visualization of a lower-molecular-weight protein band than for the wild-type protein. Relatively large gene fragments (2–4 kb) can be analyzed using PTT.

Examples of Applications of PTT

1. Duchenne muscular dystrophy diagnosis
2. *BRCA1* and *BRCA2* mutation detection[51]
3. *APC* mutations in colorectal cancer[52]

Other Forms of In Vitro Nucleic Acid Amplification

PCR is widely used in the clinical laboratory. The proprietary nature of PCR prompted other in vitro diagnostic companies to develop alternative methods of in vitro nucleic acid amplification. Several are described here: ligase chain reaction (LCR); transcription mediated amplification (TMA), strand displacement amplification (SDA); and nucleic acid sequence–based amplification (NASBA).

Ligase Chain Reaction

Ligase chain reaction (LCR)[53,54] is initiated when a mixture of target DNA, thermostable DNA ligase, four oligonucleotide probes, and NAD$^+$ or ATP is heated to denature dsDNA (both target and complementary probes) in the reaction mixture. Two pairs of complementary probes are used, and, of necessity, their correct design demands a priori knowledge of the sequence of the DNA target. After denaturation and subsequent reaction cooling, the four probes present in the reaction mixture hybridize to their complementary sequences on each target DNA sister strand. The two probes that hybridize to one sister strand and the two probes that bind to the other sister strand are designed such that when hybridized, the 3′ hydroxyl end of the upstream probe is immediately adjacent to the 5′ phosphate end of the downstream probe. Thermostable DNA ligase enzymatically ligates the two bound probes, thus achieving a "doubling" of the mass of target DNA in the reaction. As the temperature cycling proceeds, a theoretical exponential amplification of the mass of target DNA in the original reaction occurs because the resultant ligated amplicons also serve as targets for probe hybridizations. In practice, amplification is less than exponential, but sufficient to achieve target DNA identification by various detection methods.

There is a tendency for target-independent blunt-end ligation of the probes in the reaction to occur in LCR, which can cause unacceptably high levels of background signal, limiting the assay's sensitivity and specificity. This problem has been solved by use of gap LCR (G-LCR). In G-LCR, the probes are designed such that they cannot be ligated in a target-independent manner because they are not blunt ended. When G-LCR probes hybridize to target DNA, a gap of one or more bases exists between the probes

hybridized to the same target strand. This gap is then biochemically "filled" in vitro, thus providing a suitable substrate for DNA ligase, which then performs target-dependent ligation.

Examples of Applications of LCR

1. *Chlamydia trachomatis* detection
2. *Neisseria gonorrhoeae* detection

Transcription-Mediated Amplification

Transcription-mediated amplification (TMA) uses RNA as the template, two primers and two enzymes: reverse transcriptase and RNA polymerase. One primer contains a promoter sequence that binds RNA polymerase. As the amplification process begins, the promoter-containing primer hybridizes to the target RNA at a complementary site (Figure 2-5). Reverse transcriptase then synthesizes a cDNA copy of the target RNA template by extension of the 3′ end of the promoter-primer. The result is an RNA:DNA duplex. The RNA component is degraded by the activity of the enzyme RNase H inherent in reverse transcriptase. The other primer in the reaction mixture hybridizes to the DNA

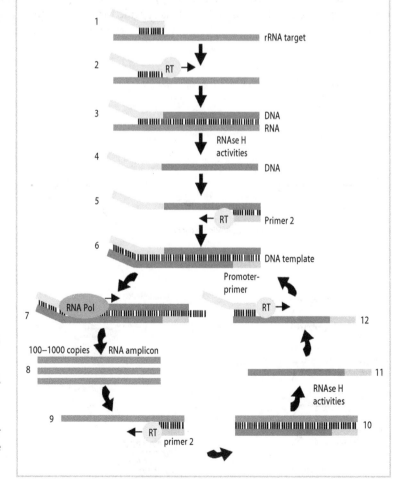

Figure 2-5. Transcription-mediated amplification cycle (TMA):
Step 1. Promoter-primer binds to rRNA target.
Step 2. Reverse transcriptase (RT) creates DNA copy of rRNA target.
Step 3. RNA:DNA duplex.
Step 4. RNAse H activities of RT degrades the rRNA.
Step 5. Primer 2 binds to the DNA and RT creates a new DNA copy.
Step 6. Double-stranded DNA template with a promoter sequence.
Step 7. RNA polymerase (RNA Pol) initiates transcription of RNA from DNA template.
Step 8. 100 to 1000 copies of RNA amplicon are produced.
Step 9. Primer 2 binds to each RNA amplicon and RT creates a DNA copy.
Step 10. RNA:DNA duplex.
Step 11. RNAse H activities of RT degrades the rRNA.
Step 12. Promoter-primer binds to the newly synthesized DNA. RT creates a double-stranded DNA and the autocatalytic cycle repeats, resulting in a billion-fold amplification.

(Reprinted with permission from Gen-Probe.)

copy, and a new DNA strand is synthesized from the end of the primer by RT, generating a dsDNA molecule. The other enzyme in the mixture, RNA polymerase, binds the promoter sequence in the DNA template and initiates transcription. Each of the resulting newly synthesized RNA amplicons reenters the TMA cycle, serving as a template for a new round of replication and exponential expansion of the RNA target. Each DNA template can generate 10^2 to 10^3 copies of RNA amplicon, with the potential for 10^8- to 10^9-fold amplification in less than 1 hour. The process is autocatalytic and isothermal. Acridinium ester–labeled DNA probes are added on completion of the reaction to initiate detection and quantitation based on chemiluminescence.

Examples of Applications of TMA

1. *Chlamydia trachomatis* detection[55]
2. *Neisseria gonorrhoeae* detection
3. HCV detection (qualitative)[56]

Strand Displacement Amplification

Strand displacement amplification (SDA) is an isothermal in vitro nucleic acid amplification technique.[57] Hemimodified DNA is polymerized by using three conventional dNTPs and one containing a 5′-[alpha-thio]triphosphate. The primer(s) is designed with an RE recognition site in the 5′ overhang end. The recognition site is specific for an RE that can nick the unmodified DNA strand at a double-stranded hemiphosphorothioate recognition site, that is, when the newly synthesized strand incorporates the 5′-[alpha-thio]triphosphate nucleotide in the recognition sequence. DNA polymerase lacking 5′ to 3′ exonuclease activity is used to extend the 3′ end at the nick and displace the downstream strand. Nicking and polymerization with re-formation of the hemiphosphorothioate recognition site continuously cycle, generating complementary copies of the DNA target. Linear amplification (called target-generation SDA) occurs when a single primer is used. Exponential amplification (exponential SDA) is achieved by using two primers complementary to opposite DNA strands, with both primers containing RE recognition sites in the 5′ overhang end. Strand displacement amplification has been used in a microarray format,[58] which may become a clinically useful method to combine amplification of low copy number targets with the multiple features of microarray in a format that can be automated.

Examples of Applications of SDA

1. *Chlamydia trachomatis* detection
2. *Neisseria gonorrhoeae* detection

Nucleic Acid Sequence–Based Amplification

Nucleic acid sequence–based amplification (NASBA) is an isothermal method for amplifying nucleic acids using two sequence-specific primers (P1, antisense, and P2, sense; see Figure 2-6), and the coordinated activities of three

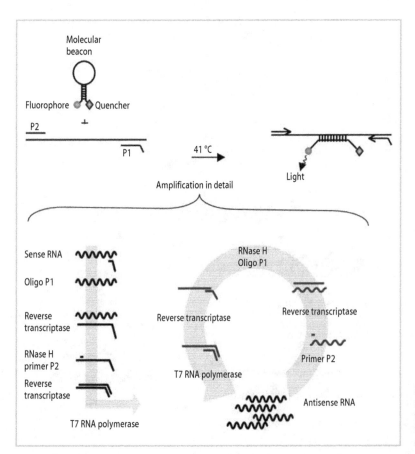

Figure 2-6. Schematic of NASBA reaction. Two primers are used: P1 (antisense) and P2 (sense). The P1 overhang is a promoter sequence for T7 RNA polymerase. A molecular beacon (with fluorophore and quencher, by definition) serving as probe with reporter molecules coupled to NASBA generates a real-time detection system.

enzymes, avian myeloblastosis virus reverse transcriptase (AMV-RT), RNase H, and T7 RNA polymerase.[59] A primer with a T7 RNA polymerase recognition sequence at its 5′ end is used by AMV-RT to transcribe cDNA from the RNA template. The RNA template is destroyed by RNase H. AMV-RT then uses the second primer to synthesize dsDNA. The T7 RNA polymerase uses the dsDNA to synthesize multiple antisense RNA transcripts, and the cycle is repeated. Generally, amplification is approximately 10^{12}-fold in 1 to 2 hours.

In NASBA, nucleic acids serve as amplification templates only if they are single stranded and contain primer-binding regions. NASBA is performed isothermally at 41°C, so RNA is preferentially amplified, because at this temperature genomic DNA remains double stranded and does not bind primers. It is therefore possible to detect RNA in a genomic DNA background without getting false-positive results. Specific DNA amplification using NASBA may be done by introducing a denaturation step before amplification.

Quantitative detection of target nucleic acids is achieved by use of an internal calibrator added at RNA isolation. The calibrator is included at a known concentration, is coamplified during the NASBA process, and is subsequently identified along with the target RNA. Quantitation is based on the analysis of signals generated in real time (one color for calibrator and another for target).

Examples of Applications of NASBA

1. HIV quantitation
2. CMV detection

Amplicon Carryover Contamination

Vast numbers of target DNA copies are generated when PCR and other in vitro nucleic acid amplification techniques are used. By contrast, signal amplification methods (see below) do not generate vast quantities of amplicon and so do not create the potential for amplicon carryover contamination of the laboratory workspace. Amplicons from previous reactions inadvertently introduced into new amplification reactions for the same amplicon are suitable substrates for amplification. Clinical molecular laboratories must therefore take precautions to prevent generation of false-positive results from amplicon carryover contamination.

Amplicon contamination and false-positive results are prevented by using physical barriers and chemical and ultraviolet techniques to destroy amplicons or make them unsuitable for amplification. The physical barriers include large-scale separation of nucleic acid isolation, PCR setup, thermal cycling, and post-PCR analysis in separate areas of the laboratory (different rooms). Air flow is controlled such that air pressure is positive, that is, flows out of the room, in the isolation and PCR setup rooms and is negative in the thermal cycling and post-PCR analysis rooms. Hoods are another way of providing physical separation of

the different PCR steps. Small-scale physical separation techniques include the use of barrier pipette tips, frequent glove changes, designated lab coats that do not leave the pre- or post-PCR areas of the laboratory, and PCR tube openers or careful, slow opening of tubes to prevent aerosolization of contents. Real-time PCR reduces the chances of amplicon contamination since the PCR product can be detected and quantified without opening the real-time PCR reaction vessel after PCR.

Chemical techniques include thorough cleansing with bleach of work areas and instruments before and after use. Ultraviolet lights are frequently placed in hoods and work areas. Ultraviolet light creates thymine dimers within amplicons, rendering the amplicons unsuitable as substrates for further amplification. The introduction of isopsoralens in PCR reactions allows DNA cross-linking of amplicons by UV light, also rendering them unsuitable for further amplification. Deoxyuridine may be used in lieu of thymidine in the reaction mixture. Use of deoxyuridine has minimal effect on amplification or product detection, but amplicons with uracil are substrates for uracil-N-glycosylase (UNG). UNG has no effect on DNA that contains only thymidine residues (new patient DNA in subsequent reactions) but digests the uracil-containing amplicons, allowing removal of amplicons before PCR proceeds.[62] So-called UNG sterilization may therefore be performed prior to PCR to rid the reaction of any amplicon contaminants that may be present.

Signal Amplification Methods

Branched DNA Method

The branched DNA method (bDNA)[63,64] is carried out in microwells and begins with the addition of a lysis buffer to a small volume of serum, plasma, or culture supernatant containing cells or virus. The lysis reagent contains detergent to release target nucleic acid, inhibitors to prevent target degradation, and multiple capture extenders (oligonucleotides) that hybridize to specific areas of the target RNA or DNA. In the case of the HIV bDNA assay, the capture extenders hybridize to multiple sequences in the *pol* gene. A common sequence on the capture extenders interacts with capture probes immobilized on the surface of 96-microwell plates, thereby anchoring the target nucleic acid to the plate.

Multiple target probes are added that hybridize to different, conserved sequences on the target RNA or DNA. In the HIV bDNA assay, more than 80 target probes covering a large portion of the 3000 bp of the *pol* gene are used. The target probes contain key sequences that form the foundation for signal amplification, accomplished via the sequential addition of preamplifier (complementary to a region of the target probes), amplifier (complementary to a region of the preamplifier molecule), and alkaline-phosphatase-modified label probes (complementary to portions of the amplifier molecule).

Preamplifier, amplifier, and label probes, as well as the preamplifier region of the binding probes, contain the nonnatural nucleotides 5-methyl-2'-deoxyisocytidine (iso^{Me}C) and 2'-deoxyisoguanosine (isoG). These isomers of natural bases can participate in Watson-Crick base pairing with each other but not with cytosine or guanine residues in probes or in DNA or RNA sequences. Incorporation of nonnatural bases into the synthetic probe molecules increases the specificity of hybridization by decreasing nonspecific probe interactions, and increases the sensitivity of the assay since higher concentrations of probes can be used.

The series of probes results in formation of large hybridization complexes on the target RNA or DNA. For example, if each hybridization step was 100% efficient in the HIV bDNA assay, each target molecule would be labeled with more than 10,000 alkaline phosphatase molecules. Addition of dioxetane substrate for the alkaline phosphatase results in steady-state chemiluminescence. The luminescent signal is proportional to the amount of target RNA or DNA present in the sample. The amount of target RNA or DNA in a specimen may be calculated by interpolation from a standard curve generated by signals produced from calibrators that contain known concentrations of the specific viral, bacterial, or cellular RNA or DNA. A schematic of this technology is shown in Figure 2-7.

Examples of Applications of bDNA method

1. HIV quantitation[65,66]
2. Hepatitis B virus (HBV) quantitation[67-70]
3. HCV quantitation[71,72]

Hybrid Capture

Hybrid capture (HC) is a signal amplification system based on antibody binding of RNA:DNA hybrids. The first step of HC is the hybridization of unlabeled RNA probes with denatured target DNA. The resulting RNA:DNA hybrids are captured to the surface of microplate wells by an immobilized antibody that recognizes RNA:DNA hybrids. A second anti-RNA:DNA monoclonal antibody conjugated to alkaline phosphatase then is added. Many secondary antibodies bind to each RNA:DNA hybrid. Dioxetane-based substrate is added, which is cleaved by the alkaline phosphatase, producing a chemiluminescent signal. The signal is measured using a microplate luminometer and is proportional to the amount of target DNA in the specimen.[73] The sensitivity of HC can be increased by using a precipitation buffer and high-speed centrifugation.

Examples of Applications of HC

1. Human papilloma virus detection
2. CMV quantitation[74]
3. *Chlamydia trachomatis* and *Neisseria gonorrhoeae* detection[75]
4. HBV quantitation[76]
5. HSV detection[77]

Fluorescence In Situ Hybridization

Fluorescence in situ hybridization (FISH) uses fluorescently tagged DNA or RNA probes to identify genomic

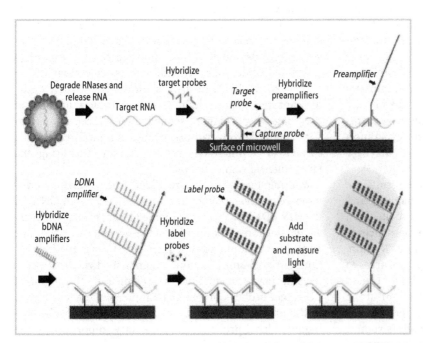

Figure 2-7. Diagram of branched DNA (bDNA) method. (Reprinted with permission of Bayer Healthcare.)

sequences of interest.[78,79] The major advantages of FISH are the ability to utilize FFPE tissue sections, allowing correlation of probe hybridization with tissue morphology, and the increased resolution provided by FISH for identification of specific abnormalities when partnered with conventional cytogenetics. The number and location of the fluorescent signal(s) can identify chromosomal abnormalities including gene amplification, gene deletion, or structural rearrangements such as translocations.

FISH is similar to Southern blot in that sequential steps of denaturation, hybridization, and washing are involved. Slides are prepared in the cytogenetic or histology laboratory. Probe(s) are then applied to the slide along with a nuclear counterstain and reagents to enhance denaturation and reduce background. The slides are sealed and incubated (usually overnight) in a humid environment at high temperature. These conditions denature the probe and patient DNA, allowing hybridization to occur between the probe and its complementary DNA sequence without binding to nonspecific sites. Excess nonspecifically bound probe is washed away, and the pattern of fluorescence is read by fluorescence microscopy. The fluorescent signal(s) can be enhanced by the use of a digital imaging system and computer software.

The specificity of FISH is largely based on the selection of the probe. Ideally, the probe is complementary to the gene of interest; however, if the disease gene is unknown, satellite probes that identify a chromosomal region linked to the disease may be used. Labeled bacterial or yeast artificial chromosomes (BAC or YAC, respectively) are typically used as FISH probes, but short oligonucleotides also can be used with signal amplification techniques. Probes that identify individual whole chromosomes or chromosomal arms are often called "painting probes" due to the colorful patterns they generate. Other probes that hybridize to a specific gene can be used for the detection of deletions or duplications and are called single-copy gene probes. Probes that hybridize to the alpha-satellite regions near centromeres are used in clinical cytogenetics to identify and count individual chromosomes. Probes that hybridize to the subtelomeric portions of chromosomes are used to identify cryptic telomeric abnormalities such as translocations.

Dual-color FISH (dFISH) employs two probes with different fluorescence wavelengths to identify structural chromosomal rearrangements. Each probe generates a characteristic color by itself (split signal) and a third color when the two probes are juxtaposed (fusion signal). A fusion signal indicating chromosomal rearrangement is used to identify disease-causing mutations that predictably involve only two partner genes, for example, BCR and ABL. However, when a particular gene with multiple potential translocation partners is tested, it is more efficient to have both probes bind to the 5′ and 3′ ends of the particular gene such that the normal allele shows the fusion signal and the rearranged allele shows two split signals. This is the technique used for the MLL gene, which is rearranged to over 30 different partner genes in various types of leukemia.

Spectral karyotyping (SKY) and multiplex FISH (M-FISH) are relatively new advancements of conventional FISH that utilize multiple fluorochromes, specialized optics, and image analysis that can simultaneously identify all chromosomes.[80] Comparative genomic hybridization (CGH), also called "copy number karyotyping," is a variation of FISH that detects relative gains or losses of the genome.[81] This method compares the ratios of patient specimen DNA, labeled with one fluorochrome, to that of normal DNA, labeled with a different fluorochrome when hybridized to control chromosomes. CGH is used predominantly in research to identify possible pathways involved in tumor progression, recurrence, or metastasis. Colorimetric probes are used in chromogenic in situ hybridization (CISH), which has the advantage that the signal does not fade with time or require fluorescence microscopy for analysis.

Examples of Applications of FISH

1. Detection of BCR/ABL in chronic myelogenous leukemia
2. Detection of HER2 gene amplification for breast cancer diagnosis and prognosis
3. Detection of MYCN amplification in neuroblastoma[82]

DNA Arrays and Chips

Arrays are a relatively recent phenomenon in the field of molecular pathology.[83] The term "array" is jargon for an orderly collection of molecules on solid supports ranging from nylon membranes to printed circuit board to glass slides to silicon surfaces. There are macroscopic arrays, for example, reverse line blots on nylon membranes, and microarrays, for example, DNA chips. Synonyms for microarrays include gene chip, DNA chip, genome chip, biochip, gene array, DNA array, and DNA microarray.

Though most do not think of line probe assays as belonging in a section describing DNA chips, they are indeed arrays. Line probe assays are being used to determine mutations in the HIV genome, to type HCV, and to detect CFTR mutations for cystic fibrosis.[84] The method is based on classic nucleic acid hybridization using nylon or nitrocellulose strips as a solid support matrix for hybridization and detection. Generally, reverse hybridization is employed. Oligonucleotide probes specific for mutations or polymorphisms of interest are bound to the membrane strip in a parallel line format. Patient specimen DNA is amplified with biotinylated primers, thereby labeling the amplicon, which is hybridized to probes on the membrane. After hybridization, alkaline phosphatase-labeled streptavidin is added and binds to the biotin of the bound amplicons. Detection is colorimetric following incubation with a specific chromogen, generating a purple-brown precipitate. The resulting colored lines are read as positive results, hence the name of the assay.

DNA chips, such as those produced by Affymetrix, Nanogen, Clinical Micro Sensors, and other companies, may be thought of as miniaturized ASOH platforms with multiple oligonucleotide probe assays. In one model, the oligonucleotides are synthesized directly onto a solid support, for example, glass or silicon, that is, the "chip." Some companies' chips can hold thousands of unique sequences. The sample DNA is labeled with fluorescent dye, denatured, and hybridized with the oligonucleotides on the chip. The chip is then scanned and the fluorescence patterns are measured with the aid of computer analysis to determine the presence of mutant or wild-type sequences. Gene expression chips use probes that bind to many different cDNA species (up to 33,000 in one array at the time of this writing) to quantitate the level of each cDNA isolated in a sample. Gene expression microarrays with large densities are appropriate for analysis of differential patterns of gene expression between normal and diseased tissues.

Clinical molecular laboratory diagnostic applications for DNA chips currently are limited to those with clinically appropriate density, in the range of 10 to 200. Utility for these platforms is found in SNP and mutation detection[85] as well as pathogen identification. Chips with densities in the thousands have limited, if any, use in clinical laboratories at this time. So much data are generated that more analysis needs to be done to winnow down the numbers to a relevant few genes or transcripts that can be used in clinical assays. This work is progressing well. Furthermore, the informatics software currently being used to analyze these data requires simplification and modification so that useful algorithms for data analysis can be employed for disease diagnosis or prognosis. While these are certainly considerable challenges, it should be noted that DNA array chip technology benefits enormously from robotic manufacturing techniques and rapidly advancing computer software. This has greatly decreased the costs per array feature of DNA chips, giving DNA microarrays enormous potential in the clinical molecular laboratory of the near future.

Examples of Applications of Arrays

1. Line probe assay for HCV genotyping
2. DNA chips for detection of polymorphisms in cytochrome P450 genes for pharmacogenetics

Acknowledgments

The authors thank Zed Penn, Cepheid; Tiffany Murphy, Beckman Coulter; H. James Hnatyszyn, Bayer; Paul van de Wiel and Mike Cronin, bioMerieux; Steve Geiner and Irma Alfaro, Digene; and Andrew Olson and Carl Hilliker, Roche, for their help with different sections of this chapter.

References

1. Kessler HH, Muhlbauer G, Stelzl E, Daghofer E, Santner BI, Marth E. Fully automated nucleic acid extraction: MagNA Pure LC. *Clin Chem.* 2001;47:1124–1126.
2. Fiebelkorn KR, Lee BG, Hill CE, Caliendo AM, Nolte FS. Clinical evaluation of an automated nucleic acid isolation system. *Clin Chem.* 2002;48:1613–1615.
3. Williams SM, Meadows CA, Lyon E. Automated DNA extraction for real-time PCR. *Clin Chem.* 2002;48:1629–1630.
4. Davies J, Reznikoff WS, eds. *Milestones in Biotechnology: Classic Papers on Genetic Engineering.* Boston: Butterworth-Heinemann; 1992.
5. Wasserman LM. A nested reverse-transcriptase-polymerase chain reaction assay to detect *BCR/ABL*. In: Killeen AA, ed. *Methods in Molecular Medicine Molecular Pathology Protocols.* Totowa, NJ: Humana Press; 2001:105–114.
6. Sanger F, Nicklen S, Coulson AR. DNA sequencing with chain-terminating inhibitors. *Proc Natl Acad Sci U S A.* 1977;74:5463–5467.
7. Esch RK. Basic nucleic acid procedures. In: Coleman WB, Tsongalis GJ, eds. *Molecular Diagnostics for the Clinical Laboratorian.* Totowa, NJ: Humana Press; 1997:55–58.
8. Schmaizing D, Koutny L, Salas-Solano O, Adourian A, Matsudaira P, Ehrlich D. Recent developments in DNA sequencing by capillary and microdevice electrophoresis [review]. *Electrophoresis.* 1999;20:3066–3077.
9. Farkas DH. Specimen procurement, processing, tracking, and testing by the Southern blot. In: Farkas DH, ed. *Molecular Biology and Pathology: A Guidebook for Quality Control.* San Diego: Academic Press; 1993:51–75.
10. Farkas DH. Quality control of the B/T cell gene rearrangement test. In: Farkas DH, ed. *Molecular Biology and Pathology: A Guidebook for Quality Control.* San Diego: Academic Press; 1993:77–101.
11. Mullis K, Faloona F, Schart S, Saiki R, Horn G, Erlich H. Specific enzymatic amplification of DNA *in vitro*: the polymerase chain reaction. *Cold Spring Harb Symp Quant Biol.* 1986;51:263–273.
12. Farkas DH. Thermal cyclers. In: *Laboratory Instrument Evaluation Verification and Maintenance Manual.* Northfield, IL: College of American Pathologists; 1998:130–133.
13. Loeffelholz MJ, Lewinski CA, Silver SR, et al. Detection of *Chlamydia trachomatis* in endocervical specimens by polymerase chain reaction. *J Clin Microbiol.* 1992;30:2847–2851.
14. DiDomenico N, Link H, Knobel R, et al. COBAS AMPLICOR™: fully automated RNA and DNA amplification and detection system for routine diagnostic PCR. *Clin Chem.* 1996;42:1915–1923.
15. Greenfield L, White TJ. Sample preparation methods. In: Persing DH, Smith TF, Tenover FC, White TJ, eds. *Diagnostics Molecular Microbiology Principles and Applications.* Washington, DC: American Society for Microbiology; 1993:126–127.
16. Liu XY, Nelson D, Grant C, Morthland V, Goodnight SH, Press RD. Molecular detection of a common mutation in coagulation factor V causing thrombosis via hereditary resistance to activated protein C. *Diagn Mol Pathol.* 1995;3:191–197.
17. Linderman R, Hu SP, Volpato F, Trent RJ. Polymerase chain reaction mutagenesis enabling rapid nonradioactive detection of common β-thalassaemia mutations in Mediterraneans. *Br J Haematol.* 1991; 78:100.
18. Sorscher EJ, Huang Z. Diagnosis of genetic disease by primer-specified restriction map modification, with application to cystic fibrosis and retinitis pigmentosa. *Lancet.* 1991;11:1115–1118.
19. Khanna M, Park P, Zirvi M, et al. Multiplex PCR/LDR for detection of K-*ras* mutations in primary colon tumors. *Oncogene.* 1999;18: 27–38.
20. McMillin DE, Muldrow LL, Laggette SJ. Simultaneous detection of toxin A and toxin B genetic determinants of *Clostridium difficile* using the multiplex polymerase chain reaction. *Can J Microbiol.* 1992;38:81–83.

21. Sugita T, Nakajima M, Ikeda R, Niki Y, Matsushima T, Shinoda T. A nested PCR assay to detect DNA in sera for the diagnosis of deep-seated trichosporonosis. *Microbiol Immunol.* 2001;45:143–148.

22. Ferrie RM, Schwarz MJ, Robertson NH, et al. Development, multiplexing, and application of ARMS tests for common mutations in the CFTR gene. *Am J Hum Genet.* 1992;51:251–262.

23. Bugawan TL, Begovich AB, Erlich HA. Rapid HLA-DPB typing using enzymatically amplified DNA and nonradioactive sequence-specific oligonucleotide probes. *Immunogenetics.* 1990;32:231–241.

24. Nickerson DA, Kaiser R, Lappin S, Stewart J, Hood L, Landegren U. Automated DNA diagnostics using an ELISA-based oligonucleotide ligation assay. *Proc Natl Acad Sci U S A.* 1990;87:8923–8927.

25. Jarvius J, Nilsson M, Landegren U. Oligonucleotide ligation assay. *Methods Mol Biol.* 2003;212:215–228.

26. Howell WM, Jobs M, Gyllensten U, Brookes AJ. Dynamic allele-specific hybridization. *Nat Biotechnol.* 1999;17:87–88.

27. Baltimore D. Viral RNA-dependent DNA polymerase. *Nature.* 1970;226:1209–1211.

28. Bustin SA. Absolute quantification of mRNA using real-time reverse transcription polymerase chain reaction assays. *J Mol Endocrinol.* 2000;25:169–193.

29. Lay MJ, Wittwer CT. Real-time fluorescence genotyping of factor V Leiden during rapid-cycle PCR. *Clin Chem.* 1997;43:2262–2267.

30. Bernard PS, Wittwer CT. Real-time PCR technology for cancer diagnostics. *Clin Chem.* 2002;48:1178–1185.

31. Olek A, Oswald J, Walter JAA. A modified and improved method of bisulfite based cytosine methylation analysis. *Nucleic Acids Res.* 1996;24:5064–5066.

32. Herman JG, Graff JR, Myöhänen S, Nelkin BD, Baylin SB. Methylation specific PCR: a novel PCR assay for methylation status of CpG islands. *Proc Natl Acad Sci U S A.* 1996;93:9821–9826.

33. Lo Y, Wong I, Zhang J, Tein M, Ng M, Hjelm N. Quantitative analysis of aberrant p16 methylation using real-time quantitative methylation-specific polymerase chain reaction. *Cancer Res.* 1999;59:3899–3903.

34. Fodde R, Losekoot M. Mutation detection by denaturing gradient gel electrophoresis (DGGE). *Hum Mutat.* 1994;3:83–94.

35. Lerman LS, Beldjord C. Comprehensive mutation detection with denaturing gradient gel electrophoresis. In: Cotton RGH, Edkins E, Forrest S, eds. *Mutation Detection: A Practical Approach.* Oxford: Oxford University Press; 1998:35–59.

36. Rosenbaum V, Riesner D. Temperature-gradient gel electrophoresis: thermodynamic analysis of nucleic acids and proteins in purified form and in cellular extracts. *Biophys Chem.* 1987;26:235–246.

37. Riesner D, Henco K, Steger G. Temperature-gradient gel electrophoresis: a method for the analysis of conformational transitions and mutations in nucleic acids and proteins. *Adv Electrophoresis.* 1991;4:169–250.

38. van der Luijt RB, Khan PM, Vasen HF, et al. Molecular analysis of the APC gene in 105 Dutch kindreds with familial adenomatous polyposis: 67 germline mutations identified by DGGE, PTT, and Southern analysis. *Hum Mutat.* 1997;9:7–16.

39. De Braekeleer M, Mari C, Verlingue C, et al. Complete identification of cystic fibrosis transmembrane conductance regulator mutations in the CF population of Saguenay Lac-Saint-Jean (Quebec, Canada). *Clin Genet.* 1998;53:44–46.

40. Alkan S, Cosar E, Ergin M, Hsi E. Detection of T-cell receptor-gamma gene rearrangement in lymphoproliferative disorders by temperature gradient gel electrophoresis. *Arch Pathol Lab Med.* 2001;125:202–207.

41. Nagamine CM, Chan K, Lau YF. A PCR artifact: generation of heteroduplexes. *Am J Hum Genet.* 1989;45:337–339.

42. Bhattacharyya A, Lilley DM. The contrasting structures of mismatched DNA sequences containing looped-out bases (bulges) and multiple mismatches (bubbles). *Nucleic Acids Res.* 1989;17:6821–6840.

43. Orita M, Iwahana H, Kanazawa H, Hayashi K, Sekiya T. Detection of polymorphisms of human DNA by gel electrophoresis as single-strand conformation polymorphisms. *Proc Natl Acad Sci U S A.* 1989;86:2766–2770.

44. Hayashi, K. PCR-SSCP: a simple and sensitive method for detection of mutations in the genomic DNA. *PCR Methods Appl.* 1991;1:34–38.

45. Liu Q, Feng J, Buzin C, et al. Detection of virtually all mutations-single stranded conformational polymorphisms (DOVAM-S): a rapid method for mutation scanning with virtually 100% sensitivity. *Biotechniques.* 1999;26:932–942.

46. Widjojoatmodjo MC, Fluit AC, Verhoef J. Molecular identification of bacteria by fluorescence-based PCR-single-strand-conformation polymorphism of the 16S rRNA gene. *J Clin Microbiol.* 1995;33:2601–2606.

47. Liu W, Smith DI, Rechtzigel KJ, Thibodeau SN, James CD. Denaturing high performance liquid chromatography (DHPLC) used in the detection of germline and somatic mutations. *Nucleic Acids Res.* 1998;26:1396–1400.

48. O'Donovan MC, Oefner PJ, Roberts SC, et al. Blind analysis of denaturing high-performance liquid chromatography as a tool for mutation detection. *Genomics.* 1998;52:44–49.

49. Wagner T, Stoppa-Lyonnet D, Fleischmann E, et al. Denaturing high-performance liquid chromatography detects reliably BRCA1 and BRCA2 mutations. *Genomics.* 1999;62:369–376.

50. Roest PA, Roberts RG, Sugino S, van Ommen GJ, den Dunnen JT. Protein truncation test (PTT) for rapid detection of translation-terminating mutations. *Hum Mol Genet.* 1993;2:1719–1721.

51. Pohlreich P, Stribna J, Kleibl Z, et al. Mutations of the *BRCA1* gene in hereditary breast and ovarian cancer in the Czech Republic. *Med Princ Pract.* 2003;12:23–29.

52. Zajac V, Kovac M, Kirchhoff T, Stevurkova V, Tomka M. The most frequent APC mutations among Slovak familial adenomatous polyposis patients. *Neoplasma.* 2002;49:356–361.

53. Laffler TG, Carrino JJ, Marshall RL. The ligase chain reaction in DNA-based diagnosis. *Ann Biol Clin (Paris).* 1993;51:821–826.

54. Burczak JD, Ching S, Hu H-Y, Lee HH. Ligase chain reaction for the detection of infectious agents. In: Wiedbrauk DL, Farkas DH, eds. *Molecular Methods for Virus Detection.* San Diego: Academic Press; 1995:315–328.

55. Mahony J, Chong S, Jang D, et al. Urine specimens from pregnant and nonpregnant women inhibitory to amplification of *Chlamydia trachomatis* nucleic acid by PCR, ligase chain reaction, and transcription-mediated amplification: identification of urinary substances associated with inhibition and removal of inhibitory activity. *J Clin Microbiol.* 1998;36:3122–3126.

56. Gorrin G, Friesenhahn M, Lin P, et al. Performance evaluation of the VERSANT HCV RNA qualitative assay by using transcription-mediated amplification. *J Clin Microbiol.* 2003;41:310–317.

57. Walker GT, Little MC, Nadeau JG, Shank DD. Isothermal *in vitro* amplification of DNA by a restriction enzyme/DNA polymerase system. *Proc Natl Acad Sci U S A.* 1992;89:392–396.

58. Westin L, Xu X, Miller C, Wang L, Edman CF, Nerenberg M. Anchored multiplex amplification on a microelectronic chip array. *Nat Biotechnol.* 2000;18:199–204.

59. Sooknanan R, van Gemen B, Malek LT. Nucleic acid sequence-based amplification. In: Wiedbrauk DL, Farkas DH, eds. *Molecular Methods for Virus Detection.* San Diego: Academic Press; 1995:261–285.

60. Polstra AM, Goudsmit J, Cornelissen M. Development of real-time NASBA assays with molecular beacon detection to quantify mRNA coding for HHV-8 lytic and latent genes. *BMC Infect Dis.* 2002;2:18.

61. Baeumner AJ, Cohen RN, Miksic V, Min J. RNA biosensor for the rapid detection of viable *Escherichia coli* in drinking water. *Biosens Bioelectron.* 2003;18:405–413.

62. Spadoro JP, Dragon EA. Quality control of the polymerase chain reaction. In: Farkas DH, ed. *Molecular Biology and Pathology: A*

Guidebook for Quality Control. San Diego: Academic Press; 1993: 149–158.

63. Wilber JC. Branched DNA for quantification of viral load. *Immunol Invest.* 1997;26:9–13.

64. Nolte FS. Branched DNA signal amplification for direct quantitation of nucleic acid sequences in clinical specimens. *Adv Clin Chem.* 1998;33:201–235.

65. Elbeik T, Alvord WG, Trichavaroj R, et al. Comparative analysis of HIV-1 viral load assays on subtype quantification: Bayer Versant HIV-1 RNA 3.0 versus Roche Amplicor HIV-1 Monitor version 1.5. *J Acquir Immune Defic Syndr.* 2002;29:330–339.

66. Gleaves CA, Welle J, Campbell M, et al. Multicenter evaluation of the Bayer VERSANT HIV-1 RNA 3.0 assay: analytical and clinical performance. *J Clin Virol.* 2002;25:205–216.

67. Hann HW, Fontana RJ, Wright T, et al. A United States compassionate use study of lamivudine treatment in nontransplantation candidates with decompensated hepatitis B virus-related cirrhosis. *Liver Transpl.* 2003;9:49–56.

68. Hendricks DA, Stowe BJ, Hoo BS, et al. Quantitation of HBV DNA in human serum using a branched DNA (bDNA) signal amplification assay. *Am J Clin Pathol.* 1995;104:537–546.

69. Martinot-Peignoux M, Boyer N, Colombat M, et al. Serum hepatitis B virus DNA levels and liver histology in inactive HBsAg carriers. *J Hepatol.* 2002;36:543–546.

70. Pawlotsky JM, Bastie A, Hezode C, et al. Routine detection and quantification of hepatitis B virus DNA in clinical laboratories: performance of three commercial assays. *J Virol Methods.* 2000;85: 11–21.

71. Beld M, Sentjens R, Rebers S, et al. Performance of the new Bayer VERSANT HCV RNA 3.0 assay for quantitation of hepatitis C virus RNA in plasma and serum: conversion to international units and comparison with the Roche COBAS Amplicor HCV Monitor, Version 2.0, assay. *J Clin Microbiol.* 2002;40:788–793.

72. Trimoulet P, Halfon P, Pohier E, Khiri H, Chene G, Fleury H. Evaluation of the VERSANT HCV RNA 3.0 assay for quantification of hepatitis C virus RNA in serum. *J Clin Microbiol.* 2002;40:2031–2036.

73. Lorincz A, Anthony J. Hybrid capture: a system for nucleic acid detection by signal amplification technology. In: Van Dyke C,

Woodfork K, eds. *Luminescence Biotechnology: Instruments and Applications.* Boca Raton, FL: CRC Press; 2002:149–158.

74. Mazzulli T, Drew LW, Yen-Lieberman B, et al. Multicenter comparison of the Digene hybrid capture CMV DNA assay (version 2.0), the pp65 antigenemia assay, and cell culture for detection of cytomegalovirus viremia. *J Clin Microbiol.* 1999;37:958–963.

75. Schachter J, Hook EW III, McCormack WM, et al. Ability of the Digene hybrid capture II test to identify *Chlamydia trachomatis* and *Neisseria gonorrhoeae* in cervical specimens. *J Clin Microbiol.* 1999;37:3668–3671.

76. Kessler HH, Pierer K, Dragon E, et al. Evaluation of a new assay for HBV DNA quantitation in patients with chronic hepatitis B. *Clin Diagn Virol.* 1998;9:37–43.

77. Lorincz A. Hybrid capture method for detection of human papilloma virus DNA in clinical specimens. *Pap Rep.* 1996;7:1–5.

78. Guan X-Y, Zhang H, Bittner M, Jiang Y, Meltzer P, Trent J. Chromosome arm painting probes. *Nature Genet.* 1996;12:10–11.

79. Dyanov HM, Dzitoeva SG. Method for attachment of microscopic preparations on glass for *in situ* hybridization, PRINS, and *in situ* PCR studies. *Biotechniques.* 1995;18:823–826.

80. Schrock E, du Manoir S, Veldman T, et al. Multicolor spectral karyotyping of human chromosomes. *Science.* 1996;273:494–497.

81. du Manoir S, Speicher MR, Joos S, et al. Detection of complete and partial chromosome gains and losses by comparative genomic *in situ* hybridization. *Hum Genet.* 1993;90:590–610.

82. Hachitanda Y, Toyoshima S, Akazawa K, Tsuneyoshi M. N-myc gene amplification in rhabdomyosarcoma detected by fluorescence in situ hybridization: its correlation with histologic features. *Mod Pathol.* 1998;11:1222–1227.

83. Ekins R, Chu FW. Microarrays: their origins and applications. *Trends Biotechnol.* 1999;17:217–218.

84. Descamps D, Calvez V, Collin G, et al. Line probe assay for detection of human immunodeficiency virus type 1 mutations conferring resistance to nucleoside inhibitors of reverse transcriptase: comparison with sequence analysis. *J Clin Microbiol.* 1998;36:2143–2145.

85. Evans JG, Lee-Tataseo C. Determination of the factor V Leiden single-nucleotide polymorphism in a commercial clinical laboratory by use of NanoChip microelectronic array technology. *Clin Chem.* 2002;48:1406–1411.

Chapter 3

Human Immunodeficiency Virus Type 1

Angela M. Caliendo

Human immunodeficiency virus types 1 and 2 (HIV-1 and HIV-2), the causative agents of the acquired immunodeficiency syndrome (AIDS), are RNA viruses belonging to the genus *Lentivirus* of the family Retroviridae. Like all retroviruses, replication involves reverse transcription of the RNA genome into a double-stranded DNA molecule, with subsequent integration into the host genome. This integrated retroviral DNA is referred to as the provirus. Due to this complex replicative cycle, molecular assays used in the diagnosis and management of HIV-1 infection may target either HIV-1 RNA or proviral DNA.

HIV-1 is a very genetically diverse virus; two distinct genetic groups have been identified, the major (M) and outlier (O) groups. Viruses in the M group are further divided into eight subtypes or clades, designated A through H, based on the sequence diversity within the HIV-1 *gag* and *env* genes. The nucleotide sequence of the *env* gene may differ by as much as 25% among the different clades, while viruses within the same clade generally differ by less than 15%.[1] Group M virus is found worldwide, with clade B predominating in Europe and North America. The genetic diversity of HIV-1 plays an important role in the design and interpretation of viral load and resistance tests.

The uses of molecular tests in the clinical management for persons with HIV-1 infection are many and diverse and include diagnosis of infection, monitoring response to therapy, and assessing the efficacy of a treatment regimen. Here we review the available assays and their clinical utility.

Clinical Utility

HIV-1 Viral Load Testing

The clinical utility of HIV-1 viral load testing, which refers to the quantification of HIV-1 RNA, has been well documented. HIV-1 viral load assays are very useful in determining when to initiate antiretroviral therapy, in monitoring response to therapy, and in predicting time to progression to AIDS. With the availability of commercial assays and their proven clinical utility, viral load testing quickly became the standard of care in the clinical management of persons with HIV-1 infection. Clinical guidelines have been established for the initiation of antiretroviral therapy, and viral load levels are among the parameters used in this decision. Initiation of therapy may be considered in patients with a high plasma viral load even if the patient is without symptoms and the CD4 cell count is above 350 cells/mm³.[2]

HIV-1 viral load is a strong predictor of the rate of progression to AIDS that is independent of CD4 cell count.[3] A study of homosexual men in which the time of seroconversion was documented showed that an initial viral load of 100,000 equivalents/ml of plasma soon after seroconversion was associated with a greater than ten-fold increase in the risk of developing AIDS. However, persons who had a viral load of <1,000 equivalents/ml did not progress to AIDS during the next 5 years.[3] A study of hemophiliacs found similar results; the level of HIV-1 RNA early during chronic infection was a strong predictor of clinical outcome.[4] The same association between viral load level and progression to AIDS is seen in patients for whom the duration of HIV-1 infection is unknown. Mellors et al. showed that HIV-1 seropositive men with a baseline RNA level of <4,530 molecules/ml had a median time to progression to AIDS of >10 years, compared to 3.5 years with a baseline viral load of >36,270 molecules/ml.[5]

Monitoring response to therapy is another key use of viral load testing. The magnitude of the decrease in viral load in response to therapy is dependent on the specific combinations of antiretroviral drugs used. For example, when zidovudine (AZT) or lamivudine (3TC) are used as monotherapy, the decrease in viral load is in the range of 0.5 to $1.0 \log_{10}$ copies/ml. But when these two drugs are used in combination, the drop in viral load is $1.5 \log_{10}$ copies/ml and this decrease in viral load is sustained for a longer period of time.[6] When AZT, 3TC, and the protease inhibitor indinavir are used in combination, the decrease in viral load is 2.0 to $2.8 \log_{10}$ copies/ml and this regimen slowed the progression of HIV-1 disease in patients with ≤200 CD4 cells/mm^3.[7] Decreases in viral load of approximately $2\log_{10}$ have been reported with other combination regimens.[8–10] Based on these findings, the current standard for treating HIV-1 infected individuals is to use combinations of protease inhibitors or nonnucleoside reverse transcriptase inhibitors with nucleoside analogs.[2] This combination therapy is often referred to as highly active antiretroviral therapy or HAART.

The ultimate goal of therapy is to achieve a viral load below the limit of detection of the assay, as studies have shown suppression of plasma viral load to below 20 copies/ml was associated with a longer response to antiretroviral therapy compared with that achieved when the viral load was suppressed to below 500 copies/ml.[11] However, this may not be possible in all cases, particularly in those patients with very high pretreatment viral load levels or in those who have failed prior therapeutic regimens. Guidelines for the use of HIV-1 RNA levels in clinical practice have been published[12] (AIDSinfo [http://aidsinfo.nih.gov/], International AIDS Society–USA [http://www.iasusa.org]). In general, a plasma HIV-1 RNA level should be measured at baseline, immediately before beginning therapy, and then again at 2 to 8 weeks after the start of therapy to determine the initial response. Testing then is repeated at 3- to 4-month intervals to evaluate continued effectiveness of the regimen. Any increase in viral load should be confirmed with repeat testing, as a variety of clinical illnesses can lead to a transient rise in viral load. Once a significant increase in viral load has been documented, HIV-1 resistance testing should be considered.

HIV-1 viral load testing also has proven useful in the diagnosis of acute HIV-1 infection, although the Food and Drug Administration (FDA) has not approved the assays for this indication. Acute HIV-1 infection, also referred to as acute retroviral syndrome, is defined as the "window period" after exposure to the virus prior to seroconversion, when the ELISA and western blot tests are negative or indeterminate. In this "window period," patients often are symptomatic with a mononucleosis-type syndrome, which may include fever, fatigue, rash, lymphadenopathy, and oral ulcers.[13] During acute HIV-1 infection, the level of RNA is very high, usually 10^5 to 10^7 copies/ml of plasma, making viral load measurement a very useful diagnostic tool. A recent study compared the utility of p24 antigen and viral load testing for identifying patients with acute HIV-1 infection.[14] Viral load testing was found to be more sensitive, while p24 antigen testing was more specific. However, the majority of viral load testing in the study was done using the Versant HIV-1 RNA assay (Bayer Diagnostics Corporation, Tarrytown, NY), a signal amplification method, which is known to have a lower specificity compared to target amplification methods. There were no false positives when the Amplicor reverse transcription–polymerase chain reaction (RT-PCR) assay (Roche Diagnostics, Indianapolis, IN) was used, although the sample size was small. When molecular assays for the diagnosis of HIV-1 infection are used,

the possibility of a false-positive result must be considered. Patients must be educated about the limitations of these tests and must give informed consent prior to testing. To minimize the likelihood of reporting a false-positive result, an HIV1/2 ELISA should be obtained at the time of viral load testing, and repeat viral load testing should be done on all positive specimens. It is critical to remember that patients with acute retroviral syndrome should have very high levels of HIV-1 RNA. Requiring laboratory approval for HIV-1 diagnostic testing is a prudent approach to ensure that the patient has signs and symptoms consistent with acute HIV-1 infection prior to testing.

Molecular tests are useful in the diagnosis of acute HIV-1 infection in neonates. Since maternal IgG crosses the placenta, an uninfected infant may be seropositive into the second year of life. Studies have established the utility of both qualitative proviral DNA and viral load assays for the diagnosis of HIV-1 infection in newborns.[15–17] HIV-1 viral load testing appears to be more sensitive than proviral DNA testing for the diagnosis of acute HIV-1 infection in newborns.[16,17] Current guidelines for the diagnosis of neonatal HIV-1 infection recommend that the molecular testing be performed at two separate time points, and that testing cord blood samples be avoided.[18]

HIV-1 Drug Resistance Testing

The replication cycle of HIV-1 is error prone because the reverse transcriptase (RT) does not have proofreading activity. As a result, about one error occurs with each replicative cycle. This error rate coupled with a replication rate that produces about one billion viral particles per day gives rise to viral quasispecies. Therefore, a patient has a high probability of having a virus with a drug-resistance mutation in the quasispecies prior to drug exposure. Treatment with an antiretroviral drug leads to selection pressure that allows a resistant virus to predominate. As a result, monotherapy has been found to be ineffective and the standard of care is to treat patients with a combination of antiretroviral drugs. Currently, there are four general classes of antiretroviral drugs that are used in clinical care, nucleoside reverse transcriptase inhibitors (NRTIs), non-nucleoside reverse transcriptase inhibitors (NNRTIs), protease inhibitors (PIs), and a new class of drug, fusion inhibitors. Viral resistance can occur with each of these classes of drug, particularly when viral replication is not maximally suppressed while the patient is on therapy. The current standard of care is to use regimens that contain a combination of drugs, usually a PI or NNRTI with several NRTIs, since resistance is less likely to occur on these complex regimens than on monotherapy.

The clinical utility of resistance testing in the management of HIV-1-infected persons has been studied in several prospective randomized clinical trials. Two early studies focused on the clinical utility of genotypic resistance testing, while more recent studies also have assessed the role of phenotypic resistance testing. The early clinical trials evaluating resistance testing evaluated the use of genotyping in establishing the treatment regimen in patients who had failed therapy with PIs and NRTIs.[19–21] In the control arm, the salvage regimen was determined based on prior antiretroviral drug use, while patients in the genotype arm received therapy based on the results of a genotyping test. In both studies, patients in the genotype arm showed an improved response to therapy compared to the control group, as measured by either the decrease in viral load or the percentage of patients with an undetectable viral load. To clarify the role of expert advice, the Havana trial evaluated the clinical utility of genotyping and expert advice.[22] As with earlier studies, genotyping was found to improve virologic outcomes. In addition, the use of expert advice showed a virologic benefit in patients with two previous treatment regimen failures. A recent study showed that use of genotypic resistance testing to determine the next regimen following treatment failure is cost-effective.[23] In addition, the use of resistance testing to guide the initial treatment regimen appears to be cost-effective if the prevalence of primary genotypic resistance in the population is at least 4%.[23]

The VIRA3001 study was a prospective randomized trial that compared standard of care to phenotypic drug resistance testing in patients who failed a PI-containing regimen. At week 16, an intention-to-treat analysis showed that patients in the phenotype arm had a greater drop in viral load, and a greater proportion of the patients in the phenotype arm had an undetectable viral load compared to the standard-of-care arm.[24] However, not all clinical trials of resistance testing have shown an improved clinical outcome compared to standard of care. The NARVAL trial compared phenotypic testing or genotypic testing to standard of care for choosing an antiretroviral regimen after treatment failure. As with previous studies, the patients had failed therapy that contained a PI. Overall, the resistance assays did not demonstrate a benefit over standard of care. However in patients with the most limited PI use, a significant benefit was observed in the genotyping arm.[25] The California Collaborative Treatment Group Study 575 (CCTG575) randomized patients who had experienced treatment failure to receive phenotypic testing or

standard of care. At both 6 and 12 months there was not a significant difference in either reduction in viral load or in the proportion of patients with a viral load of <400 copies/ml. However, in a subgroup of patients with resistance to three or more PIs at baseline, a statistically greater number of patients achieved a viral load of <400 copies/ml at 6 months in the phenotype arm compared to the standard-of-care arm.[26,27]

An International AIDS Society–USA panel of experts has established clinical guidelines for the use of HIV-1 resistance testing in adults.[28] Either genotypic or phenotypic drug resistance testing is recommended in patients who fail an initial antiretroviral regimen or in those who fail after numerous regimens. Treatment failure usually refers to failure to achieve the desired drop in viral load or rebound in viral load after achieving an initial response. Resistance testing also is recommended in pregnant women to optimize treatment and in hopes of minimizing transmission of HIV-1 infection to the neonate. Resistance testing should be considered prior to initiating therapy in patients with primary HIV-1 infection or in treatment of naive persons with established HIV-1 infection.

Assays and Their Performance

Viral Load Assays

Currently, four HIV-1 viral load test kits have been approved by the FDA for clinical use (Table 3-1). Additional tests are under development and are expected to be available within the next few years. The available assays differ in their limit of quantification and linear range. Both the standard and ultrasensitive Amplicor RT-PCR assays are needed to cover the clinically important range of viral load values. Of note, the Amplicor RT-PCR version 1.0 test has been replaced by the version 1.5 test. The lower limit of quantification is a key characteristic of viral load assays, and how this parameter is defined is equally important. For example, the NucliSens NASBA assay can detect as few as 25 copies/ml when 1 ml of plasma is used, but this level is detected in less than 50% of replicates. The limit of quantification is best defined as the amount of nucleic acid

Table 3-1. Commercially Available HIV-1 Viral Load Assays

Test Kit	Method	Manufacturer	Gene Target	Range* (copies/ml)	Specimen Volume
Amplicor HIV-1 monitor test, standard	RT-PCR	Roche Diagnostics (Indianapolis, IN)	HIV-1 *gag*	400–750,000	200 µl
Amplicor HIV-1 monitor test, ultrasensitive	RT-PCR	Roche Diagnostics (Indianapolis, IN)	HIV-1 *gag*	50–100,000	500 µl
Versant HIV-1 RNA 3.0 assay	Branched DNA	Bayer Diagnostics Corporation, (Tarrytown, NY)	HIV-1 *pol*	75–500,000	1 ml
NucliSens HIV-1 QT assay	NASBA	bioMerieux (Durham, NC)	HIV-1 *gag*	176–3,470,000	1 ml†

*See text for a detailed discussion of the dynamic range of the assays.
†Can accommodate volumes between 50 µl and 2 ml.
RT-PCR, reverse transcription–polymerase chain reaction; NASBA, nucleic acid sequence-based amplification.

that can be verified in 95% of replicate samples. Using this definition, the ultrasensitive Amplicor RT-PCR assay has a sensitivity of 50 copies/ml, followed by the Versant bDNA assay at 75 copies/ml, and the NucliSens HIV-1 QT assay (bioMerieux, Durham, NC) at 176 copies/ml.[29-31] It is unclear whether there is a clinical difference when the viral load is decreased to less than 50 copies/ml compared to reduction below 100 copies/ml.[29]

The ability to detect the various subtypes of HIV-1 RNA also differs among the various viral load assays. Though the majority of HIV-1 infections in North America and Europe are subtype B,[32] infections with non-B subtypes are becoming more common in the United States and certainly represent an important cause of HIV-1 infection globally. The Versant bDNA assay accurately quantifies HIV-1 subtypes A through G, while the Amplicor RT-PCR version 1.0 assay underquantifies HIV-1 subtypes A, E, and F by 1–2 $\log_{10}$ copies/ml.[33] This problem has been resolved with the FDA approval of the Amplicor RT-PCR version 1.5 assay, which has modified primer sequences that allow accurate quantification of subtypes A through H.[32-34] For the NucliSens NASBA assay, studies have shown decreased quantification of subtype G.[32,33,35] None of the currently available assays are recommended for quantification of group O viruses. An assay is under development that can detect all types of HIV-1 as well as HIV-2 RNA, but it is not available for clinical use at this time.[36]

The viral load values obtained with the different assays may not be comparable because each uses a different molecular technique and may use a different HIV-1 RNA standard. The viral load values obtained with the standard Amplicor RT-PCR (version 1.0) are reported to be about two-fold higher than levels obtained with either version 2.0 of the Versant bDNA assay[37,38] or the NucliSens NASBA assay.[39] The viral load levels obtained with version 3.0 of the Versant bDNA assay and the Amplicor RT-PCR assay (version 1.5) were highly correlated in one study, with differences between the two assays within the coefficients of variation for the assays.[40] The Amplicor version 1.0 and 1.5 assays have been reported to generate comparable values on matched clinical specimens.[41] Although the differences in viral load levels obtained with the different assays are narrowing, it is still best to use the same assay when monitoring patients over time.

Proper collection and processing of blood samples are essential to assure accurate assessment of viral load levels; the key is to minimize RNA degradation. For both the Versant bDNA and Amplicor RT-PCR assays, EDTA is the preferred anticoagulant for blood collection. Blood anticoagulated with acid citrate dextrose (ACD) also is acceptable, but the viral load will be decreased approximately 15% due to the volume of anticoagulant.[42-44] Blood anticoagulated with heparin is unacceptable for the Versant bDNA or Amplicor RT-PCR assays. Due to the extraction method used with the NucliSens NASBA assay, any anticoagulant can be accommodated, though EDTA is most commonly used.[45]

To ensure minimal degradation of RNA, plasma must be separated from blood cells within 4 to 6 hours of collection. Delays in processing may lead to a falsely decreased viral load due to RNA degradation. Plasma specimens can be stored at 4°C for several days without significant degradation of RNA. Moreover, HIV-1 RNA remains stable after three cycles of freezing (−70°C) and thawing.[43] For long-term storage, plasma samples should be frozen at or below −70°C.[44] Vacutainer Plasma Preparation Tubes (PPT) also can be used for the collection of blood specimens for viral load testing. The PPT contain a gel barrier, which, after centrifugation, physically separates plasma from the cellular components.[42] Whole blood collected in PPT can be held at room temperature for as long as 6 hours after collection and shipped as plasma (in the original tube) at ambient temperature or on wet or dry ice without affecting the HIV-1 viral load.[46] Freezing PPTs (after separating the plasma) prior to testing can give higher viral load values compared to those obtained when the plasma is separated and stored at 4°C. For this reason freezing PPTs is not recommended. The PPTs provide a closed sample collection system, which is a safe, convenient, and practical approach to shipping specimens collected at sites remote from the laboratory.

Although measuring viral load in plasma is the standard of care in clinical practice, these assays have been adapted for use with other specimens, most notably serum, dried blood spots, cerebrospinal fluid (CSF), seminal fluid or semen, or cervical secretions. When serum specimens are used, the viral load is decreased approximately 50% compared to plasma.[44] Both blood and plasma dried spots can be used for viral load testing; in fact, viral load levels from dried plasma spots are equivalent to those obtained from fresh frozen plasma specimens. HIV-1 RNA in dried plasma spots remains stable for up to 16 days when stored at 4°C or ambient temperature.[47] Similarly, HIV-1 RNA from dried whole blood spots, corrected for hematocrit, yields viral load results comparable to those obtained from plasma.[48] The measurement of HIV-1 viral load in genital secretions has been done with the Amplicor and NucliSens assays, although this testing is largely reserved for research studies.[44,49] Viral load levels in CSF have been used in the evaluation of patients with AIDS dementia.

Proviral DNA Assays

Qualitative proviral DNA assays are used primarily for the diagnosis of neonatal or acute HIV-1 infections. Currently, there is one commercial test kit available, the Amplicor DNA test; however, it is not FDA approved. The assay uses the same primers as version 1.5 of the Amplicor RT-PCR assay, thus allowing reliable detection of subtypes A through H. Due to the limited availability of commercial proviral DNA assays, many laboratories have developed their own tests using either standard or real-time amplification methods. The performance characteristics of laboratory-developed assays can vary, and performance characteristics to consider include sensitivity, specificity, reproducibility, and the ability to detect non-B subtypes of HIV-1 proviral DNA.

Drug Resistance Assays

Antiretroviral resistance can be detected using either genotypic or phenotypic assays. HIV-1 genotypic assays identify mutations or changes in the nucleotide sequence known to confer decreased susceptibility to antiretroviral drugs. The effective use of genotypic resistance testing in clinical practice requires an extensive understanding of the genetics of antiretroviral resistance. Phenotype, on the other hand, refers to a viral trait or behavior resulting from the expression of a specific genotype. HIV-1 phenotypic assays measure viral replication in the presence of antiretroviral drugs. Results of phenotypic assays are typically reported as the inhibitory concentration of a drug that reduces in vitro HIV-1 replication by 50% (IC_{50}). The IC_{50} is usually reported as the fold change in IC_{50} relative to a wild-type strain. A "virtual phenotype" also is available commercially for assessing HIV-1 drug resistance. With a virtual phenotype, a phenotypic assay is not performed directly; rather, the information is inferred from the genotypic assay. The results of the genotypic assay are entered into a database containing matching genotypic and phenotypic results from thousands of clinical specimens, and the closest matching phenotypic results are averaged and reported as the virtual phenotype.

There are several methods used for genotypic resistance assays, including automated dideoxynucleotide terminator cycle sequencing, DNA hybridization using high-density microarrays, and reverse hybridization to mutation-specific probes. The initial step in all these genotypic assays is the extraction of HIV-1 RNA from a clinical specimen, which is usually plasma. This is followed by reverse transcription and PCR amplification of the entire protease gene and most of the RT gene (Figure 3-1). The amplified products then are analyzed using one of the methods mentioned above. The vast majority of genotypic resistance testing used for clinical management decisions is done by automated dideoxynucleotide terminator cycle sequencing. These methods are complex, requiring sequence alignment and editing, mutation detection by comparison to a standard wild-type sequence, and interpretation of the significance of the mutations identified. Two FDA-cleared assays are available that include reagents for sequencing and software programs to assist with sequence alignment and interpretation (Trugene HIV-1 Genotyping Kit and OpenGene DNA Sequencing System, Bayer Diagnostics Corporation, Tarrytown, NY; and ViroSeq HIV-1 Genotyping System, Abbott Molecular, Des Plaines, IL). In addition to these commercial assays, several laboratories have developed automated cycle sequencing assays for HIV-1 resistance testing. The currently available commercial assays do not amplify the envelope gene, so mutations that lead to resistance to the

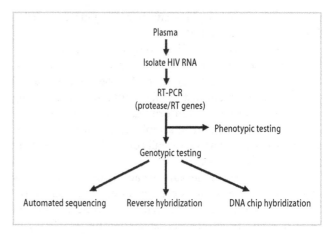

Figure 3-1. Overview of HIV-1 resistance testing.

fusion inhibitor drugs are not detected. However, this testing is available from reference laboratories.

HIV-1 sequencing also can be done by DNA hybridization of the amplified viral genes to defined oligonucleotide probes using high-density microarrays followed by automated base calling and mutation detection. One such method, GeneChip (Affymetrix, Santa Clara, CA), provides the nucleotide sequence of the entire HIV-1 protease gene and most of the RT gene.[50] Although several studies found good overall concordance (<97%) of sequence data between cycle sequencing and the GeneChip method,[51–53] problems were noted in the ability to detect mixtures of mutant and wild-type virus.[51] However, with continued improvements in DNA chip technology, it is possible that this technology will prove to be successful in the future for detection of resistance mutations.

A reverse hybridization method, the line probe assay (LiPA, manufactured for Bayer Diagnostics Corporation, Tarrytown, NY, by Innogenetics, Gent, Belgium), can rapidly and simultaneously determine the presence of drug resistance mutations in preselected codons rather than the entire gene sequence.[54] The amplified portions of the RT and protease genes are hybridized to nitrocellulose strips containing probes that are complementary to target sequences containing specific mutations. The strips also contain probes complementary to corresponding wild-type target sequences. This method can identify specific mutations but will not provide information about the entire gene sequence. A discordance rate of 8% between LiPA and automated sequencing for the RT gene was noted in one study.[53] Although hybridization failures for some codons exceeded 10% in another study, LiPA appeared to be more sensitive than automated sequencing in detecting minority mutant populations.[55] To date, the LiPA assay has been designed to identify primary resistance mutations only. The nitrocellulose strips will require constant updating as new drugs become available and new mutations are identified. However, because of the relative ease of use, and with ongoing improvements, genotypic methods that rely on reverse hybridization will likely remain important for clinical and research applications.

There have been few direct comparisons of the various automated sequencing assays used in clinical practice. A study comparing the Trugene and ViroSeq assays showed that both tests identified similar mutations after taking into account differences in drug databases and reference strains.[56] Nineteen of the 21 samples tested were equivalent in the two assays, with an overall concordance of 99% (249 of 252 mutation sites).

Phenotypic assays measure the ability of HIV-1 to grow in the presence of various concentrations of an antiretroviral drug. Results are expressed as the concentration of drug needed to inhibit viral replication by 50% (IC_{50}) or 90% (IC_{90}) compared with a drug-susceptible control virus (Figure 3-2). Initially, phenotypic assays required isolation of infectious HIV-1 from a blood specimen. However, now phenotypic assays are performed using high-throughput automated assays based on recombinant DNA technology. HIV-1 phenotypic resistance testing is available from two different commercial laboratories. For one assay, PhenoSense (ViroLogic, South San Francisco, CA), the protease and RT genes are amplified using RT-PCR and inserted into a modified HIV-1 vector that has a luciferase reporter gene in place of the viral envelope gene. Viral replication, in the presence of various drugs, is measured by quantification of luciferase expression.[57] The reproducibility of the assay is such that increases in IC_{50} of greater than 2.5-fold can be reliably detected in the assay. The second assay, Antivirogram (Virco, Mechelen, Belgium), combines patient and HIV-1 vector sequences using in vitro recombination. Viral replication is measured using a reporter gene system.[58]

There is little data directly addressing specimen collection and processing for HIV-1 resistance testing. These assays are very sensitive to RNA degradation because the methods require the amplification of a large portion of the viral genome (1,200 to 1,600 base pairs). Current recommendations for resistance testing are to follow guidelines established for viral load testing regarding collection, processing, and storage of specimens. The method of RNA extraction can be altered depending on the viral load of the specimen. For specimens with a low viral load (<1,000 to 5,000 copies/ml plasma), the most common approach to improve the yield of RNA is to concentrate virions from a larger specimen volume by high-speed centrifugation (23,000 × g or higher) prior to RNA extraction. Typically a viral load of 1,000 copies/ml or greater is required for reliable results from automated sequencing assays. However, using methods to concentrate virus from a larger volume of plasma, it is possible to obtain sequencing data on specimens with a viral load of <1,000 copies/ml.[56] Considering the cost of these assays and the variability of viral load measurements near the limit of quantification, it may be best to avoid resistance testing until the viral load in the plasma is >1,000 copies/ml. Both the Trugene and ViroSeq assays have been used successfully to genotype non-B subtypes of HIV-1.[59,60]

Interpretation

Viral Load Assays

HIV-1 viral load assays have become the standard of care for monitoring response to antiretroviral therapy. To effectively use viral load assays in clinical practice there must be an understanding of which changes in viral load re-present a clinically important change in viral replication. This requires knowledge of both viral biology and assay performance. The available viral load assays have an intra-assay variability of 0.12 to $0.2 \log_{10}$ on repeated testing of individual samples,[44,61] with the bDNA assay showing the lowest intra-assay variability. Biologically, HIV-1 RNA levels are fairly stable in individuals who are not receiving therapy; the biological variation is approximately $0.3 \log_{10}$.[12] Therefore, changes in HIV-1 RNA levels must exceed $0.5 \log_{10}$ (3-fold) to represent biologically relevant changes in viral replication. For all the viral load assays, the intra-assay variability is even greater near the lower limit of quantification, so for HIV-1 RNA values less than $3 \log_{10}$ (1,000 copies/ml), it is particularly important not to overinterpret small changes in viral load. Reporting viral load levels as $\log_{10}$-transformed data assists in preventing clinicians from overinterpreting small changes in viral load.

Several clinical illnesses, including herpes simplex virus (HSV) infections, acute infections, and opportunistic infections, as well as vaccinations for influenza, tetanus, or pneumonococcal infection, can lead to transient increases in HIV-1 RNA levels.[62-64] For some individuals these increases in viral load may be quite dramatic, $\geq 1 \log_{10}$; however, HIV-1 RNA levels usually return to baseline within a month of the acute event. For this reason it is recommended that viral load measurements be avoided during acute illness or within a month of vaccination.

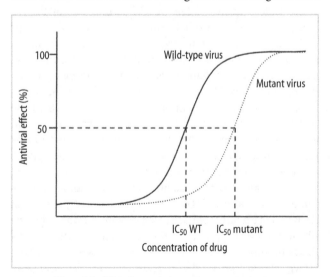

Figure 3-2. HIV-1 phenotypic drug resistance testing results.

False-positive results can occur with HIV-1 viral load assays and are attributed to carryover contamination with amplicons, limitations in assay chemistry, or cross-contamination of specimens during specimen processing. Carryover contamination of amplified products is a problem for the Amplicor RT-PCR and NucliSens NASBA assays, as both are target amplification methods. The Amplicor RT-PCR assay has been designed to minimize this problem; specifically, the assay uses dUTP and the DNA repair enzyme uracil-N-glycosylase (UNG) to destroy carryover amplicons before amplification. Carryover contamination will become less of a problem when real-time RT-PCR versions of these assays are used, since the sample is not manipulated after the amplification step. An advantage of the Versant bDNA assay is that carryover contamination does not occur, since it is a signal amplification method. However, the Versant bDNA assay chemistry involves complex hybridization of nucleic acid probes and there can be nonspecific hybridization leading to false-positive results. The assay has a specificity of approximately 98% when testing specimens from HIV-1-negative individuals.[14] Most of the false-positive samples have viral load values of less than 2000 copies/ml. Contamination with HIV-1 RNA during specimen processing can lead to false-positive results with any of the three assays.

Drug Resistance Assays

Interpretation of genotypic resistance testing is very complex and requires a detailed understanding of the genetics of resistance. For many drugs, the mutations associated with resistance have been well characterized when used as monotherapy. However, when drugs are used in combination, as is the standard of care for HIV-1-infected individuals, interactions may occur between mutations, which may increase or decrease drug susceptibilities. These interactions, although complex, must be understood to accurately interpret genotypic results. In general, viral mutations make the virus less fit for replication. The terms "primary" and "secondary" may be used when referring to resistance mutations. Primary mutations are relatively drug specific and may decrease viral susceptibility to the drug. Drug-resistant mutants may have a reduced replication capacity or viral fitness compared to wild-type virus. Secondary mutations alone may have no effect on viral drug susceptibility but may improve viral fitness, allowing a virus with a primary mutation to improve its replicative capacity.[65] A current and comprehensive discussion of the specific mutations associated with each antiretroviral drug and the interactions of mutations is available from a variety of sources,[28] including Los Alamos National Laboratory HIV Databases (http://hiv-web.lanl.gov), International AIDS Society–USA (http://www.iasusa.org), and Stanford University HIV Drug Resistance Database (http://hivdb.stanford.edu).

The proper interpretation of genotypic drug resistance assays involves two independent processes, identification of resistance mutations and interpretation of how these mutations alter viral susceptibility to specific antiretroviral drugs. An error in either process will lead to an inaccurate genotyping interpretation. While establishing appropriate quality control guidelines for the technical aspect of an assay is common practice, the complex interpretation of HIV-1 genotyping assays represents a new challenge for clinical laboratory personnel. Since interpretation of genotypic assays is so complex and critical to patient care, both of the FDA-cleared assays provide software programs that assist in base calling, sequence alignment, and identification of the resistance mutations by comparing the sequence to that of a wild-type virus.

After identifying the resistance mutations, a "rule-based" software program is used to interpret the meaning of the various mutations. For example, with the OpenGene system (Bayer Diagnostics Corporation), the rules are established by an independent panel of experts and updated regularly as new information becomes available. A computer algorithm has been developed based on these rules that accounts for primary and secondary mutations, cross resistance, and interactions of mutations. In addition to listing the mutations identified in the RT and protease genes, an interpretative report is provided that lists each drug and provides a designation of either "no evidence of resistance," "possible resistance," "resistance," or "insufficient evidence."[66] "No evidence of resistance" is used if no known mutations are detected or if reduced susceptibility to a specific drug has not been associated with the identified mutation(s). "Possible resistance" is used when the mutations detected have been associated with diminished virologic response in some but not all patients, or if the mutation has been associated with an intermediate decrease in susceptibility to the drug. "Resistance" refers to mutations that have been associated with a maximum reduction in susceptibility to the drug. If there is inadequate evidence to determine susceptibility, the term "insufficient evidence" is used.[66] A similar approach is used in the ViroSeq assay (Abbott Molecular), though the interpretation of all mutations may not be identical for both systems. These rule-based interpretation systems are essential for providing clinicians with results in a user-friendly format that is easily understood and clinically useful without the need for an extensive knowledge of the genetics of HIV-1 resistance. Ideally, one rule-based system would be used for the interpretation of all genotypic assays. These databases require frequent updates as new data regarding drug resistance become available and new drugs are available for clinical use. Clinically, resistance results must be interpreted in the context of the treatment history of each patient.

Mutations in HIV-1 are reported with a specific nomenclature in which amino acids are reported using single-letter abbreviations. The wild-type amino acid encoded by the nucleotide triplet is followed by the location of the mutation (codon number) and then the mutant amino acid. For example, K103N indicates that the lysine (wild

Table 3-2. Example of Genotypic Resistance Report

Drug	Interpretation
Nucleoside RT Inhibitor Mutations: D67N, K70R, M184V, K219E	
Zidovudine	Resistance
Didanosine	Possible resistance
Zalcitabine	Possible resistance
Lamivudine/emtricitabine	Resistance
Stavudine	Possible resistance
Abacavir	Possible resistance
Tenofovir	No evidence of resistance
Nonnucleoside RT Inhibitor Mutations: K103N	
Nevirapine	Resistance
Delavirdine	Resistance
Efavirenz	Resistance
Protease Inhibitor Mutations: D30N	
Saquinavir	No evidence of resistance
Indinavir	No evidence of resistance
Ritonavir	No evidence of resistance
Nelfinavir	Resistance
Amprenavir/fosamprenavir	No evidence of resistance
Lopinavir and ritonavir	No evidence of resistance
Atazanavir	No evidence of resistance

type) at codon 103 is replaced by an asparagine (mutant). Genotyping reports include a list of the mutations identified as well as the effect of the mutations on antiretroviral drug susceptibility (Table 3-2).

An important issue for the interpretation of HIV-1 phenotypic assays is defining the cutoff change in IC_{50} that is associated with resistance. Initially, this cutoff was established based on the technical performance of the assays, which is the increase in IC_{50} that could be reliably detected when compared to wild-type virus. For the PhenoSense assay, this was established at a 2.5-fold increase in IC_{50}, while for the Antivirogram assay this was set at a 4-fold increase in IC_{50}. More recently there has been a move to define the cutoffs in relationship to the likelihood of a clinical response. Clinically important increases in IC_{50} have been defined for some drugs, and these cutoffs can vary with different drugs. For example, with abacavir, stavudine, and lopinavir the fold change in IC_{50} that is clinically important is 4.5, 1.7, and 10, respectively.[67] However, with NNRTIs, 4- to 10-fold increases in IC_{50} values in therapy-naive subjects were not associated with a poor virologic outcome.[68] It is likely that IC_{50} cutoffs will continue to be modified as more clinical outcomes data become available. Reports of phenotypic assay results include not only the change in IC_{50} value but also an interpretation of whether there is an increase or decrease in susceptibility compared to wild-type virus.

A standard of care has not been established for the preferential use of genotypic or phenotypic resistance testing. Some clinicians prefer phenotypic testing because it is a direct measure of viral susceptibility. Others prefer genotypic testing because the development of a mutation may precede phenotypic expression of resistance. In addition,

genotypic testing can be completed in 1 to 2 days, compared to 1 to 2 weeks for phenotypic testing. Another important factor is that phenotypic testing is significantly more expensive than genotypic testing. Due to issues of availability and cost, providers often use genotypic testing routinely and rely on phenotypic testing for patients who have failed multiple regimens and have very complex genotypic results. If both assays are used, it is key to remember that the results of both assays may not agree, as the presence of a resistance mutation does not assure its expression in a phenotypic assay. Depending on the drug regimen, genotypic and phenotypic testing may provide complementary information.[67]

The currently available genotypic and phenotypic methods can detect a mutant virus only if it comprises at least 20% of the total viral population. So resistance testing is best used to predict failure of a regimen rather than ensure success, because a mutant may be present at a concentration below the detection limit of the assay. The one exception is the LiPA assay, which can detect mutants that comprise as little as 4% of the total viral population,[51,54] though this test is not widely used in clinical laboratories. Detection of these minor mutants is important because, in the presence of drug selection pressure, these minority populations will quickly predominate. Likewise, drug selection pressure is required for mutations to persist, and in the absence of drug selection pressure the viral population can revert back to wild type. One study showed that this reversion back to wild type can occur within several weeks of withdrawing the antiretroviral drug.[69] Although the virus may appear susceptible to the specific drug, reintroducing the drug will select for resistance again. For this reason, it is recommended that specimens for resistance testing be obtained while the patient is on antiretroviral therapy.

Laboratory Issues

With the proven clinical utility and the availability of commercial assays, viral load testing for HIV-1 is performed routinely in many clinical laboratories. Three companies have FDA-approved test kits; the appropriate choice of a viral load assay will vary depending on the laboratory. Issues to consider include available space, volume of testing, turnaround time, expertise of technologists, and cost of reportable result. Each of the viral load assays has its strengths and weaknesses. The Versant bDNA assay has the advantages of high throughput and a broad dynamic range, without concern for carryover contamination of amplified product. The System 340 instrument for the Versant bDNA assay allows for a greater level of automation. However, the assay does not have an internal control to compensate for loss of RNA during nucleic acid extraction, and false-positive results have been reported.[14] The Amplicor RT-PCR assay has good specificity, but the dynamic range is limited, requiring the use of both a standard and an ultrasensitive version of the assay, and adequate space is needed for proper laboratory design to separate the pre- and post-PCR steps of analysis. The Cobas Amplicor instrument, which automates the amplification and detection steps of the test, is available. However, the throughput of the instrument is limited, requiring 6 hours to test 24 specimens. The NASBA assay has a broad dynamic range and can accommodate a wide range of clinical specimen types and specimen volumes, but the assay is slightly less sensitive than the other available assays. The MiniMag and EasyMag are instruments that automate the nucleic acid extraction step of the NucliSens assay and have greatly reduced the hands-on time needed to perform the test.

The initial step in some genotypic and all phenotypic assays involves amplification of viral RNA using RT-PCR technology. As a result, strict precautions must be followed to avoid contamination of specimens with amplified products and to prevent contamination between specimens during processing and amplification. Genetic fingerprinting programs are a very important tool to assist the laboratory in detecting contamination or sample mix-up. Each sequence that is generated is compared to a laboratory-specific database that contains the sequences of other specimens and controls. The database then displays the prior sequences most closely related to the current sample. Due to the variation in the HIV-1 sequence, there should not be an exact or a highly similar match within the database unless it is an earlier specimen from the same patient. If different patients are found to have highly similar sequences, this can be a clue to problems with contamination in the laboratory. This genetic fingerprinting function is included in the Trugene System, allowing all sequenced specimens to be checked against the fingerprinting database. The ViroSeq system uses UTP and uracil N-glycosylase (UNG), which is a very effective method to control for contamination of amplified products. As with viral load testing, extreme care must be taken to avoid cross contamination of specimens during processing.

The College of American Pathologists(CAP) Surveys Program offers proficiency testing for HIV-1 viral load measurements (HIV/HV2 survey) three times per year. The Centers for Disease Control and Prevention (CDC) offers laboratory performance evaluations twice a year (the CDC Model Performance Evaluation).

Phenotypic resistance testing, which requires culture of HIV-1, is not performed in clinical laboratories but is available from two commercial laboratories (Virologic and Virco). Genotypic assays that rely on automated sequencing technology are performed in clinical laboratories; the testing is very complex and challenging for laboratories because quality control is required for both the generation of sequence and the subsequent interpretation of the results. An international HIV-1 genotyping proficiency program (ENVA-3)[70] distributed five plasma samples to 175 laboratories. One sample in the panel contained a 50:50 mixture of wild-type and mutant HIV-1 with mutations in various resistance codons. For this specimen, at least eight of the nine resistance mutations were detected by 55% of the laboratories using ViroSeq, 62% of the laboratories using Trugene, and 33% of the laboratories using laboratory-developed assays. Overall these results are quite disappointing considering that sequencing technology is reported to detect mutants that comprise as little as 20% of the total viral population. In addition to difficulties identifying resistance mutations, there was extensive variation between laboratories in the interpretation of the significance of the mutations.[71] These results clearly point out the need for proficiency testing for both identification and interpretation of resistance mutations.

The interpretation of an assay as complex as HIV-1 genotyping presents a new challenge for clinical laboratories. Many laboratories rely on databases and algorithms provided by commercial companies, since experts in the interpretation of resistance testing may not be available locally. One problem with this approach is that the laboratory has no control over how frequently these databases are updated. In addition, the databases may use different reference strains, base-calling algorithms, or resistance reference files, leading to different interpretations of the same resistance mutations. Standardization of these test components is needed to minimize misinterpretation of genotyping results. FDA clearance has been an important step for genotyping assays, but standardization of interpretive criteria is needed.

Proficiency testing for HIV-1 genotyping is available from the College of American Pathologists (Northfield, IL) Surveys Program (HIV/HV2 surveys), with three challenges per year. To date, this proficiency program has focused on identification of specific resistance mutations, rather than interpretation of these mutations. In the future, proficiency programs will need to include mutation identification as well as interpretation challenges.

An important advance for HIV-1 drug resistance testing has been the establishment of CPT codes for both phenotypic (87903) and genotypic (87901) testing. However, reimbursement rates vary greatly from state to state and may be below the cost of performing the tests. Adequate reimbursement is essential to assure access to resistance testing for all HIV1-infected individuals.

The Future

The use of HAART in combination with HIV-1 viral load and drug resistance assays has revolutionized the management of HIV-1-infected persons. Future advancements for these tests will likely focus on improved assay performance and automation. Real-time RT-PCR methods, which allow the simultaneous amplification and detection of amplified product, offer many improvements over the current assays. The technical time to perform the assay and time to result will be decreased. The risk of contamination due to carryover of amplified product will be greatly reduced since there is no postamplification handling of the sample. Analysis is done early in the log phase of amplification, thus decreasing differences in amplification efficiency between samples. Real-time HIV-1 viral load assays are under development that are ultrasensitive (20 to 50 copies/ml) with a $6\log_{10}$ linear range. Some of these assays also quantify group O virus.

The currently available genotypic drug resistance assays are very labor-intensive. Future assays will need to be much more automated with a higher throughput. With advances in DNA chip technology, this approach may prove to be applicable to complex genotypic assays. Other needed improvements include standardization of databases and interpretive algorithms, optimization of assay performance to improve detection of minor mutant populations, and establishing appropriate quality control and quality assurance programs. HIV-1 drug resistance assays will need to be very flexible to accommodate new antiretroviral drugs that target other genes such as *gag, integrase,* or *envelope.* Finally, the clinical correlation between genotypic and phenotypic assays needs to be better defined.

In the future, the clinical management of HIV-1 infected individuals may include therapeutic drug monitoring, and pharmacogenomic testing to identify individuals with altered metabolism of drugs or those at risk for adverse reactions to antiretroviral drugs. The use of these types of assays may allow for better individualization of antiretroviral therapy and improved clinical outcomes.

References

1. Connor R, Ho D, Kuritzkes DR, Richman D. Human Immunodeficiency Virus. In: *Clinical Virology,* 1st ed. Richman DD, Whitley RJ, and Hayden FG (eds.) Churchill Livingstone, New York; 1997:707–754.
2. Yeni PG, Hammer SM, Hirsch MS, et al. Treatment for adult HIV infection: 2004 recommendations of the International AIDS Society–USA Panel. *JAMA.* 2004;292:251–265.
3. Mellors JW, Kingsley LA, Rinaldo CR Jr, et al. Quantitation of HIV-1 RNA in plasma predicts outcome after seroconversion. *Ann Intern Med.* 1995;122:573–579.
4. O'Brien TR, Blattner WA, Waters D, et al. Serum HIV-1 RNA levels and time to development of AIDS in the Multicenter Hemophilia Cohort Study. *JAMA.* 1996;276:105–110.
5. Mellors JW, Rinaldo CR Jr, Gupta P, White RM, Todd JA, Kingsley LA. Prognosis in HIV-1 infection predicted by the quantity of virus in plasma. *Science.* 1996;272:1167–1170.
6. Eron JJ, Benoit SL, Jemsek J, et al. Treatment with lamivudine, zidovudine, or both in HIV-positive patients with 200 to 500 CD4+ cells per cubic millimeter. *N Eng J Med.* 1995;333:1662–1669.
7. Hammer SM, Squires KE, Hughes MD, et al. A controlled trial of two nucleoside analogues plus indinavir in persons with human immunodeficiency virus infection and CD4 counts of 200 per cubic millimeter or less. *N Eng J Med.* 1997;337:725–739.
8. Cameron DW, Heath-Chiozzi M, Danner S, et al. Randomised placebo-controlled trial of ritonavir in advanced HIV-1 disease. The Advanced HIV Disease Ritonavir Study Group. *Lancet.* 1998;351:543–549.
9. Ho DD, Neumann AU, Perelson AS, Chen W, Leonard JM, Markowitz M. Rapid turnover of plasma virions and CD4+ lymphocytes in HIV-1 infection. *Nature.* 1995;373:123–126.
10. Wei X, Ghosh SK, Taylor ME, et al. Viral dynamics in human immunodeficiency virus type 1 infection. *Nature.* 1995;373:117–122.
11. Raboud JM, Montaner JS, Conway B, et al. Suppression of plasma viral load below 20 copies/ml is required to achieve a long-term response to therapy. *AIDS.* 1998;12:1619–1624.
12. Saag MS, Holodniy M, Kuritzkes DR, et al. HIV viral load markers in clinical practice. *Nature Med.* 1996;2:625–629.
13. Kahn JO, Walker BD. Acute human immunodeficiency virus type 1 infection. *N Eng J Med.* 1998;339:32–39.
14. Daar ES, Little S, Pitt J, et al. Diagnosis of primary HIV-1 infection. Los Angeles County Primary HIV Infection Recruitment Network. *Ann Intern Med.* 2001;134:25–29.
15. Young NL, Shaffer N, Chaowanachan T, et al. Early diagnosis of HIV-1-infected infants in Thailand using RNA and DNA PCR assays sensitive to non-B subtypes. *J Acquir Immune Defic Syndr.* 2000;24:401–407.
16. Cunningham CK, Charbonneau TT, Song K, et al. Comparison of human immunodeficiency virus 1 DNA polymerase chain reaction and qualitative and quantitative RNA polymerase chain reaction in human immunodeficiency virus 1-exposed infants. *Pediatr Infect Dis J.* 1999;18:30–35.
17. Steketee RW, Abrams EJ, Thea DM, et al. Early detection of perinatal human immunodeficiency virus (HIV) type 1 infection using HIV RNA amplification and detection. *J Infect Dis.* 1997;175:707–711.
18. Centers for Disease Control. 1994 Revised classification system for human immunodeficiency virus infection in children less than 13 years of age. *MMWR Morb Mortal Wkly Rep.* 1994;43:(RR-12):1–11.
19. Durant J, Clevenbergh P, Halfon P, et al. Drug-resistance genotyping in HIV-1 therapy: the VIRADAPT randomised controlled trial. *Lancet.* 1999;353:2195–2199.
20. Clevenbergh P, Durant J, Halfon P, et al. Persisting long-term benefit of genotype-guided treatment for HIV-infected patients failing HAART. The VIRADAPT study: week 48 follow-up. *Antivir Ther.* 2000;5:65–70.
21. Baxter JD, Mayers DL, Wentworth DN, et al. A randomized study of antiretroviral management based on plasma genotypic antiretroviral resistance testing in patients failing therapy. *AIDS.* 2000;14:F83–F93.
22. Tural C, Ruiz L, Holtzer C, et al. Clinical utility of HIV-1 genotyping and expert advice—the Havana trial. *AIDS.* 2002;16:209–218.
23. Weinstein MC, Goldie SJ, Losina E, et al. Use of genotypic resistance testing to guide HIV therapy: clinical impact and cost-effectiveness. *Ann Intern Med.* 2001;134:440–450.
24. Cohen CJ, Hunt S, Sension M, et al. A randomized trial assessing the impact of phenotypic resistance testing on antiretroviral therapy. *AIDS.* 2002;16:579–588.
25. Meynard J-L, Vray M, Morand-Joubert L, et al. Phenotypic or genotypic resistance testing for choosing antiretroviral therapy after treatment failure: a randomized trial. *AIDS.* 2002;16:727–736.
26. Miller V. HIV drug resistance: overview of clinical data. *J HIV Ther.* 2001;6:68–72.
27. Haubrich RH, Kemper CA, Hellmann NS, et al. A randomized, prospective study of phenotype susceptibility testing versus standard of care to manage antiretroviral therapy: CCTG 575. *AIDS.* 2005;19:295–302.
28. Hirsch MS, Conway B, D'Aquila RT, et al. Antiretroviral drug resistance testing in adults with human immunodeficiency virus type 1: 2003 recommendations of an International AIDS Society–USA panel. *Clin Infect Dis.* 2003;37:113–128.
29. Erice A, Brambilla D, Bremer J, et al. Performance characteristics of the QUANTIPLEX HIV-1 RNA 3.0 assay for detection and quantitation of human immunodeficiency virus type 1 RNA in plasma. *J Clin Microbiol.* 2000;38:2837–2845.
30. Sun R, Ku J, Jayakar H, et al. Ultrasensitive reverse transcription-PCR assay for quantitation of human immunodeficiency virus type 1 RNA in plasma. *J Clin Microbiol.* 1998;36:2964–2969.
31. Witt DJ, Kemper M, Stead A, Ginocchio C, Caliendo AM. Relationship of incremental specimen volumes and enhanced detection of

human immunodeficiency virus type 1 RNA with nucleic acid amplification technology. *J Clin Microbiol.* 2000;38:85–89.

32. Parekh B, Phillips S, Granade TC, Baggs J, Hu DJ, Respess R. Impact of HIV type 1 subtype variation on viral RNA quantitation. *AIDS Res Hum Retroviruses.* 1999;15:133–142.

33. Jagodzinski LL, Wiggins DL, McManis JL, et al. Use of calibrated viral load standards for group M subtypes of human immunodeficiency virus type 1 to assess the performance of viral RNA quantitation tests. *J Clin Microbiol.* 2000;38:1247–1249.

34. Pasquier C, Sandres K, Salama G, Puel J, Izopet J. Using RT-PCR and bDNA assays to measure non-clade B HIV-1 subtype RNA. *J Virol Methods.* 1999;81:123–129.

35. Nkengasong JN, Bile C, Kalou M, et al. Quantification of RNA in HIV Type 1 subtypes D and G by NucliSens and Amplicor Assays in Abidjan, Ivory Coast. *AIDS Res Hum Retroviruses.* 1999;15:495–498.

36. Abravaya K, Esping C, Hoenle R, et al. Performance of a multiplex qualitative PCR LCx assay for detection of human immunodeficiency virus type 1 (HIV-1) group M subtypes, group O, and HIV-2. *J Clin Microbiol.* 2000;38:716–723.

37. Nolte FS, Boysza J, Thurmond C, Clark WS, Lennox JL. Clinical comparison of an enhanced-sensitivity branched-DNA assay and reverse transcription-PCR for quantitation of human immunodeficiency virus type 1 RNA in plasma. *J Clin Microbiol.* 1998;36:716–720.

38. Segondy M, Izopet J, Pellegrin I, et al. Comparison of the Quantiplex HIV-1 RNA 2.0 assay with the Amplicor HIV-1 monitor 1.0 assay for quantitation of levels of human immunodeficiency virus type 1 RNA in plasma of patients receiving stavudine-didanosine combination therapy. *J Clin Microbiol.* 1998;36:3392–3395.

39. Dyer JR, Pilcher CD, Shepard R, Schock J, Eron JJ, Fiscus SA. Comparison of NucliSens and Roche Monitor assays for quantitation of levels of human immunodeficiency virus type 1 RNA in plasma. *J Clin Microbiol.* 1999;37:447–449.

40. Elbeik T, Charlebois E, Nassos P, et al. Quantitative and cost comparison of ultrasensitive human immunodeficiency virus type 1 RNA viral load assays: Bayer bDNA quantiplex versions 3.0 and 2.0 and Roche PCR Amplicor Monitor version 1.5. *J Clin Microbiol.* 2000;38:1113–1120.

41. Triques K, Coste J, Perret JL, et al. Efficiencies of four versions of the AMPLICOR HIV-1 MONITOR test for quantification of different subtypes of human immunodeficiency virus type 1. *J Clin Microbiol.* 1999;37:110–116.

42. Ginocchio CC, Wang XP, Kaplan MH, et al. Effects of specimen collection, processing, and storage conditions on stability of human immunodeficiency virus type 1 RNA levels in plasma. *J Clin Microbiol.* 1997;35:2886–2893.

43. Sebire K, McGavin K, Land S, Middleton T, Birch C. Stability of human immunodeficiency virus RNA in blood specimens as measured by a commercial PCR-based assay. *J Clin Microbiol.* 1998;36:493–498.

44. Lew J, Reichelderfer P, Fowler M, et al. Determinations of levels of human immunodeficiency virus type 1 RNA in plasma: reassessment of parameters affecting assay outcome. TUBE Meeting Workshop Attendees. Technology Utilization for HIV-1 Blood Evaluation and Standardization in Pediatrics. *J Clin Microbiol.* 1998;36:1471–1479.

45. Boom R, Sol C, Salimans M, Jansen C, Wertheim-van Dillen PM, van derNoordaa J. Rapid and simple method for purification of nucleic acids. *J Clin Microbiol.* 1990;28:495–503.

46. Holodniy M, Rainen L, Herman S, Yen-Lieberman B. Stability of plasma human immunodeficiency virus load in VACUTAINER PPT plasma preparation tubes during overnight shipment. *J Clin Microbiol.* 2000;38:323–326.

47. Cassol S, Gill MJ, Pilon R, et al. Quantification of human immunodeficiency virus type 1 DNA from dried plasma spots collected on filter paper. *J Clin Microbiol.* 1997;35:2795–2801.

48. Fiscus SA, Brambilla D, Grosso L, Schock J, Cronin M. Quantitation of human immunodeficiency virus type 1 RNA in plasma by using blood dried on filter paper. *J Clin Microbiol.* 1998;36:258–260.

49. Bremer J, Nowicki M, Beckner S, et al. Comparison of two amplification technologies for detection and quantitation of human immunodeficiency virus type 1 RNA in the female genital tract. *J Clin Microbiol.* 2000;38:2665–2669.

50. Kozal MJ, Shah N, Shen N, et al. Extensive polymorphisms observed in HIV-1 clade B protease gene using high-density oligonucleotide arrays. *Nat Med.* 1996;2:753–759.

51. Gunthard HF, Wong JK, Ignacio CC, Havlir DV, Richman DD. Comparative performance of high-density oligonucleotide sequencing and dideoxynucleotide sequencing of HIV type 1 pol from clinical samples. *AIDS Res Hum Retroviruses.* 1998;14:869–876.

52. Hanna GJ, Johnson VA, Kuritzkes DR, et al. Comparison of sequencing by hybridization and cycle sequencing for genotyping of human immunodeficiency virus type 1 reverse transcriptase. *J Clin Microbiol.* 2000;38:2715–2721.

53. Wilson JW, Bean P, Robins T, Graziano F, Persing DH. Comparative evaluation of three human immunodeficiency virus genotyping systems: the HIV-Genotype R method, the HIV PRT GeneChip assay, and the HIV-1 RT line probe assay. *J Clin Microbiol.* 2000;38:3022–3028.

54. Stuyver L, Wyseur A, Rombout A. Line probe assay for rapid detection of drug-selected mutations in the human immunodeficiency virus type 1 reverse transcriptase gene. *Antimicrob Agents Chemother.* 1997;41:284–291.

55. Servais J, Lambert C, Fontaine E, et al. Comparison of DNA sequencing and a line probe assay for detection of human immunodeficiency virus type 1 drug resistance mutations in patients failing highly active antiretroviral therapy. *J Clin Microbiol.* 2001;39:454–459.

56. Erali M, Page S, Reimer LG, Hillyard DR. Human immunodeficiency virus type 1 drug resistance testing: a comparison of three sequence-based methods. *J Clin Microbiol.* 2001;39:2157–2165.

57. Petropoulos CJ, Parkin NT, Limoli KL. A novel phenotypic drug susceptibility assay for human immunodeficiency virus type 1. *Antimicrob Agents Chemother.* 2000;44:920–928.

58. Hertogs K, de Bethune MP, Miler V, et al. A rapid method for simultaneous detection of phenotypic resistance to inhibitors of protease and reverse transcriptase in recombinant human immunodeficiency virus type 1 isolates from patients treated with antiretroviral drugs. *Antimicrob Agents Chemother.* 1998;42:269–276.

59. Mracna M, Becker-Pergola G, Dileanis J, et al. Performance of the Applied Biosystems ViroSeq HIV-1 genotyping system for sequence-based analysis of non-subtype B human immunodeficiency virus type 1 from Uganda. *J Clin Microbiol.* 2001;39:4323–4327.

60. Rozenbaum W, Charpentier C, Delphin N, et al. Comparative performance evaluation of a kit-based HIV-1 genotyping assay and a laboratory developed "home-brew" genotyping assay with samples of varying viral loads and non-B subtypes of group M virus [abstract 171]. *Antiviral Therapy, 5th International Workshop on HIV Drug Resistance & Treatment Strategies.* Scottsdale, AZ; 2001;6:130.

61. Brambilla D, Leung S, Lew J, et al. Absolute copy number and relative change in determinations of human immunodeficiency virus type 1 RNA in plasma: effect of an external standard on kit comparisons. *J Clin Microbiol.* 1998;36:311–314.

62. Donovan RM, Bush CE, Markowitz NP, Baxa DM, Saravolatz LD. Changes in virus load markers during AIDS-associated opportunistic diseases in human immunodeficiency virus-infected persons. *J Infect Dis.* 1996;174:401–403.

63. O'Brien WA, Grovit-Ferbas K, Namazi A, et al. Human immunodeficiency virus-type 1 replication can be increased in peripheral blood of seropositive patients after influenza vaccination. *Blood.* 1995;86:1082–1089.

64. Staprans SI, Hamilton BL, Follansbee SE, et al. Activation of virus replication after vaccination of HIV-1-infected individuals. *J Exp Med.* 1995;182:1727–1737.

65. Hirsch MS, Conway B, D'Aquila RT, et al. Antiretroviral drug resistance testing in adults with HIV infection. *JAMA.* 1998;279:1984–1991.

66. D'Aquila RT. Incorporating antiretroviral resistance testing into clinical practice. Medscape HIV/AIDS CME Circle. Web MD Medscape Health Network. 2002. Available at: http://www.medscape.com.

67. Parkin N, Chappey C, Maroldo L, Bates M, Hellmann NS, Petropoulos CJ. Phenotypic and genotypic HIV-1 drug resistance assays provide complementary information. *J Acquir Immune Defic Syndr.* 2002;31:128–136.

68. Van Houtte M. Update on resistance testing. *J HIV Ther.* 2001;6:61–64.

69. Devereux HL, Youle M, Johnson MA, Loveday C. Rapid decline in detectability of HIV-1 drug resistance mutations after stopping therapy. *AIDS.* 1999;13:F123–F127.

70. Keulen W, Brambilla D, Buimer M, et al. A study on HIV-1 genotyping proficiency in 125 laboratories, using the ENVA-3 panel [abstract 166]. *Antiviral Therapy, 5th International Workshop on HIV Drug Resistance & Treatment Strategies.* Scottsdale, AZ; 2001;6:127.

71. Wensing AM, Keulen W, Buimer M, Brambilla D, Schuurman R, Boucher C. Analysis of the world-wide evaluation study on HIV-1 genotype interpretation: ENVA-3 [abstract 133]. *Antiviral Therapy, 5th International Workshop on HIV Drug Resistance & Treatment Strategies,* Scottsdale, AZ; 2001;6:101.

Chapter 4

Hepatitis B and C Viruses

Frederick S. Nolte

Introduction

Viral hepatitis is believed to have existed in antiquity, with references traced back to the fifth century BC. A new era in viral hepatitis was ushered in by the landmark discovery of Australia antigen, subsequently renamed hepatitis B surface antigen (HbsAg) by Blumberg and coworkers in 1965.[1] What followed was a rapid growth in information about the hepatitis B virus (HBV), development of serologic and molecular tests for HBV, understanding of the natural history and pathogenesis of infection, development and approval of antiviral therapies, and most importantly, the development of effective vaccines for prevention of HBV infection.

Although non-A, non-B hepatitis was thought to have a viral etiology since 1974, the virus eluded investigators for more than a decade. It was discovered in 1989 by a brute force application of molecular cloning techniques through the joint efforts of the Centers for Disease Control and Prevention (CDC) and the Chiron Corporation, and was named the hepatitis C virus (HCV).[2] This discovery led rapidly to the development of serologic screening assays for HCV infection prior to blood donation, which dramatically reduced the incidence of posttransfusion chronic hepatitis. Sequencing of the HCV genome also provided impetus for the development of molecular assays for detection, quantitation, and characterization of HCV. Although there has been explosive growth in information about this medically important virus since its discovery, much remains to be learned about its pathogenesis, treatment, and prevention.

The key characteristics of HBV and HCV are summarized in Table 4-1. Both viruses represent major global public health problems, with an estimated 350 million and 170 million persons chronically infected with HBV and HCV, respectively. Although clinical characteristics and risk factors for infection may give some indication of the specific etiology of viral hepatitis, the diagnosis is laboratory based. Laboratory diagnosis is based on serologic and molecular tests because cell culture techniques for isola-

tion of HBV and HCV are not effective. This chapter reviews the molecular tests that are available to detect, quantitate, and characterize HBV and HCV and how these tests can be used for effective diagnosis and clinical management of patients.

HEPATITIS B VIRUS

The HBV genome is a 3.2 kilobase (kb), relaxed circular, partially double-stranded DNA molecule. It has four partially overlapping open reading frames encoding the viral envelope (pre-S and S), nucleocapsid (precore and core), polymerase, and X proteins. Although HBV is a DNA virus, it replicates by a reverse transcriptase that lacks proofreading activity and, as a result, is prone to errors. The overlapping open reading frames of the genome limit the types of mutations that can be tolerated. However, variations in HBV sequences have been detected in almost all regions of the genome. Consequently, HBV exists as quasispecies, and different patients may be infected with different strains and genotypes.

There are seven phylogenetic genotypes (A through G), most of which have distinct geographic distribution. Genotypes are defined by intergroup divergence of greater than 8% in the complete genome nucleotide sequence. Genotypes A and D are common in the United States and Europe; genotypes B and C are most frequent in China and Southeast Asia. There is insufficient data to determine whether differences in clinical outcome or response to treatment correlate with virus genotype.

Clinical Utility

Serologic assays with high levels of sensitivity, specificity, and reproducibility have been developed to detect HBV antigens and their respective antibodies. This complicated system of serologic markers is used for diagnosis of HBV infection and to define the phase of infection, degree of infectivity, prognosis, and immune status. The presence of

Table 4-1. Characteristics of Hepatitis B Virus and Hepatitis C Virus

Characteristic	Hepatitis B Virus	Hepatitis C Virus
Type of virus	Hepadnavirus	Hepacivirus
Viral genome	3.2 kb, relaxed circular, partially double-stranded DNA	9.5 kb, positive-sense, single-stranded RNA
Routes of transmission	Parenteral Sexual Injection drug use Perinatal	Parenteral Injection drug use Blood products before 1990 Perinatal (infrequent) Sexual (infrequent)
Frequency of acute icteric disease	Common in adults Uncommon in children	Uncommon
Frequency of evolution to chronic disease	Infrequent (<10%) in adults Common in children	Frequent (>80%)
Estimated number of acute infections/yr in the United States	185,000	38,000
Estimated number of chronically infected persons in the United States	1,250,000	2,700,000
Estimated number of chronically infected persons in the world	350,000,000	170,000,000
Treatment	Interferon-α Lamivudine	Interferon-α with ribavirin
Prophylaxis	Recombinant vaccine Hepatitis B immune globulin	None

Source: Adapted from Lauer GM, Walker BD. Hepatitis C virus infection. *N Engl J Med.* 2001;345:41–52.

HBV DNA in the serum is a marker of viral replication in the liver and has replaced hepatitis Be antigen (HBeAg) as the most sensitive marker of viral replication. Efforts are currently under way to develop HBV DNA tests for screening blood donors as an early marker of infection.

The initial evaluation of patients found to have HBsAg in serum should include routine liver tests and a variety of virologic tests including HBV DNA tests.[3] Chronic HBV infection is a disease of variable course, and it is important to establish baseline laboratory values. Monitoring disease activity in chronically HBV-infected patients is best done by measuring aminotransferase (ALT) levels at 6-month intervals. Serial HBV DNA testing is not necessary.

The determination of HBV DNA levels (viral load) is important in the pretreatment evaluation and monitoring of therapeutic response in patients with chronic infection.[3]

Currently, therapy for HBV infection is difficult and has limited long-term efficacy. The decision to treat should be based on ALT elevations, presence of HBeAg or high HBV DNA levels or both, presence of moderate disease activity and fibrosis on liver biopsy, and virologic testing to exclude concurrent infections with hepatitis D virus (HDV), HCV, and human immunodeficiency virus (HIV). Currently, the only two approved therapies for HBV infection are interferon-α (IFN) and lamivudine. Several factors predict a favorable response to IFN treatment, the most important being high ALT and low serum HBV DNA levels, which are indirect markers of immune clearance.

Lamivudine is an orally administered nucleoside analog, which is a potent inhibitor of HBV DNA synthesis. A 1-year course has been shown in clinical trials to be as effective as a 16-week course of IFN but is better tolerated by patients.[4,5] The antiviral response appears to be durable, although most treated patients had detectable serum HBV DNA when sensitive tests were used in follow-up studies. A major problem with lamivudine is the development of drug-resistant mutants. Genotypic resistance has been reported in 15% to 25% of patients treated for 1 year, increasing to 49% of patients treated for 3 years. The development of resistance usually is associated with a rebound in viral load. However, in many patients the viral load and ALT level remain lower than pretreatment values because the mutations that occur in the viral polymerase affect viral replication efficiency. The two most common mutations are a methionine-to-valine or -isoleucine substitution at codon 552 (M552V/I) and a leucine-to-methionine substitution at codon 528 (L528M) in the HBV polymerase gene.[6]

Although the ideal goal of therapy is to eradicate the virus, this is not always achievable because of the difficulty of eliminating the covalently closed circular form of the HBV genome from the liver and the existence of extrahepatic reservoirs of HBV. Endpoints of treatment have traditionally been clearance of HBeAg, development of anti-HBe antibodies, and undetectable serum HBV DNA using insensitive hybridization assays with detection limits of approximately 10^6 genome copies/ml. Achieving these endpoints usually is accompanied by remission of liver disease as evidenced by normalization of the ALT level and decreased histologic activity on liver biopsy. The response usually is sustained at long-term follow-up. Nevertheless, most responders continue to have detectable HBV DNA when a sensitive nucleic acid amplification test is used.

Several variations in the nucleotide sequence of HBV have important clinical consequences. An important mutation in the S gene is a glycine-to-arginine substitution at codon 145 (G145R) in the conserved "a" determinant, which causes decreased affinity of the HBsAg for anti-HBs antibodies.[7] HBV with this mutation has been found in children of HBsAg-positive mothers in whom HBV infection develops despite vaccination and an adequate anti-HBs antibody response after vaccination, as well as in liver transplant recipients who have recurrent infection despite administration of HBV immune globulin.[8,9] These immune escape mutants have raised concern about vaccine efficacy and serologically silent infections. The G145R mutation has been reported in many countries and is responsible for 2% to 40% of vaccine failures. Although there is diminished binding to anti-HBs antibodies, the vast majority of S mutants can be readily detected with the current generation of HBsAg tests. Thus, the initial concern that widespread use of HBV immune globulin and vaccination would result in HBV mutants that would escape detection in the HBsAg test was unfounded.

Core promoter and precore mutants produce virions that do not produce HBeAg. The most common core promoter mutation has a dual change of A to T at nucleotide (nt) 1762 and G to A at nt 1764 that diminishes the amount of mRNA and hence HBeAg secretion.[10] The predominant mutation is a G-to-A change at nt 1896 (A1896), which leads to premature termination of the precore protein at codon 28, thus preventing the production of HBeAg.[11] The A1896 mutation is infrequent in North America and western Europe but is geographically widespread. This geographic variability in frequency is related to the predominant genotypes in a geographic region because the mutation is found only in genotypes B, C, D, and E.

The A1896 mutation was first reported in patients with chronic active hepatitis or fulminant hepatitis. However, the A1896 mutation also can be present in asymptomatic carriers and viruses with this mutation replicate no more efficiently than wild-type HBV. Thus, the pathophysiologic significance of this mutation is unclear.[12] However, the clinical picture of persistent HBV replication and active liver disease in HBeAg-negative patients appears to be increasingly prevalent, and in some regions the A1896-mutant virus may be more prevalent than wild-type virus.

Available Assays

HBV DNA Detection and Quantitation

The commercially available tests for quantitation of HBV DNA in serum and plasma are listed in Table 4-2. These tests employ either signal or target amplification. All of these assays are available as research-use-only kits or analyte-specific reagents, since the Food and Drug Administration (FDA) has not cleared any of these reagents for diagnostic use. In addition, a number of laboratory-developed conventional and real-time polymerase chain reaction (PCR) tests have been described.[4,13-15] All of the quantitative HBV DNA test formats have been used in monitoring the status of HBV infection before and after treatment.

The Hybrid Capture tests (Digene, Gaithersburg, MD) are liquid hybridization assays employing full-length genomic RNA probes and antibodies that bind to DNA-RNA hybrids to quantitate HBV DNA in serum and plasma specimens. The dynamic ranges of the Standard and Ultra-sensitive Hybrid Capture II assays are 200,000 to 2 billion genome copies/ml and 5,000 to 60 million genome copies/ml, respectively.

The Versant HBV assay (Bayer Corp, Tarrytown, NY) uses branched DNA (bDNA) technology for HBV DNA quantitation. The virus is concentrated from 1 ml of serum by ultracentrifugation to achieve greater sensitivity. Quantitation of HBV DNA in clinical samples is determined from a standard curve generated with each run using a set of HBV DNA standards included as part of the kit. The Versant HBV assay has a dynamic range of 700,000 to 5 billion copies/ml.

The Amplicor HBV Monitor Test (Roche Diagnostics, Indiannapolis, IN) uses PCR for HBV DNA quantitation[16] and has the greatest sensitivity of all the available assays, detecting as few as 200 HBV genome copies/ml. The PCR primers are biotin labeled and target conserved sequences in the precore/core region of the HBV genome. A known number of copies of a quantitation standard (QS) are added to each specimen aliquot prior to DNA isolation. The QS is a DNA fragment with 5' and 3' sequences that are complementary to the HBV PCR primers with a unique internal sequence. After PCR amplification, the HBV and QS amplicons are detected using specific probes for internal sequences of the target and QS in a solid phase assay with an avidin-enzyme conjugate and a colorimetric substrate. HBV DNA in the serum sample is quantitated by reference to the QS signal. The amplification, hybridiza-

Table 4-2. Commercially Available HBV DNA Tests

Test Kit	Method	Manufacturer	Gene Target	Dynamic Range*
Standard Hybrid Capture II	Liquid hybridization	Digene (Gaithersburg, MD)	Full-length RNA probe†	2×10^5 to 2×10^9
Ultra-Sensitive Hybrid Capture II	Liquid hybridization	Digene (Gaithersburg, MD)	Full-length RNA probe†	5×10^3 to 6×10^7
Versant HBV	Branched DNA	Bayer Corp (Tarrytown, NY)	Multiple probes	7×10^5 to 5×10^9
Amplicor HBV Monitor	PCR	Roche Diagnostics (Indiannapolis, IN)	Precore/core	2×10^2 to 2×10^5
TaqMan HBV Analyte-Specific Reagent	Real-time PCR	Roche Diagnostics (Indiannapolis, IN)	Precore/core	2×10^2 to 2×10^7

*Genome copies/ml.
†Genotypes A and D.

tion, and detection steps can be performed using the COBAS Amplicor analyzer.[17]

A real-time PCR assay for HBV DNA based on TaqMan chemistry is available from Roche Diagnostics as an analyte-specific reagent (ASR). This assay combines the analytical sensitivity of conventional PCR with the broad dynamic range of the Hybrid Capture and Versant bDNA tests, and simplifies the analytical process relative to the PCR tests by combining the amplification and detection steps.

HBV Genotyping

The only commercially available test for genotyping HBV is a line probe assay (Innogenetics, Ghent, Belgium) for mutations in the HBV polymerase gene associated with resistance to lamivudine.[18] A 341 base pair (bp) PCR product from the polymerase gene is amplified with primers biotinylated at their 5′ ends. The PCR product is denatured and hybridized to probes immobilized on a nitrocellulose strip. The assay uses 38 probes to cover codon positions 528, 552, and 555 of the polymerase gene in 19 different probe lines on a nitrocellulose strip. The hybrids are visualized on the strip after addition of streptavidin-alkaline phosphatase and colorimetric substrate. The mutations are identified by the colored patterns of PCR product hybridization to the probes.

Interpretation of Test Results

The availability of clinical molecular tests for detection and quantitation of HBV DNA in serum has improved our understanding of the clinical manifestations and natural history of HBV infection and facilitated the monitoring of response to therapy. However, the use of increasingly sensitive tests for this purpose has led to new questions and dilemmas. For example, most patients with chronic HBV infection have detectable HBV DNA in serum when sensitive PCR assays are used, even in HBsAg carriers without apparent disease. This leads to the question of what serum level of HBV DNA should be used to determine the need for treatment. Likewise, because of the limitations of currently available therapies, most treatment responders continue to have HBV DNA detectable in serum when the most sensitive assays are used.[19] This raises the questions of when to stop treatment and how virologic treatment response should be defined.

Early studies using insensitive hybridization assays demonstrated that most patients who developed spontaneous or treatment-induced anti-HBeAg seroconversion with undetectable serum HBV DNA have normal ALT levels, reduced histologic activity, decreased risk of hepatic decompensation, and improved survival.[20] The majority, however, have detectable HBV DNA when PCR assays are used. Therefore, it seems that patients with low serum HBV

DNA levels may not require treatment. Although there appears to be a level of serum HBV DNA below which hepatitis B is inactive and nonprogressive, this level may range from 10^4 to 10^6 genome copies/ml and may vary with the patient and the assay used to determine the levels. There is poor agreement between HBV DNA results generated with the different assays.[15,21]

Laboratory Issues

The major laboratory issue in HBV DNA quantitation is the widely divergent results obtained with the different assays. To address interassay differences, the World Health Organization (WHO) developed an international standard for HBV DNA, designated 97/746.[22] The WHO standard is a lyophilized plasma specimen that has been analyzed by several laboratories using different nucleic acid tests and has an assigned potency of 10^6 international units (IU)/ml. In the future, all new assays for HBV DNA should be calibrated against the WHO standard and the results reported in IU/ml. In the interim, laboratories should be aware of the substantial interassay differences in quantitative results.

The lack of FDA-cleared test kits for HBV DNA places increased burden on laboratories to verify the test performance characteristics. Unfortunately, there are no formal proficiency surveys for HBV nucleic acid tests, although control and reference materials are available from several companies.

Serum and plasma, with EDTA or citrate dextrose as an anticoagulant, are acceptable specimens for most nucleic acid tests for HBV. In the absence of stability data, samples for nucleic acid testing should be processed to separate blood cells from the plasma or serum within 6 hours of collection and either tested within 24 hours or stored at −70°C. In one study HBV DNA was stable in separated serum samples for at least 5 days when specimens were stored at 4°C.[23]

Future Directions

As more antiviral agents for treatment of HBV are developed, the key surrogate endpoints that will be used are suppression of serum HBV DNA levels and prevention of the development of antiviral resistance. Long-term suppression of viral replication is associated with both biochemical and histological improvement in liver disease. These factors make the development, clinical evaluation, and availability of reliable, standardized quantitative tests for HBV DNA a major priority for the near future. Similarly, increased emphasis will be placed on characterization of drug resistance mutants and HBV genotyping to assist with clinical management of patients as new drugs are developed.

HEPATITIS C VIRUS

HCV is an RNA virus with a positive-sense, single-stranded genome of approximately 9500 nt encoding a single polyprotein of about 3000 amino acids. The long open reading frame is flanked at each end by a short untranslated region (UTR). The genome structure is most similar to viruses of the family Flaviviridae, which includes many of the arthropod-borne viruses. As in other flaviviruses, the three N-terminal proteins of HCV (core, envelope 1, and envelope 2) are probably structural and the four C-terminal proteins (nonstructural 2, 3, 4, and 5) are thought to function in viral replication.

The 5′ UTR is a highly conserved region of 341 nt and has a complex secondary structure. It contains an internal ribosome entry site and presumably is important in the translation of the long open reading frame. The 3′ UTR contains a short region that varies in sequence and length, followed by a polypyrimidine stretch of variable length, and finally a highly conserved sequence of 98 nt, which constitutes the terminus of the genome. The function of the 3′ UTR is not known but is thought to be essential for viral replication.

The envelope 1 (E1) and 2 (E2) regions of HCV are the most variable regions within the genome at both the nucleotide and amino acid levels. Two regions in the E2, called hypervariable regions 1 and 2 (HVR1 and HRV2), show extreme sequence variability, which is thought to result from selective pressure by antiviral antibodies. E2 also contains the binding site for CD81, the putative HCV receptor or coreceptor.

The nonstructural regions 2 (NS2) and 3 (NS3) contain a Zn-dependent autoprotease that cleaves the polyprotein at the NS2-NS3 junction. The aminoterminal portion of the NS3 protein also is a serine protease that cleaves the polyprotein at several sites. The carboxyterminal portion of the NS3 protein has helicase activity, which is important for HCV replication. The NS4A protein is a cofactor for NS3 serine protease. The NS5B region encodes the RNA-dependent RNA polymerase, which replicates the viral genome. A region in NS5A has been linked to response to IFNα and is therefore called the IFNα-sensitivity determining region (ISDR).

HCV Genotypes

The first complete HCV genome sequence was reported by Choo et al. in 1991.[24] As additional genome sequences from isolates from different parts of the world were determined and compared, it was evident that HCV exists as distinct genotypes with as much as 35% sequence diversity over the whole viral genome.[25] Much of the early literature on genotyping is confusing because investigators developed and used their own classification schemes. However, a consensus nomenclature system was developed in 1994. In this system the genotypes are numbered using Arabic numer-

Table 4-3. Terms Describing Genomic Heterogeneity of HCV

Term	Definition	% Nucleotide Similarity*
Genotype	Heterogeneity among different viruses	66–69
Subtype	Closely related viruses within each genotype	77–80
Quasispecies	Complex of genetic variants within individual viruses	91–99

Source: Adapted from Zein NN. Clinical significance of hepatitis C virus genotypes. *Clin Microbiol Rev.* 2000;13:223–235.
*Full-length genome sequence identity.

als in order of their discovery, and the more closely related strains within some types are designated as subtypes with lowercase letters. The complex of genetic variants found within an individual isolate is termed the "quasispecies." The quasispecies result from the accumulation of mutations that occur during viral replication in the host. The terminology and degree of nucleotide similarity that define the relationships of HCV variants are given in Table 4-3.

Six major HCV genotypes have been identified. Sequence analysis of the E1 region suggested that HCV could be grouped into six major genotypes and 12 subtypes.[26] The same investigators sequenced 573 nt of the core region of the same isolates to confirm this classification scheme.[27] Simmonds et al.[28] also were able to classify HCV isolates into the same six major genotypes and numerous subtypes using sequence analysis of the NS5B region. Analyses of full-length open reading frame sequences have confirmed the original classification scheme based on analyses of individual gene regions.[29]

Genome sequence analysis of HCV isolates from Southeast Asia have led some authors to propose new major genotypes 7, 8, 9, 10, and 11.[30,31] However, other investigators suggested that these variants could be classified within the six major genotypes originally described.[32] Under this scheme, genotype 10 is a divergent subtype of genotype 3, and genotypes 7, 8, 9, and 11 are divergent subtypes of genotype 6.

HCV genotypes 1, 2, and 3 are found throughout the world, but there are clear differences in their distribution.[33] HCV subtypes 1a, 1b, 2a, 2b, 2c, and 3a are responsible for more than 90% of infections in North and South America, Europe, and Japan. In the United States, type 1 accounts for approximately 70% of the infections with equal distribution between subtypes 1a and 1b. In Japan, subtype 1b causes more than 70% of HCV infections. Although subtypes 2a and 2b have wide distributions in North America, Europe, and Japan, subtype 2c is widespread in a region of northern Italy. HCV subtype 3a is common among intravenous drug users in the United States and Europe. Other subtypes of genotype 3 are common in Nepal, Bangladesh, India, and Pakistan.

Genotype 4 is prevalent in North Africa and the Middle East, and genotypes 5 and 6 are limited to South Africa and Hong Kong, respectively.[28] Subtype 4a constitutes the majority of infections in Egypt, and this and other subtypes of genotype 4 are found in Zaire and Gabon. Subtype 5a is a particular problem in South Africa, where some reports indicate that it is responsible for more than 50% of infections. Subtype 6a infections are common in Hong Kong. The isolates classified as genotypes 7, 8, and 9 by some investigators have been found only in Vietnamese patients.[31] Putative genotypes 10 and 11 have been identified only in patients from Indonesia.[30]

The retrospective nature of most of the studies makes it difficult to determine the role of genotype as a risk factor for disease progression and to separate it from other known risk factors, such as older age at infection, male gender, alcohol consumption, and concurrent viral infection. However, in two prospective studies, viral genotype did not correlate with disease progression.[34,35]

Clinical Utility

HCV RNA Detection and Quantitation

Detection of HCV RNA in serum or plasma by nucleic acid amplification methods is important for confirming the diagnosis of HCV, distinguishing active from resolved infection, assessing the virologic response to therapy, and screening the blood supply. These tests are incorporated into diagnostic algorithms for HCV proposed by the National Institutes of Health,[36] the CDC,[37] European Association of the Study of the Liver,[38] and National Academy of Clinical Biochemistry.[39]

The detection of HCV RNA in the plasma or serum is the earliest marker of infection, appearing 1 to 2 weeks after infection and weeks before the appearance of alterations in liver enzyme levels or anti-HCV antibodies. Approximately 80% of individuals infected with HCV will be chronically infected with the virus. In antibody-positive individuals, HCV RNA tests can distinguish active from resolved infections. In patients with a high pretest probability of infection, a positive serological screening test is usually "confirmed" with a qualitative test for HCV RNA rather than the supplemental recombinant immunoblot assay (RIBA). This strategy is cost-effective and more informative than using the RIBA to confirm positive antibody screening tests in a diagnostic setting. It is important to remember that the RIBA confirms the presence of antibody, whereas an HCV RNA test detects the presence of the virus.

The CDC recently developed guidelines for HCV antibody testing in which the signal to cutoff (s/co) ratio of the serological screening test can be used effectively to determine which screening test results need supplemental testing for confirmation.[40] Screening enzyme-linked immunoassay results with s/co ratios ≥3.8 predict a RIBA-positive result >95% of the time in all populations tested. Consequently, supplemental testing is required only for those screening tests with low s/co ratios. Either a RIBA or an HCV RNA test can be used for confirmation, but all negative HCV RNA tests should be followed by a RIBA since a single negative RNA test does not rule out infection. Confirmation of an HCV antibody screening test is important to ensure that further clinical evaluation is limited to those patients who are truly antibody positive and to reduce psychological stress on patients who test falsely positive for antibody.

HCV RNA testing also is helpful for the diagnosis of infection in infants born to HCV-infected mothers, due to persistence of maternal antibody, and in immuno-compromised or debilitated patients who may have blunted serological responses. A qualitative HCV RNA test also should be used for patients suspected of having an acute infection and in patients with hepatitis of no identifiable cause.

Qualitative HCV RNA tests are the most reliable means of identifying patients with active HCV infection. A negative HCV RNA test in a serologically positive individual may indicate that the infection has resolved or that the viremia is intermittent. Up to 15% of chronically infected individuals may have intermittent viremia and, as a result, a single negative HCV RNA determination may not be sufficient to exclude active infection when the index of clinical suspicion is high.[41] In these individuals a second specimen should be collected and tested.

IFN-based regimens, either IFN in combination with ribavirin or IFN monotherapy for those patients who cannot tolerate ribavirin, are the standard treatment for patients with chronic HCV infection. Because these regimens produce sustained virological responses in only about half of the patients treated, are of long duration (24 to 48 weeks), and are associated with significant adverse events, early identification of patients who are likely or unlikely to respond to treatment is desirable.

Early clearance of HCV RNA as assessed with a sensitive assay or a rapid decline in HCV RNA levels during the early treatment period is predictive of sustained virological response among patients receiving either standard or pegylated IFN alone, and pegylated IFN plus ribavirin.[42,43] Patients who have detectable or less than a $2 \log_{10}$ decrease in viral RNA levels after 12 weeks of treatment have a minimal chance of achieving a sustained virological response (negative predictive value of 98%).

In contrast, early viral kinetics are less predictive of sustained virological response among patients treated with standard IFN and ribavirin because late responses are seen in some patients. Thus, discontinuing therapy in patients based on a positive HCV RNA test early in treatment would deny the treatment to a substantial number of patients who would achieve a sustained response. The virological response to combination therapy with IFN and ribavirin should be assessed after 24 weeks of therapy with a sensitive (≤50 IU/ml) qualitative assay for HCV RNA.[44] Individuals with a positive qualitative RNA test after week 24 of therapy are considered treatment failure and therapy is discontinued. Therapy also can be safely stopped at 24 weeks in patients infected with HCV genotypes 2 and 3 who have a negative HCV RNA test, because there is no benefit to longer therapeutic regimens. However, an additional 24 weeks of therapy is recommended for patients infected with other genotypes, even with a negative qualitative HCV RNA test. In addition, a qualitative HCV RNA test should be performed 24 weeks after completion of treatment in all patients to establish if a sustained virological response was achieved regardless of the treatment regimen.

The use of anti-HCV antibody tests to screen the blood supply has dramatically reduced the risk of transfusion-associated HCV infection in developed countries. The risk in the United States from blood that is negative for anti-HCV antibodies is less than 1 in 103,000 transfused units.[45] To drive the risk of infection even lower, blood donor pools are currently tested for the presence of HCV RNA.[46] The serologic screening tests for HCV have a 70-day window period of seronegativity, and antigen detection tests are not yet available for blood bank screening. It is estimated that HCV RNA testing will reduce the detection window by 25 days and reduce the number of infectious units from 116 to 32 per year.[47]

An enzyme immunoassay (EIA) for the detection and quantitation of total HCV core antigen in serum has recently been developed and is available as a research-use-only test (Ortho Trak C, Ortho Clinical Diagnostics, Raritan, NJ). This test significantly shortens the serologically silent window period using seroconversion panels, and its performance correlates closely with RNA detection tests in blood donors.[48,49] However, the analytical sensitivity is less than most RNA tests, at approximately 20,000 IU/ml. The analytical sensitivity of the core antigen test is too high to be used in the monitoring of late events during and after treatment.[50] Antigen detection may represent a cost-effective alternative to HCV RNA testing to distinguish active from resolved infections in resource-poor settings.

HCV viral load testing is useful in pretreatment evaluations of patients being considered for therapy, since a viral load of less than 2×10^6 copies/ml (800,000 IU/ml) is one of several predictors of achieving a sustained virological response.[51,52] Other factors associated with achieving a sustained response to therapy include the absence of cirrhosis, age less than 40 years, female gender, white race, and viral genotype other than 1. Viral load testing also can be used in an early assessment of viral kinetics in patients treated with IFN alone or with pegylated IFN plus ribavirin.[42,43] Patients who fail to achieve less than a 2 $\log_{10}$ decline in viral load with treatment have little chance of achieving a sustained virological response to these therapies.

HCV viral load does not predict disease progression and is not associated with severity of liver disease.[53] This is in sharp contrast to HIV-1, in which the viral load is the principal factor determining the rate of disease progression. Monitoring HCV viral load in untreated patients is not warranted and should be discouraged.

HCV Genotyping

Sequence analysis of variable regions of the HCV genome has been used to investigate outbreaks of infection and to study modes of transmission. Two large outbreaks of infection associated with contaminated lots of anti-rhesus D immunoglobulin (anti-D) in Ireland and Germany were investigated using molecular typing.[54,55] In both studies, sequence analysis showed that the virus infecting the women was the same as that found in the implicated batches of anti-D. In another report, sequencing part of the NS3 region provided evidence of patient-to-patient transmission during colonoscopy.[56] Sequence analysis also is becoming a routine part of investigations of HCV infections associated with blood transfusions. In addition, molecular analysis has been used to study vertical and sexual transmission of HCV.[57-60]

Although a number of baseline factors are predictive of response to treatment of chronic hepatitis C infection, HCV genotype is the strongest and most consistent predictor for achieving a sustained virological response. In the large clinical trials of combination therapy with IFN and ribavirin, only 30% of patients infected with genotype 1 had a sustained response compared to 65% of patients infected with genotypes 2 or 3.[51,52] Too few patients infected with genotypes 4, 5, and 6 were included in the clinical trials to adequately assess the likelihood of therapeutic response with these genotypes.

In practice, HCV genotype can be used in tailoring the duration of therapy to individual patients. In an algorithm proposed by Poynard et al.,[44] the five independent predictors of sustained virological response are considered at the end of 24 weeks of combination therapy. The predictors of sustained response are HCV genotype other than 1, viral load of <2,000,000 copies/ml, age <40 years, female gender, and no or only portal fibrosis on liver biopsy. If HCV RNA is still detectable in the serum at the end of 24 weeks of therapy, then the patient is unlikely to benefit from an additional 24 weeks of IFN and ribavirin, and therapy can be stopped. However, if the HCV RNA is undetectable after 24 weeks of therapy and the patient has fewer than four favorable factors, then therapy should be continued for an additional 24 weeks since these patients may obtain benefit from additional therapy. Conversely, therapy can be safely stopped if the patient has four or five favorable factors and is HCV RNA undetectable at 24 weeks. This algorithm ensures that only those patients who may benefit from 48 weeks of therapy have to endure it.

There is considerable interest in identifying isolates within a genotype that exhibit different responses to IFN. For example, Enomoto et al.[61] found that genotype 1b isolates in Japan identical to the HCV-J prototype strain within the carboxyterminal part of the NS5A protein were resistant to IFN. In contrast, patients infected with genotype 1b strains with mutations within this region had a better response to IFN. This region of amino acids 2209 to 2248 in the NS5A protein has been termed the interferon-sensitivity-determining region (ISDR). The same group recently confirmed and extended their observations. They found that sustained response rates correlated with the number of mutations in the ISDR with a larger group of patients and identified the mutation sites within the ISDR that were significantly associated with sustained response.[62] Although these results have been confirmed for Japanese isolates, in studies of patients from other countries the majority of IFN-sensitive isolates showed no or only a few mutations in the ISDR.[5,63,64] The reasons for the different findings are not clear but may involve racial, virological, or other factors.

Available Assays

A variety of test kits for detection or quantitation of HCV RNA are available commercially (Table 4-4). These assays are based on traditional reverse transcription–polymerase chain reaction (RT-PCR), transcription-mediated amplification (TMA), bDNA, or, most recently, real-time RT-PCR technologies.

• Qualitative Detection HCV Assays

There are currently two FDA-cleared qualitative HCV RNA test kits available for diagnostic use, the Amplicor HCV test v2.0 (Roche) and the Versant HCV RNA qualitative test (Bayer).

The Amplicor HCV test v2.0 is based on RT-PCR amplification of a portion of the 5′ UTR and has an analytical sensitivity of 50 IU/ml.[65] The test incorporates an internal control to detect PCR inhibitors and deoxyuridine triphosphate (dUTP) and uracil-N-glycosylase in the reaction mixture to prevent false positives due to amplicon carryover. The test is available in two formats, a manual microwell plate assay and a semiautomated assay designed for the COBAS instrument. The performance characteristics of the Amplicor HCV tests are well established[66] and are the most commonly used qualitative HCV RNA tests in clinical laboratories participating in the proficiency-testing surveys of the College of American Pathologists.

The Versant HCV RNA qualitative test also targets the 5′ UTR but uses TMA to amplify the targeted region. The analytical sensitivity of the Versant HCV RNA assay is 5 IU/ml. The increase in analytical sensitivity over the Amplicor tests is due in part to the larger sample volume (500 μl versus 200 μl) and the use of a specific target capture step to isolate HCV RNA rather than total RNA precipitation. This test also employs an internal control RNA to detect the presence of amplification inhibitors.

The Versant HCV RNA assay can detect residual serum HCV RNA in some patients with no detectable HCV RNA as determined by the Amplicor v2.0 assay at the end of treatment with IFN and subsequently experienced virological relapse.[67,68] However, this difference was not observed with end-of-treatment samples from patients treated with pegylated IFN.[69] The two qualitative HCV RNA assays demonstrated excellent concordance in a study designed

Table 4-4. Commercially Available HCV RNA Tests

Test Kit	Method	Manufacturer	Lower Limit of Detection (IU/ml)	Dynamic Range	Clinical Application
Qualitative					
Amplicor HCV Test v2.0*	RT-PCR	Roche Diagnostics (Indiannapolis, IN)	50	NA	Diagnose active infection and assess response to therapy
Versant HCV RNA Assay*	TMA	Bayer Corp, (Tarrytown, NY)	5	NA	Diagnose active infection and assess response to therapy
Ampliscreen HCV Test v2.0*	RT-PCR	Roche Diagnostics (Indiannapolis, IN)	<50	NA	Blood screening
Procleix HIV-1/ HCV Assay*	TMA	GenProbe, San (Diego, CA)	<50	NA	Blood screening
Quantitative					
Amplicor HCV Monitor Test v2.0	RT-PCR	Roche Diagnostics (Indiannapolis, IN)	600	$2.9\log_{10}$	Determine duration of therapy and early prediction of therapy failure
Versant HCV RNA Assay v3.0*	bDNA	Bayer Corp (Tarrytown, NY)	615	$4.1\log_{10}$	Determine duration of therapy and early prediction of therapy failure
TaqMan HCV Analyte Specific Reagent	Real-time RT-PCR	Roche Diagnostics (Indiannapolis, IN) Abbott Molecular (Des Plaines, IL)	10	$6.0\log_{10}$	Diagnose active infection, assess response to therapy, determine duration of therapy, and early prediction of therapy failure

*FDA-cleared tests.
NA, not applicable.

to compare the performance characteristics with specimens submitted for HCV diagnosis.[70] The difference in analytical sensitivity between the two tests does not result in any meaningful difference in clinical sensitivity when the tests are used diagnostically, because it is rare for patients with chronic hepatitis C infection to present for initial evaluation with viral loads of less than 10^5 copies/ml.

The Procleix HIV-1/HCV test (GenProbe, San Diego, CA) also uses TMA technology and is approved by the FDA for the screening of blood products.[71] The Ampliscreen HCV RNA test v2.0 is an RT-PCR assay (Roche) designed for blood screening that is based on the Amplicor HCV test. Both assays have analytical sensitivities of less than 50 IU/ml.

Quantitative HCV Assays

Currently there are several commercially available and proprietary laboratory-developed methods used to quantitate HCV RNA levels in patients. The Versant HCV RNA Assay v3.0 (Bayer Corp.),[72] which is FDA approved, and the Amplicor HCV Monitor Test v2.0 (Roche Diagnostics)[65] are the most widely used commercially available assays. The HCV Superquant is a proprietary RT-PCR assay developed by National Genetics Institute (Los Angeles, CA), which has been used by many investigators in clinical trials of treatment for HCV.

The Amplicor HCV Monitor test v2.0 is a quantitative RT-PCR assay that amplifies the same target region as the qualitative Amplicor HCV test. The assay uses an internal quantitation standard to calculate the amount of HCV RNA in a sample. The assay has a sensitivity of 600 IU/ml and a 2.9 $\log_{10}$ dynamic range. Specimens with values greater than the upper limit of quantitation (500,000 IU/ml) can be diluted 100-fold and retested as recommended by the manufacturer. The Amplicor HCV Monitor test is available in both manual microwell plate and semiautomated COBAS instrument formats.

The Versant HCV RNA Assay v3.0 is based on bDNA technology. The sensitivity of the Versant HCV RNA Assay v3.0 is 615 IU/ml, with a 4.1 $\log_{10}$ dynamic range. A number of changes to the design of the v3.0 test improved both the sensitivity and specificity over the v2.0 test. These include an increased number of capture probes, improved probe design, the use of nonnatural synthetic nucleotides in detection probes, and redesigned label extenders. The System 340 bDNA analyzer automates all incubations, wash steps, readings, and data analysis. The instrument can process two 96-microwell plates per run.

Overall, the results of the Versant HCV RNA Assay v3.0 and the Amplicor HCV Monitor Test v2.0 have been found to be in substantial agreement.[72,73] The results of the Amplicor Monitor test are reported as IU/ml and those of the Versant assay are reported as either copies/ml or IU/ml. Both tests are free of significant HCV genotype bias and have similar analytical sensitivities. The Versant

results tend to be more precise than the Amplicor Monitor results, but the Amplicor Monitor test is better able to discriminate low-positive from negative specimens. The Versant assay has a much greater dynamic range than the Amplicor Monitor test; however, a pretest sample dilution permits quantification of high viral load specimens by the Amplicor Monitor test. The throughput and level of automation are much greater with the Versant assay than with the Amplicor Monitor test.

A number of TaqMan RT-PCR assays for detection and quantitation for HCV RNA have been described.[74] These tests have sensitivities comparable to qualitative tests, have a broad dynamic range, and provide precise quantitation of viral load. These tests also generate results more rapidly than conventional RT-PCR assays and are not prone to amplicon carryover contamination since the amplification and detection steps are combined in a single closed tube. With the development of real-time RT-PCR, clinical laboratories will no longer need to have separate qualitative and quantitative assay formats for HCV RNA to achieve both high sensitivity and broad dynamic range. Roche and Abbott manufacture TaqMan HCV analyte-specific reagents that contain the necessary HCV-specific primers, dual-labeled fluorescent HCV and HCV quantitation standard specific probes, enzyme, and dNTPs for the detection and quantitation of HCV RNA.[75,76]

HCV Genotyping Assays

A variety of laboratory-developed and commercial assays are used for HCV genotyping. The methods include nucleic acid sequencing, reverse hybridization, subtype-specific PCR, DNA fragment length polymorphism, heteroduplex mobility analysis, melting curve analysis and serological genotyping. The FDA has not cleared any of these methods for clinical diagnostic use.

A commercially available reverse hybridization line probe assay is the most commonly used method for genotyping HCV among clinical laboratories participating in the HCV proficiency-testing surveys of the College of American Pathologists. This reverse hybridization assay was developed by Innogenetics to genotype HCV and is now marketed as the Versant HCV Genotype Assay by Bayer. In this line probe assay (LiPA), biotinylated PCR products from the 5′ UTR are hybridized under stringent conditions with 19 type- and subtype-specific oligonucleotide probes attached to a nitrocellulose strip. Hybridized PCR products are detected with a streptavidin-alkaline phosphatase conjugate. The second-generation assay discriminates among genotypes 1a, 1b, 2a/c, 2b, 3a, 3b, 3c, 4a–h, 5a, and 6a.[77] The results from the Versant HCV Genotype LiPA Assay correlate well with results obtained by direct sequencing assays of the 5′ UTR and other genes in published evaluations, but may not distinguish between genotypes 1a and 1b in 5% to 10% of cases, and does not distinguish between genotypes 2a and 2c.[32,59,78,79] The LiPA is the most common method used in clinical laboratories for HCV genotyping because it can be used with amplicons from both the qualitative and quantitative Amplicor HCV tests, and is easy to perform and interpret. Mixed genotype infections are easily recognized as unusual patterns of hybridization with the typing probes. However, the LiPA requires a considerable amount of amplicon for typing, and the assay may regularly fail when the viral load is less than 10^4 copies/ml.

Sequence analysis of amplified subgenomic sequences is the most definitive way to genotype HCV strains. Genotyping schemes based on sequencing variable genes such as E1, C, and NS5B provide enough resolution to determine types and subtypes.[26-28] The 5′ UTR is too highly conserved to discriminate all subtypes reliably.[59] Genotyping methods targeting highly variable regions have higher failure rates due to primer mismatches and failed amplification reactions. Sequencing reactions can be performed directly on PCR products or on cloned amplicons. Mixed infections with multiple genotypes may be missed with direct sequence analysis. Definitive detection of mixed infections requires analysis of a large number of clones. Cloning may, however, emphasize artifactual nucleotide substitutions introduced by the DNA polymerase during amplification or by selection during the cloning procedure,[80] and is generally not practical for the clinical laboratory.

A standardized direct sequencing system has been recently developed for clinical use by Visible Genetics (Suwanee, GA) and now marketed by Bayer. The Trugene HCV 5′NC genotyping kit targets the 5′ UTR (nt 96 to 282) and employs proprietary single-tube chemistry that is robust and highly sensitive. This method can be used with the 244 bp amplicon generated by either the Roche Amplicor HCV or Amplicor HCV Monitor tests as the sequencing template after a column purification step.[81] The sequencing chemistry produces bidirectional sequences. The software acquires the sequence data in real time, and each pair of forward and reverse sequences is combined. A reference sequence library module contains approximately 200 sequences from the six major genotypes and 24 subtypes of HCV. The software automatically aligns the patient HCV sequence with the reference sequences in the library and reports type, subtype, and closest isolate determinations. The Trugene HCV 5′NC genotyping system is a rapid and reliable method for determining HCV genotypes but, like all approaches targeting the conserved 5′ UTR, cannot reliably distinguish all HCV subtypes.[36,48,81,82]

The practice of using sequence analysis of a single subgenomic region for HCV genotyping has recently been challenged by the description of a naturally occurring intergenotypic recombinant of two HCV genotypes.[83] This virus was found in patients in St Petersburg, Russia, and was assigned to two different genotypes, 2 and 1, by sequence analysis of the 5′ UTR and the NS5B region, respectively. The crossover point for the genome was mapped within the NS2 region. The extent to which such viruses occur in other patient populations is largely unknown.

A DNA EIA (Sorin Biomedica, Saluggia, Italy) for HCV genotyping is based on hybridization of denatured amplicon from the core region to genotype-specific probes that are bound to the wells of a microtiter plate. Mouse monoclonal antibodies to double-stranded DNA are used to detect the hybrids. The results of the DNA EIA were highly concordant with the results of other genotyping methods in two evaluations.[79,81]

A variety of laboratory-developed methods have been used to genotype HCV, including subtype-specific PCR,[25] primer-specific and mispair extension analysis,[84] nested restriction site–specific PCR,[85] restriction fragment length polymorphism,[86] heteroduplex mobility analysis,[87] and melting-curve analysis with fluorescence resonance energy transfer probes.[88,89]

Genotype-specific antibodies directed against the immunodominant epitopes in NS4 have been used to develop serotyping or serological genotyping tests. Two serological genotyping tests are commercially available. An NS4 recombinant immunoblot assay (Chiron Corporation, Emeryville, CA) uses synthetic proteins from the NS4 and core regions to discriminate among HCV genotypes 1, 2, and 3.[90] The competition enzyme-linked immunoassay (Murex Diagnostics Ltd, Dartford, UK) uses eight branched synthetic peptides to detect genotype-specific anti-NS4 antibodies to discriminate among HCV genotypes 1 to 6.[14] The high degree of cross reactivity among genotypes to these synthetic peptides necessitates absorbing the cross-reacting antibodies with an excess of heterologous peptides in solution prior to use. Both of these serologic assays lack sensitivity and specificity as compared with direct sequencing or the Versant HCV Genotype LiPA Assay for HCV genotyping; however serological genotyping is inexpensive, is simple to perform, and lends itself well to large epidemiological studies. It is the only way to determine the genotype of a virus in patients with low-level viremia or who have cleared their infection, as well as for specimens in which the RNA has been destroyed by improper handling.

Interpretation of Test Results

The presence of HCV RNA in serum or plasma defines active infection, and HCV RNA is usually detectable within the first week after exposure. However, a single negative HCV RNA test result does not exclude the possibility of active infection because viremia may be intermittent in some chronically infected patients. An HCV RNA test may be the only evidence of infection in individuals with false-negative antibody tests. False-negative HCV antibody tests can occur in HIV-1 infected individuals, patients undergoing hemodialysis, and patients with HCV-associated essential mixed cryoglobulinemia.[91-93]

In addition to HCV diagnosis, qualitative HCV RNA tests are used to assess virological response to therapy. A negative HCV RNA test at the completion of therapy defines an end-of-treatment response (ETR), and a negative test 6 months after the completion of therapy defines a sustained virological response (SVR).

HCV RNA quantitation is useful in planning duration of therapy and in predicting the likelihood of response to treatment. Patients with high HCV RNA levels tend to respond less well to IFN and ribavirin, but lengthening the course of therapy from 24 to 48 weeks more than doubles the response rate. Patients with viral loads greater than 800,000 IU/ml are considered to have high HCV RNA levels. HCV viral load does not predict disease progression, is not correlated with disease severity, and, consequently, should not be routinely monitored in untreated patients.

Viral load testing can be used in an early assessment of viral kinetics in patients undergoing treatment with IFN and ribavirin. Patients who fail to achieve at least a 2 $\log_{10}$ decline in viral load after 12 weeks of treatment have little chance of an SVR and therapy should be discontinued.

Viral genotyping, like viral load, helps predict the outcome of therapy and determine its duration. Currently, the only clinically relevant distinction for patients undergoing therapy is between genotype 1 and other genotypes. Patients with a genotype 1 infection require higher doses of ribavirin and treatment for 48 weeks rather than 24 weeks to increase the likelihood of an SVR. There is no proven association between genotype and disease progression or severity, so genotyping should be reserved for those patients being considered for treatment. Routine determination of HCV subtypes (e.g., 1a or 1b), other than for epidemiological purposes, is not warranted.

In summary, a qualitative HCV test is used for the initial evaluation of HCV antibody-positive individuals to distinguish active from resolved infections. Before initiating treatment, HCV viral load and genotype tests are performed to determine the dosing and length of treatment. After 12 weeks of treatment, the HCV viral load is measured to confirm at least a 2 $\log_{10}$ decline in viral load, which will be used to decide whether to continue or terminate treatment. At the end of either 24 or 48 weeks of treatment, a negative qualitative HCV test defines an ETR, and a negative qualitative test 6 months after the end of treatment defines an SVR. Assays with a limit of detection of ≤50 IU/ml should be used to define ETR and SVR to avoid misclassifying therapeutic outcomes. For patients not achieving an SVR, there is little experience with retreatment.

Laboratory Issues

The use of internal controls for a test increases the confidence in negative HCV RNA test results and eliminates concerns that the test is falsely negative because of the presence of amplification inhibitors in the sample or poor recovery of the viral RNA. In a large clinical trial of the Amplicor HCV test v2.0, the failure rate for the internal control was only 1.1%.[66] False-negative results may occur with PCR-based tests if blood samples are collected through central lines due to contamination with heparin. False-negative HCV RNA results also may occur if the specimen was not processed or stored appropriately due to the lability of the viral RNA. Serum or plasma should be separated from the cellular components of blood within 6 hours of collection to avoid significant loss of HCV RNA. Once separated, the sample is stable for 3 days at 4°C. Storage for longer periods should be at −70°C.

False-positive HCV RNA tests can result from contamination of the sample with HCV target RNA or amplicon. The widely used Amplicor HCV test employs the uracil-N-glycolase/dUTP protocol and an equivocal zone for low-level results to limit the number of false-positive test results. Real-time RT-PCR tests for HCV RNA eliminate the risk of amplicon carryover contamination because both amplification and detection are accomplished in a sealed reaction tube.

Much has been written about the lack of agreement and the genotype bias of early commercially available versions of the HCV quantitative assays. The development the WHO First International HCV RNA standard and its acceptance by the manufacturers of these assays as a calibrator was a significant advance in HCV RNA quantitation.[94] As a result, viral load values obtained with current versions of the Amplicor Monitor and Versant quantitative tests are in much better agreement and are largely interchangeable. The remaining disagreement probably results from differences in the dynamic ranges of the assays. The agreement between results for high viral load samples can be improved if the samples are diluted 1:100 prior to testing with the Amplicor Monitor assay.

Both the current versions of the Amplicor Monitor and Versant quantitative tests are free of significant genotype bias due to improvements in assay design. The Versant test is more amenable to high-volume testing and is less labor-intensive than the Amplicor Monitor test, while the Amplicor Monitor test may have advantages for laboratories with a lower test volume. Recently a sample preparation instrument, the COBAS Ampliprep, was developed to automate the cumbersome manual sample preparation method used for the Amplicor Monitor test. The automated sample preparation protocol compared favorably to the manual protocol for use with the COBAS Amplicor HCV Monitor test v2.0 in a recent clinical evaluation.[95]

Unfortunately, there is a trade-off between sensitivity and dynamic range for most of the HCV RNA tests currently used in clinical laboratories. As a result, most laboratories have separate qualitative and quantitative tests. The analytical sensitivities of the Amplicor Monitor and Versant quantitative tests are inadequate for assessing ETR or for reliable diagnostic use for some untreated chronically infected patients with low viral loads. Maintaining multiple assay formats for the same virus is costly for the laboratory and often confusing to the ordering physician. The best hope for unifying the HCV RNA assay platforms lies in the real-time PCR methods, which combine the sensitivity required for diagnosis and assessment of treatment response with the broad dynamic range required for viral load determinations.

Genotyping schemes based on variable subgenomic regions such as E1, core, and NS5B provide enough resolution to reliably determine HCV types and subtypes; however, the 5′ UTR is too conserved for accurate discrimination of all subtypes.[59] Nevertheless, the conserved nature of this region makes it the preferred target for pangenomic HCV RNA detection tests, and sequence analysis of amplicons from these tests is an efficient way to genotype HCV in a clinical laboratory since both tests can be completed with the product from a single amplification reaction. The genotyping results obtained using 5′ UTR amplicons are highly accurate at the genotype level but are not accurate for identifying different subtypes.[48,82,96]

The widespread use of tests not cleared by the FDA for HCV RNA quantitation and genotyping has placed an increased burden on clinical laboratories to verify the performance characteristics of these tests prior to clinical use. When validating HCV tests, laboratories should take advantage of the published evaluations and commercially available panels for HCV RNA quantitation and genotyping to streamline the verification process.

The College of American Pathologists has a well-established proficiency-testing program for laboratories performing tests for detection, quantitation, and characterization of HCV RNA. These surveys have shown a steady improvement in the performance of laboratories over time that probably reflects progress in both the available technologies and laboratory practices.

Future Directions

Although the incidence of new HCV infections in the United States is declining, the number of individuals infected for more than 20 years who are at risk for serious complications is expected to increase until about the year 2015. In the 15 years since the discovery of HCV, the major route of transmission through blood transfusion has all but been eliminated, improvements in therapy have resulted in better response rates, and molecular tests have proven invaluable in the diagnosis and management of patients with HCV. As new therapies evolve and laboratory assays change, the clinical relevance and use of laboratory tests will evolve.

References

1. Blumberg BS, Alter HJ, Visnich S. A "new" antigen in leukemia sera. *JAMA.* 1965;191:541–546.
2. Choo QL, Kuo G, Weiner AJ, Overby LR, Bradley DW, Houghton M. Isolation of a cDNA clone derived from a blood-borne non-A non-B viral hepatitis genome. *Science.* 1989;224:359–362.
3. Lok AS, Heathcote EJ, Hoofnagle JH. Management of hepatitis B: 2000—summary of a workshop. *Gastroenterology.* 2001;120:1828–1853.
4. Dienstag JL, Schiff ER, Wright TL, et al. Lamivudine as initial treatment for chronic hepatitis B in the United States. *N Eng J Med.* 1999;341:1256–1263.
5. Duverlie G, Khorsi H, Castelain S, et al. Sequence analysis of the NS5A protein of European hepatitis C virus 1b isolates and relation to interferon sensitivity. *J Gen Virol.* 1998;79:1373–1381.
6. Allen MI, Deslauriers M, Andrews CW, et al. Identification and characterization of mutations in hepatitis B virus resistant to lamivudine. Lamivudine Clinical Investigation Group. *Hepatology.* 1998;27: 1670–1677.
7. Carman WF, Zanetti AR, Karayiannis P, et al. Vaccine-induced escape mutant of hepatitis B virus. *Lancet.* 1990;336:325–329.
8. Hsu HY, Chang MH, Ni YH, Lin HH, Wang SM, Chen DS. Surface gene mutants of hepatitis B virus in infants who develop acute or chronic infections despite immunoprophylaxis. *Hepatology.* 1997;26:786–791.
9. McMahon G, Ehrlich PH, Moustafa ZA, et al. Genetic alterations in the gene encoding the major HBsAg: DNA and immunological analysis of recurrent HBsAg derived from monoclonal antibody-treated liver transplant patients. *Hepatology.* 1992;15:757–766.
10. Okamoto H, Tsuda F, Akahane Y, et al. Hepatitis B virus with mutations in the core promoter for an e antigen-negative phenotype in carriers with antibody to e antigen. *J Virol.* 1994;68:8102–8110.
11. Carman WF, Jacyna MR, Hadziyannis S, et al. Mutation preventing formation of hepatitis B e antigen in patients with chronic hepatitis B infection. *Lancet.* 1989;2:588–591.
12. Miyakawa Y, Okamoto H, Mayumi M. The molecular basis of hepatitis B e antigen (HBeAg)-negative infections. *J Viral Hepat.* 1997;4: 1–8.
13. Pas SD, Fries E, De Man RA, Osterhaus AD, Niesters HG. Development of a quantitative real-time detection assay for hepatitis B virus DNA and comparison with two commercial assays. *J Clin Microbiol.* 2000;38:2897–2901.
14. Pawlotsky JM, Prescott L, Simmonds P, et al. Serological determination of hepatitis C virus genotype: comparison with a standardized genotyping assay. *J Clin Microbiol.* 1997;35:1734–1739.
15. Zaaijer HL, ter Borg F, Cuypers TM, Hermus MCAH, Lelie PN. Comparison of methods for detection of hepatitis B virus DNA. *J Clin Microbiol.* 1994;32:2088–2091.
16. Gerken G, Gomes J, Lampertico P, et al. Clinical evaluation and applications of the Amplicor HBV Monitor test, a quantitative HBV DNA PCR assay. *J Virol Methods.* 1998;74:155–165.
17. Noborg U, Gusdal A, Pisa EK, Hedrum A, Lindh M. Automated quantitative analysis of hepatitis B virus DNA by using the Cobas Amplicor HBV monitor test. *J Clin Microbiol.* 1999;37:2793–2797.
18. Stuyver L, Van Geyt C, De Gendt S, et al. Line probe assay for monitoring drug resistance in hepatitis B virus-infected patients during antiviral therapy. *J Clin Microbiol.* 2000;38:702–707.
19. Lok AS, Chung HT, Liu VW, Ma OC. Long-term follow-up of chronic hepatitis B patients treated with interferon alfa. *Gastroenterology.* 1993;105:1833–1838.
20. de Jongh FE, Janssen HL, de Man RA, Hop WC, Schalm SW, van Blankenstein M. Survival and prognostic indicators in hepatitis B surface antigen-positive cirrhosis of the liver. *Gastroenterology.* 1992;103:1630–1635.
21. Pawlotsky JM, Bastie A, Hezode C, et al. Routine detection and quantification of hepatitis B virus DNA in clinical laboratories: performance of three commercial assays. *J Virol Methods.* 2000;85:11–21.
22. Saldanha J, Gerlich W, Lelie N, Dawson P, Heermann K, Heath A; WHOCSG. An international collaborative study to establish a World Health Organization international standard for hepatitis B virus DNA nucleic acid amplification techniques. *Vox Sang.* 2001;80:63–71.
23. Krajden M, Comanor L, Rifkin O, Grigoriew A, Minor JM, Kapke GF. Assessment of hepatitis B virus DNA stability in serum by the Chiron Quantiplex branched-DNA assay. *J Clin Microbiol.* 1998;36: 382–386.
24. Choo QL, Richman KH, Han JH, et al. Genetic organization and diversity of the hepatitis C virus. *Proc Natl Acad Sci USA.* 1991;88: 2451–2455.

25. Okamoto H, Kurai K, Okada S, et al. Full-length sequence of a hepatitis C virus genome having poor homology to reported isolates: comparative study of four distinct genotypes. *Virology.* 1992;188:331–341.

26. Bukh J, Purcell RH, Miller RH. At least 12 genotypes of hepatitis C virus predicted by sequence analysis of the putative E1 gene of isolates collected worldwide. *Proc Natl Acad Sci USA.* 1993;90:8234–8238.

27. Bukh J, Purcell RH, Miller RH. Sequence analysis of the core gene of 14 hepatitis C virus genotypes. *Proc Natl Acad Sci USA.* 1994;91:8239–8243.

28. Simmonds P, Holmes EC, Cha T-A, et al. Classification of hepatitis C virus into six major genotypes and a series of subtypes by phylogenetic analysis of the NS-5 region. *J Gen Virol.* 1993;74:2391–2399.

29. Bukh J, Miller RH, Purcell RH. Genetic heterogeneity of hepatitis C virus: quasispecies and genotypes. *Semin Liver Dis.* 1995;15:41–63.

30. Tokita H, Okamoto H, Iizuka H, et al. Hepatitis C virus variants from Jakarta, Indonesia classifiable into novel genotypes in the second (2e and 2f), tenth (10a) and eleventh (11a) genetic groups. *J Gen Virol.* 1996;77:293–301.

31. Tokita H, Okamoto H, Tsuda F, et al. Hepatitis C virus variants from Vietnam are classifiable into the seventh, eighth, and ninth major genetic groups. *Proc Natl Acad Sci U S A.* 1994;91:11022–11026.

32. Lau JYN, Davis GL, Prescott LE, et al. and the Hepatitis Interventional Therapy Group. Distribution of hepatitis C virus genotypes determined by line probe assay in patients with chronic hepatitis C seen at tertiary referral centers in the United States. *Ann Intern Med.* 1996;124:868–876.

33. Dusheiko G, Schmilovitz-Weiss H, Brown D, et al. Hepatitis C virus genotypes: an investigation of type-specific differences in geographic origin and disease. *Hepatology.* 1994;19:13–18.

34. Benvegnu L, Pontisso P, Cavalletto D, Noventa F, Chemello L, Alberti A. Lack of correlation between hepatitis C virus genotypes and clinical course of hepatitis C virus-related cirrhosis. *Hepatology.* 1997;25:211–215.

35. Poynard T, Bedossa P, Opolon P. Natural history of liver fibrosis progression in patients with chronic hepatitis C. The OBSVIRC, METAVIR, CLINIVIR, and DOSVIRC groups. *Lancet.* 1997;349:825–832.

36. National Institutes of Health. Management of hepatitis C. *NIH Consens Statement.* 2002;19:1–46.

37. Centers for Disease Control and Prevention. Recommendations for prevention and control of hepatitis C virus (HCV) infection and HCV-related chronic disease. *MMWR Morb Mortal Wkly Rep.* 1998;47:1–39.

38. EASL International Consensus Conference on Hepatic C. Consensus statement. *J Hepatol.* 1999;30:956–961.

39. Dufour DR, Lott JA, Nolte FS, Gretch DR, Koff RS, Seeff LB. Diagnosis and monitoring of hepatic injury. II. Recommendations for use of laboratory tests in screening, diagnosis, and monitoring. *Clin Chem.* 2000;46:2050–2068.

40. Centers for Disease Control and Prevention. Guidelines for laboratory testing and result reporting of antibody to hepatitis C virus. *MMWR Morb Mortal Wkly Rep.*. 2003;52:1–15.

41. Fanning L, Kenny-Walsh E, Levis J, et al. Natural fluctuations of hepatitis C viral load in the homogeneous patient population: a prospective study. *Hepatology.* 2000;31:225–229.

42. Fried MW, Shiffman ML, Reddy KR, et al. Peginterferon alfa-2a plus ribavirin for chronic hepatitis C virus infection. *N Eng J Med.* 2002;347:975–982.

43. Lee SS, Heathcote EJ, Reddy KR, et al. Prognostic factors and early predictability of sustained viral response with peginterferon alfa-2a (40KD). *J Hepatol.* 2002;37:500–506.

44. Poynard T, McHutchison JG, Goodman ZD, Ling M-H, Albrecht J for the ALGOVIRC Project Group. Is an "a la carte" combination interferon alfa-2b plus ribavirin regimen possible for the first line treatment in patients with chronic hepatitis C. *Hepatology.* 2000;31:211–218.

45. Schreiber GB, Busch MP, Kleinman SH, Korelitz JJ. The risk of transfusion-transmitted viral infections. The Retrovirus Epidemiology Donor Study. *N Eng J Med.* 1996;334:1685–1690.

46. Legler TJ, Riggert J, Simson G, et al. Testing of individual blood donations for HCV RNA reduces the residual risk of transfusion-transmitted HCV infection. *Transfusion.* 2000;40:1192–1197.

47. Kolk DP, Dockter J, Linnen J, et al. Significant closure of the human immunodeficiency virus type 1 and hepatitis C virus preseroconversion detection windows with a transcription-mediated-amplification-driven assay. *J Clin Microbiol.* 2002;40:1761–1766.

48. Ansaldi F, Torre F, Bruzzone BM, Picciotto A, Crovari P, Icardi G. Evaluation of a new hepatitis C virus sequencing assay as a routine method for genotyping. *J Med Virol.* 2001;63:17–21.

49. Icardi G, Ansaldi F, Bruzzone BM, et al. Novel approach to reduce the hepatitis C virus (HCV) window period: clinical evaluation of a new enzyme-linked immunosorbent assay for HCV core antigen. *J Clin Microbiol.* 2001;39:3110–3114.

50. Bouvier-Alias M, Patel K, Dahari H, et al. Clinical utility of total HCV core antigen quantification: a new indirect marker of HCV replication. *Hepatology.* 2002;36:211–218.

51. McHutchison JG, Gordon S, Schiff ER, et al. for the Hepatitis Interventional Therapy Group. Interferon alpha-2b alone or in combination of ribavirin as initial treatment for chronic hepatitis C. *N Eng J Med.* 1998;339:1485–1499.

52. Poynard T, Marcellin P, Lee SS, et al. for the International Hepatitis Interventional Therapy Group (IHIT). Randomised trial of interferon α2b plus ribavirin for 48 weeks or for 24 weeks versus interferon α2b plus placebo for 48 weeks for treatment of chronic infection with hepatitis C virus. *Lancet.* 1998;352:1426–1432.

53. McCormick SE, Goodman ZD, Maydonovitch CL, Sjogren MH. Evaluation of liver histology, ALT elevation, and HCV RNA titer in patients with chronic hepatitis C. *Am J Gastroenterol.* 1996;91:1516–1522.

54. Hohne M, Schreier E, Roggendorf M. Sequence variability in the env-coding region of hepatitis C virus isolated from patients infected during a single source outbreak. *Arch Virol.* 1994;137:25–34.

55. Power JP, Lawlor E, Davidson F, Holmes EC, Yap PL, Simmonds P. Molecular epidemiology of an outbreak of infection with hepatitis C virus in recipients of anti-D immunoglobulin. *Lancet.* 1995;345:1211–1213.

56. Bronowicki JP, Venard V, Botte C, et al. Patient-to-patient transmission of hepatitis C virus during colonoscopy. *N Eng J Med.* 1997;337:237–240.

57. Aizaki H, Saito A, Kusakawa I, et al. Mother-to-child transmission of a hepatitis C virus variant with an insertional mutation in its hypervariable region. *J Hepatol.* 1996;25:608–613.

58. Chayama K, Kobayashi M, Tsubota A, et al. Molecular analysis of intraspousal transmission of hepatitis C virus. *J Hepatol.* 1995;22:431–439.

59. Healey CJ, Smith DB, Walker JL, et al. Acute hepatitis C infection after sexual exposure. *Gut.* 1995;36:148–150.

60. Weiner AJ, Thaler MM, Crawford K, et al. A unique, predominant hepatitis C virus variant found in an infant born to a mother with multiple variants. *J Virol.* 1993;67:4365–4368.

61. Enomoto N, Sakuma I, Asahina Y, et al. Mutations in the nonstructural protein 5A gene and response to interferon in patients with chronic hepatitis C virus 1b infection. *N Eng J Med.* 1996;334:77–81.

62. Watanabe H, Enomoto N, Nagayama K, et al. Number and position of mutations in the interferon (IFN) sensitivity—determining region of the gene for nonstructural protein 5A correlate with IFN efficacy in hepatitis C virus 1b infection. *J Infect Dis.* 2001;183:1195–1203.

63. Hofgartner WT, Polyak SJ, Sullivan DG, Carithers RL, Gretch DR. Mutations in the NS5A gene of hepatitis C virus in North American patients infected with HCV genotype 1a or 1b. *J Med Virol.* 1997;53:118–126.

64. Sarrazin C, Berg T, Lee JH, et al. Improved correlation between multiple mutations within the NS5A region and virological response in

European patients chronically infected with hepatitis C virus type 1b undergoing combination therapy. *J Hepatol.* 1999;30:1004–1013.

65. Lee SC, Antony A, Lee N, et al. Improved version 2.0 qualitative and quantitative AMPLICOR reverse transcription-PCR tests for hepatitis C virus RNA: calibration to international units, enhanced genotype reactivity, and performance characteristics. *J Clin Microbiol.* 2000;38:4171–4179.

66. Nolte FS, Fried MW, Shiffman ML, et al. Prospective multicenter clinical evaluation of AMPLICOR and COBAS AMPLICOR hepatitis C virus tests. *J Clin Microbiol.* 2001;39:4005–4012.

67. Comanor L, Anderson F, Ghany M, et al. Transcription-mediated amplification is more sensitive than conventional PCR-based assays for detecting residual serum HCV RNA at end of treatment. *Am J Gastroenterol.* 2001;96:2968–2972.

68. Sarrazin C, Teuber G, Kokka R, Rabenau H, Zeuzem S. Detection of residual hepatitis C virus RNA by transcription-mediated amplification in patients with complete virologic response according to polymerase chain reaction-based assays. *Hepatology.* 2000;32:818–823.

69. Sarrazin C, Hendricks DA, Sedarati F, Zeuzem S. Assessment, by transcription-mediated amplification, of virologic response in patients with chronic hepatitis C virus treated with peginterferon alpha-2a. *J Clin Microbiol.* 2001;39:2850–2855.

70. Krajden M, Ziermann R, Khan A, et al. Qualitative detection of hepatitis C virus RNA: comparison of analytical sensitivity, clinical performance, and workflow of the Cobas Amplicor HCV test version 2.0 and the HCV RNA transcription-mediated amplification qualitative assay. *J Clin Microbiol.* 2002;40:2903–2907.

71. Jackson JB, Smith K, Knott C, et al. Sensitivity of the Procleix HIV-1/HCV assay for detection of human immunodeficiency virus type 1 and hepatitis C virus RNA in a high-risk population. *J Clin Microbiol.* 2002;40:2387–2391.

72. Beld M, Sentjens R, Rebers S, et al. Performance of the New Bayer VERSANT HCV RNA 3.0 assay for quantitation of hepatitis C virus RNA in plasma and serum: conversion to international units and comparison with the Roche COBAS Amplicor HCV Monitor, version 2.0, assay. *J Clin Microbiol.* 2002;40:788–793.

73. Germer JJ, Heimgartner PJ, Ilstrup DM, Harmsen WS, Jenkins GD, Patel R. Comparative evaluation of the Versant HCV RNA 3.0, Quantiplex HCV RNA 2.0, and COBAS Amplicor HCV Monitor version 2.0 Assays for quantification of hepatitis C virus RNA in serum. *J Clin Microbiol.* 2002;40:495–500.

74. Kleiber J, Walter T, Haberhausen G, Tsang S, Babiel R, Rosenstraus M. Performance characteristics of a quantitative, homogeneous TaqMan RT-PCR test for HCV RNA. *J Mol Diagn.* 2000;2:158–166.

75. Barbeau JM, Goforth J, Caliendo AM, Nolte F. Performance characteristics of a quantitative, TaqMan hepatitis C virus RNA analyte specific reagent. *J Clin Microbiol.* 2004:in press.

76. Caliendo AM, Valsamakis A, Zhou Y, et al. Multilaboratory comparison of hepatitis C virus viral load assays. *J Clin Microbiol.* 2006;44:1726–1732.

77. Stuyver L, Wyseur A, van Arnhem W, Hernandez F, Maertens G. Second-generation line probe assay for hepatitis C virus genotyping. *J Clin Microbiol.* 1996;34:2259–2266.

78. Andonov A, Chaudhary RK. Subtyping of hepatitis C virus isolates by a line probe assay using hybridization. *J Clin Microbiol.* 1995;33:254–256.

79. Viazov S, Zibert A, Ramakrishnan K, et al. Typing of hepatitis C virus isolates by DNA enzyme immunoassay. *J Virol Methods.* 1994;48:81–91.

80. Smith DB, McAllister J, Casino C, Simmonds P. Virus "quasispecies": making a mountain out of a molehill? *J Gen Virol.* 1997;78:1511–1519.

81. Ross RS, Viazov SO, Holtzer CD, et al. Genotyping of hepatitis C virus isolates using CLIP sequencing. *J Clin Microbiol.* 2000;38:3581–3584.

82. Halfon P, Trimoulet P, Bourliere M, et al. Hepatitis C virus genotyping based on 5′ noncoding sequence analysis (Trugene). *J Clin Microbiol.* 2001;39:1771–1773.

83. Kalinina O, Norder H, Mukomolov S, Magnius LO. A natural intergenotypic recombinant of hepatitis C virus identified in St. Petersburg. *J Virol.* 2002;76:4034–4043.

84. Hu YW, Balaskas E, Kessler G, et al. Primer specific and mispair extension analysis (PSMEA) as a simple approach to fast genotyping. *Nucleic Acids Res.* 1998;26:5013–5015.

85. Krekulova L, Rehak V, Wakil AE, Harris E, Riley LW. Nested restriction site-specific PCR to detect and type hepatitis C virus (HCV): a rapid method to distinguish HCV subtype 1b from other genotypes. *J Clin Microbiol.* 2001;39:1774–1780.

86. Davidson F, Simmonds P, Ferguson JC, Jarvis LM, et al. Survey of major genotypes and subtypes of hepatitis C virus using RFLP of sequences amplified from the 5′ non-coding region. *J Gen Virol.* 1995;76:1197–1204.

87. White PA, Zhai X, Carter I, Zhao Y, Rawlinson WD. Simplified hepatitis C virus genotyping by heteroduplex mobility analysis. *J Clin Microbiol.* 2000;38:477–482.

88. Bullock GC, Bruns DE, Haverstick DM. Hepatitis C genotype determination by melting curve analysis with a single set of fluorescence resonance energy transfer probes. *Clin Chem.* 2002;48:2147–2154.

89. Schroter M, Zollner B, Schafer P, et al. Genotyping of hepatitis C virus types 1, 2, 3, and 4 by a one-step LightCycler method using three different pairs of hybridization probes. *J Clin Microbiol.* 2002;40:2046–2050.

90. Dixit V, Quan S, Martin P, et al. Evaluation of a novel serotyping system for hepatitis C virus: strong correlation with standard genotyping methodologies. *J Clin Microbiol.* 1995;33:2978–2983.

91. Agnello V, Chung RT, Kaplan LM. A role for hepatitis C virus infection in type II cryoglobulinemia. *N Eng J Med.* 1992;327:1490–1495.

92. Cribier B, Rey D, Schmitt C, Lang JM, Kirn A, Stoll-Keller F. High hepatitis C viraemia and impaired antibody response in patients coinfected with HIV. *AIDS.* 1995;9:1131–1136.

93. Fabrizi F, Poordad FF, Martin P. Hepatitis C infection and the patient with end-stage renal disease. *Hepatology.* 2002;36:3–10.

94. Saldanha J, Lelie N, Heath A. Establishment of the first international standard for nucleic acid amplification technology (NAT) assays for HCV RNA. WHO Collaborative Study Group. *Vox Sang.* 1999;76:149–158.

95. Stelzl E, Kormann-Klement A, Haas J, et al. Evaluation of an automated sample preparation protocol for quantitative detection of hepatitis C virus RNA. *J Clin Microbiol.* 2002;40:1447–1450.

96. Nolte F, Green AM, Fiebelkorn KR, et al. Clinical evaluation of two methods for genotyping hepatitis C virus based on analysis of the 5′ noncoding region. *J Clin Microbiol.* 2003;41:1558–1564.

Chapter 5

Viral Infections in Transplant Patients

Andrea Ferreira-Gonzalez and Angela M. Caliendo

Introduction

Viruses are particularly problematic pathogens in transplant recipients. Viral infections not only can cause disease but also can enhance susceptibility to opportunistic infections by both causing tissue injury and contributing to systemic immunosuppression. Such infections have been shown to increase the rate of graft rejection and increase the risk of cancer. The outcome of viral infections in the transplant setting is the result of a balance among infection in tissues, host antiviral immune function, and the level of immunosuppression required to maintain graft function. Diagnosis of viral infections in immunocompromised patients remains a challenge due to the need to differentiate asymptomatic infection from clinically relevant disease.

The use of molecular tests has greatly enhanced the diagnosis of viral infections, in part due to the slow turnaround time or inadequate sensitivity of conventional diagnostic tests. Unlike conventional methods, which rely on viral culture or antigen detection, molecular methods detect viral nucleic acid. A number of nucleic acid–based methods have been applied to the diagnosis of viral infection in transplant patients, and the most widely used method is still the polymerase chain reaction (PCR), but other methods are used with increasing frequency. The RNA amplification methods (nucleic acid sequence–based amplification [NASBA] and transcription-mediated amplification [TMA]) and the signal-amplification methods (hybrid capture and branched DNA [bDNA]) also are available for the detection and quantitation of viral pathogens.

Molecular methods often provide increased sensitivity, a more rapid turnaround time, and, for some assays, improved specimen stability and ease of use compared to conventional methods. Even though the increased sensitivity of nucleic acid–based tests has been a major advantage, these tests also have posed some challenges. A large number of viral infections in transplant patients are due to viruses that remain in a latent state after primary infection. Nucleic acid from these viruses can be detected in patients with asymptomatic infection without evidence of clinical disease. Methods to improve clinical specificity of molecular tests have been developed and are discussed here.

One of the biggest challenges facing laboratories and clinicians is the lack of standardized molecular assays. A limited number of commercial test kits are available, and even fewer have been approved or cleared by the Food and Drug Administration (FDA). A large number of molecular assays currently in use have been developed by individual laboratories. The performance characteristics of these assays vary widely due to differences in specimen type, target sequence, limit of detection, and quantitative standard. As a result, values obtained from different laboratory-developed assays may not be comparable, which makes it very difficult to establish interpretive guidelines that can be applied broadly in clinical practice.

This chapter reviews the molecular tests that are available to detect and quantify cytomegalovirus (CMV), BK virus (BKV), hepatitis C virus (HCV), Epstein-Barr virus (EBV), and human herpes virus type 6 (HHV-6) in transplant recipients and discusses their clinical utility.

CMV

CMV remains a major cause of morbidity and mortality in solid organ transplant (SOT) and bone marrow transplant (BMT) recipients.[1] Primary CMV infection occurs during infancy, preschool age, and sexually active years. During primary infection, the virus is disseminated through the body via the bloodstream and the infection can be subclinical with diffuse organ involvement. After resolution of the primary infection, the virus remains latent in a non-replicating state or with an undetectable level of replication. However, in immunocompromised individuals, the virus can reactivate and result in clinical symptoms. CMV infection of the transplant population occurs by transmission, reactivation, or superinfection with a new strain of CMV. The clinical manifestations of CMV disease include fever, interstitial pneumonia, chorioretinitis, hepatitis, esophagitis, gastritis, and colitis. Preventive strategies have been developed for CMV disease in this patient population and include the use of CMV-seronegative blood products, CMV-seronegative donor selection whenever possible, and passive immunoprophylaxis with immunoglobulin. In recent years, prophylactic as well as preemptive treatment with antiviral drugs has been used with good success to reduce the risk of developing active CMV disease.[1]

The occurrence and severity of CMV disease in transplant recipients is influenced by the type of organ transplanted, the CMV serostatus of the organ recipient and donor, and the overall level of immunosuppression. Individuals who acquire their primary CMV infection while immunosuppressed are at risk for severe disease. Symptomatic disease can occur in CMV-seropositive recipients regardless of the serologic status of the donor. Furthermore, CMV-seronegative individuals who receive an organ from a CMV-seropositive donor are at higher risk for severe disease. The diagnostic challenge with CMV disease is distinguishing asymptomatic infection from clinically significant disease, because infectious virus, viral antigen, and viral nucleic acid can be detected in patients without clinically significant disease.[2]

CMV is a member of the Herpesviridae family and is a large, enveloped, double-stranded DNA virus. Traditionally, the detection and quantitation of CMV has relied on culture and antigen detection. Urinary shedding of CMV and even seroconversion are common but are not predictive of clinically significant CMV disease. Conventional culture methods are not sensitive enough to detect viremia in immunocompromised patients but can be useful in detecting CMV from respiratory secretions, urine, and tissue samples. However, the turnaround time for conventional culture results is slow, between 2 and 3 weeks, and as a result rarely impacts clinical care. The rapid centrifugation shell vial method has greatly reduced the time for virus detection, with positive results obtained in 24 to 48 hours, although this method lacks sensitivity for detecting viremia. The CMV antigenemia assay is limited to the detection of CMV in white blood cells and is more sensitive than conventional culture or shell vial methods. However, the antigenemia assay is labor-intensive and the sensitivity of the assay varies among different laboratories.[2-4]

Molecular biology assays have had a major impact on the rapid diagnosis of CMV disease.[5-7] The commercially available molecular tests for detection and quantitation of CMV nucleic acid are shown in Table 5-1, two of which have been cleared by the FDA. The Hybrid Capture test (Digene Corp, Gaithersburg, MD) is designed to detect CMV DNA in whole blood, while the NucliSens test (bioMerieux, Durham, NC) utilizes NASBA technology to detect CMV pp67 mRNA in whole blood. The NASBA assay is qualitative, while the Hybrid Capture assay may be either qualitative or quantitative (though it has been cleared by the FDA only as a qualitative test).

The more widely used molecular tests are based on PCR methodology, either laboratory-developed or commercially available test kits. Furthermore, analyte-specific reagents using real-time quantitative PCR (RQ-PCR) technology have recently become available. The laboratory-developed assays utilize both standard PCR and RQ-PCR methods and their performance varies due to differences in specimen type, nucleic acid extraction methods, target gene, primer sequences, quantitation standard, and detection method. These differences become quite important in the comparison of quantitative assays since viral load values may vary when the same sample is tested using different assays. Such assay variation makes comparison of results from different studies difficult, and also impedes establishment of viral load values that correlate with clinical disease. The challenges in assessing clinical performance of molecular tests include developing an understanding of the analytical performance characteristics of the

Table 5-1. Molecular Assays for the Detection of CMV

Assay	Method	Target	Lower Limit (copies/ml)	Upper Limit (copies/ml)	Test Kit	FDA Cleared
Qualitative Methods						
NucliSens CMV (bioMerieux, Durham, NC)	NASBA	pp67 mRNA	Not defined	N/A	Yes	Yes
Hybrid Capture CMV v3.0 (Digene Corp, Gaithersburg, MD)	Hybrid capture	17% of genome	1400	N/A	Yes	Yes
Laboratory-developed assays	PCR/ Real-time PCR	Variable	Variable	N/A	No	No
Quantitative Methods						
Amplicor CMV Monitor (Roche Diagnostics, Indianapolis, IN)	PCR	Pol gene	400	1×10^5	Yes	No
Hybrid Capture CMV v3.0 (Digene Corp, Gaithersburg, MD)	Hybrid capture	17% of genome	1400	600,000	Yes	No
Laboratory-developed assays and analyte specific reagents (ASR)	PCR/ Real-time PCR	Variable	Variable	Variable	No	No

N/A, not applicable.

different assays, determining what each test is measuring, and assessing the clinical implications of the results. For example, PCR assays using whole blood or leukocytes and the Hybrid Capture test detect intracellular DNA,[8] which is present in both latent and actively infected cells. On the other hand, PCR assays using plasma detect DNA in circulation that is the result of active viral replication. Furthermore, the NucliSens assay detects pp67 mRNA, which is expressed at a high level in patients with active CMV disease but is not detectable during latent infection.[9–11]

One of the primary uses of CMV molecular testing is for the diagnosis of active CMV disease, which involves distinguishing patients with asymptomatic infection from patients with clinically significant CMV disease. Early studies evaluating the clinical utility of CMV DNA tests used very sensitive qualitative assays and peripheral blood mononuclear cells (PBMC) as the specimen of choice. As a result, CMV DNA was detected in patients with CMV disease as well as in immunocompromised patients without active disease.[5,12] Several different approaches have been used in an effort to improve the clinical specificity of molecular tests for active CMV disease, including the use of quantitative assays, detecting DNA in plasma rather than whole blood or leukocytes, and detection of mRNA rather than DNA. Several studies have proven the clinical utility of quantitative PCR assays using plasma specimens.[10,13] Quantitative methods may allow the definition of threshold values that distinguish asymptomatic infection from active CMV disease. Detection of CMV DNA in plasma rather than in leukocytes may provide a better correlation with clinical disease because the detection of CMV DNA in plasma correlates with active viral replication due to the spread of virus from leukocytes and tissue to the plasma compartment.[10] The detection of CMV DNA in plasma is an early marker for active CMV disease in renal[7] and liver[14,15] transplant recipients.

Several studies have evaluated the clinical utility of laboratory-developed quantitative PCR assays for the diagnosis of CMV disease in transplant patients. Patients with active CMV disease have consistently higher viral load values than those with asymptomatic infection.[14,16] In light of these findings, cutoff values were proposed as a means to discriminate infection from clinically relevant active disease. Cutoff values associated with active disease vary by specific assay type, as well as by the type of SOT or BMT. Though these tests have proven to be very useful for individual laboratories, it has been difficult to establish broadly applicable, clinically relevant guidelines for the use of laboratory-developed CMV viral load assays.

Recently several studies have evaluated the clinical utility of two commercially available test kits, the Amplicor CMV Monitor (Roche Diagnostics, Indianapolis, IN) and the CMV Hybrid Capture (Digene Corp.). Humar et al.[15] performed a prospective study in which weekly plasma CMV viral load was measured in 97 liver transplant patients during the 12 weeks after transplantation. No

preemptive therapy was given; however, CMV-seronegative recipients who received a CMV-seropositive liver received 12 weeks of prophylactic ganciclovir (GCV). Sixty-one of the 97 patients developed CMV infection, defined as a positive laboratory test for CMV. Of these 61 patients, 21 developed documented CMV disease. Clinical manifestations of CMV disease included hepatitis, CMV viral syndrome, and esophagitis or colitis. As shown with early studies, patients with CMV disease had a statistically significant higher peak viral load than those with asymptomatic infection (median peak 55,000 copies/ml vs 1820 copies/ml, respectively). The predictive value of viral load testing also was assessed by evaluating viral load values obtained at least 3 days prior to the development of CMV disease. Using receiver-operator characteristic curves, the authors determined that the optimal viral load for detecting clinically significant CMV disease was between 2000 and 5000 copies/ml of plasma. As the viral load cutoff level for detecting CMV disease was increased, there was a loss in sensitivity but an improvement in specificity.

Two therapeutic approaches are used to prevent CMV disease in transplant patients who are at risk for CMV disease, prophylactic treatment and preemptive treatment. Prophylactic therapy is the treatment of all patients considered to be at risk for CMV disease without the use of molecular testing, without further stratification of risk. Prophylactic therapy is based on the assumption that the entire population is at substantial risk of infection and merits preventive treatment. Thus, the use of prophylactic therapy involves treatment of a large number of patients. Preemptive therapy is used for at-risk patients who are positive for CMV by a laboratory test. Molecular CMV assays are commonly used to make decisions concerning the administration of preemptive therapy.[12,15,17–21] For example, all at-risk patients would be tested for the presence of CMV DNA in their blood, and only those with a positive result would be treated. The use of preemptive therapy focuses preventive treatment on a subgroup of patients determined to be at a higher risk of CMV disease. Thus, the laboratory test is used to determine whether the level of infection makes invasive disease likely. Both these approaches provide therapy prior to the development of symptoms, hence preventing the development of active disease.

A number of studies have evaluated the clinical utility of the NucliSens CMV test (bioMerieux) for initiation of preemptive therapy.[9,18] In a prospective study by Hebart et al.,[22] a total of 33 BMT recipients at risk for CMV disease were monitored once a week for 18 months after transplantation using the NucliSens NASBA assay, a whole-blood laboratory-developed PCR assay, and viral culture. Preemptive antiviral therapy was initiated after two positive PCR results; clinical decisions were not made based on NucliSens results. The NucliSens and the PCR assays had a high level of agreement (87.9% for patients and 85.3% for samples). None of the NASBA-negative patients developed CMV disease. Sixteen of the 18 patients receiving preemptive GCV treatment also were NASBA positive. Three of the 33 patients at risk for developing CMV disease developed disease, all of whom were PCR and NASBA positive. There was no difference between assays for the time of first positive result. Ongoing studies evaluating the clinical utility of quantitative PCR assays and the NASBA assay will provide further information regarding the clinical utility of these tests for guiding preemptive antiviral therapy.

Several studies have looked at the clinical utility of quantitative molecular tests for monitoring antiviral therapy response in transplant patients.[21,23] A greater than 90% reduction in viral load, as measured by the Hybrid Capture test, has been observed after initiation of therapy for CMV infection.[5] Several studies have reported that viral loads become undetectable several weeks after initiating therapy;[7,20,21] however, the time to clear CMV is related to the viral load. Patients with low pretreatment viral loads will become undetectable for CMV more rapidly than those with high pretreatment viral load values. Failure of viral loads to decline to undetectable levels after initiation of antiviral therapy is a cause of concern because patients with documented GCV resistance have persistent CMV viral loads.[7]

Another application of molecular tests is identifying patients at risk for relapsing CMV infection.[23-25] The optimal duration of antiviral treatment for CMV infection has not been established. Relapsing episodes of CMV disease have been described in 15% to 35% of SOT patients. Although relapsing CMV disease might be due to the evolution of resistant CMV strains, it also may be the result of incomplete suppression of viral replication by antiviral treatment. In a prospective study of 24 SOT patients with CMV infection or disease, patients were treated with a 14-day course of GCV,[24] and viral load values were measured before and after treatment. Eight patients developed relapsing CMV infection and had viral load measurements prior to the initiation of therapy that were statistically higher compared to the nonrelapsing group (80,150 copies/10^6 leukocytes vs 5,500 copies/10^6 leukocytes, respectively, p = 0.007). In addition, the relapsing group had detectable viral load at the end of treatment (mean 18,800 copies/10^6 leukocytes), while viral load levels were undetectable in the nonrelapsing group. Similar results have been reported with the NucliSens assay. In one study, all six SOT recipients with detectable RNA after completing a course of therapy required further therapy for their CMV infection.[18]

The rate of decline in CMV load also is predictive of relapsing CMV infections. Fifty-two organ transplant recipients with CMV disease were monitored with the Amplicor CMV Monitor test (Roche Diagnostics), of which 12 developed relapsing CMV disease. The time to clearance of CMV DNA from plasma was 33.8 days in the group with relapsing CMV disease compared to 17.2 days in the group without recurrent disease (p = 0.002). The viral load half-life was 8.8 days compared to 3.2 days (p = 0.001) in the group with and without recurrent disease, respectively.[25]

Sequential monitoring of viral load levels after initiation of therapy may allow the identification of patients at risk of recurrent infection, thus providing the opportunity to intensify therapy and possibly prevent relapse.

Viral load measurements may be useful for individualizing treatment regimen length. Fisher et al.[26] prospectively evaluated and followed 18 SOT patients diagnosed with CMV disease. Plasma samples were obtained for viral load measurements weekly during treatment and monthly for 6 months following the end of therapy. Patients were treated with immunoglobulin for a period of time and with GCV until CMV viral load was undetectable (<100 copies/ml plasma). No patients relapsed with a mean follow-up of 16 months. This study suggests that viral load measurements have clinical utility for determining the length of time for GCV treatment. Further studies with a greater number of patients are needed to determine the utility of viral load testing for determining the duration of antiviral therapy, but this study indicates that discontinuing therapy when virus is still detectable in the plasma is a risk for relapsing infection.

Generally, transplant patients requiring treatment for CMV disease receive a lengthy course of antiviral therapy.[27-30] Such long-term treatment regimens are associated with development of antiviral drug resistance. There are currently three antiviral drugs that are FDA approved for the treatment of systemic CMV disease: GCV, cidofovir (CDV), and foscarnet (phosphonoformic acid [FOS]); of these three, GCV is the most widely used. Development of resistance does not occur very frequently because CMV is a DNA virus that replicates using a DNA polymerase that has proofreading activity, which prevents high mutation rates. Thus, selection of drug-resistant virus from the initial wild-type drug-sensitive population generally occurs only after weeks to months of therapy.

Two different types of testing are used for the detection of drug-resistant virus: phenotypic and genotypic. Phenotypic assays rely on analysis of growth characteristics of viral isolates in the presence of different concentrations of antiviral drugs and therefore require viable virus. The phenotypic assays are labor-intensive, the readout is subjective, and they require at least a month to obtain results, which is generally not therapeutically useful. The lengthy time requirement has led to development of genotypic assays based on detection of nucleotide sequence changes that are known to cause drug resistance. The currently used antiviral drugs target the UL97 gene (GCV) or the DNA polymerase gene (GCV, CDV, FOS) or both. Point mutations or short deletions in these genes confer drug resistance. GCV resistance mutations are most frequently mapped to the UL97 gene within codons 460 and 520 and either point mutations or deletions within the codon range 590 to 607.[28,29] GCV resistance due to mutations in the DNA polymerase gene appears to occur less frequently than those in the UL97 gene.[28,29] The majority of polymerase mutations conferring resistance to GCV also are cross-resistant to CDV,[30] whereas mutations in the UL97 gene confer resistance only to GCV. In general, FOS resistance mutations within the polymerase gene do not cause cross-resistance to either of the other two drugs, although a double deletion of codons 981 and 982 has been reported to confer resistance to all three drugs.[31] At least 23 sites within the polymerase gene have been mapped that confer drug resistance.[32] This covers approximately 2000 nucleotides, a much larger region than that of the UL97 gene. One caveat for genotypic assays is the presence of some normal baseline sequence variability in the UL97 and DNA polymerase genes in drug-sensitive strains. The assumption is made that the same mutation will produce resistance in all genetic backgrounds, which may not prove to be the case as more strains are examined. While phenotypic assays are biologically more relevant for detection of drug resistance because individual strains are tested for replication directly in the presence of antiviral drugs, genotypic results do correlate with the clinical drug resistance and provide rapid results not possible for the presently available phenotypic assays.[33] An advance in genotyping testing is the ability to sequence CMV DNA directly from the plasma specimens in patients failing therapy.

BKV

Since first reported, BKV-associated nephropathy has emerged as an important cause of allograft failure in renal transplant recipients. BKV is ubiquitous, with more than 90% of adults having serologic evidence of past infection. BKV is transmitted at an early age via oral or respiratory routes, and after primary infection remains latent in uroepithelial cells and circulating leukocytes. During immunosuppression, virus reactivation causes cytopathic changes in the uroepithelium, with increased shedding of BKV in the urinary tract. This in turn results in a range of clinical syndromes from viremia and viruria to ureteral ulceration or stenosis, and hemorrhagic cystitis. In renal transplant recipients, persistent active replication of BKV in the renal allograft, called BKV nephropathy, is associated with progressive graft dysfunction and graft loss due to interstitial nephritis. However, BKV nephropathy is rarely diagnosed in transplant recipients of nonrenal organs. BKV nephropathy develops in 1% to 5% of renal transplant recipients, with graft failure in as many as 45% to 67% of affected patients. Risk factors associated with BKV-associated nephritis in renal transplant patients are not well known, but most of the patients with this disorder have received the newer immunosuppressive drugs such as tacrolimus or mycophenolate mofetil.[34,35]

Antiviral treatment is not established for BK nephropathy, and control of antiviral activity is tentatively attained by reduction of immunosuppressive therapy. In patients with diminished renal allograft function and possible BKV infection, a choice must be made between increasing the level of immunosuppression to treat suspected graft rejection or reduction of immunosuppression to allow the immune system to control the BKV infection. Transplant patients with BKV nephropathy who are treated with increased levels of immunosuppressive drugs have a high incidence of graft loss. On the other hand, a reduced level of immunosuppressive therapy may stabilize the graft function but increases the risk of rejection.[36] A recent study evaluated the clinical utility of CDV for the treatment of BKV nephropathy in a limited number of patients. Results were encouraging, with all four patients clearing the viremia without graft loss.[37] Further studies are needed to confirm these findings.

Accurate diagnosis of BKV nephropathy is required to preserve graft function. Progression of BKV nephropathy often occurs without clear clinical signs or symptoms; sometimes the only indication is a rise in creatinine concentration, which occurs over a period of days to weeks before symptoms appear, although not all patients with BKV nephropathy present with an elevated creatinine. Diagnosis of BKV nephropathy is made by histological demonstration of viral infection, which is distinct from signs of rejection. In these patients, histologic examination of allograft biopsy specimens reveals extensive viral cytopathic effect, necrosis of the cells of the tubules and collecting ducts, and varying degrees of interstitial inflammation. Although renal biopsy is useful for the diagnosis of BKV nephropathy, it is an invasive procedure. A noninvasive alternative is to examine the urine for the presence of decoy cells, which contain characteristic intracellular viral inclusion bodies. Identification of decoy cells confirms that there is active replication of BKV, but this finding is not specific for BKV nephropathy.[34-36]

Using a qualitative PCR method, Randhawa et al.[38] demonstrated a positive relationship between the presence of BKV DNA in blood and impairment of renal allograft function, thus indicating that viremic patients are at high risk for progression to BKV-related interstitial nephritis. Moreover, in a recent prospective study, Hirsch et al.[39] have shown that BKV viral load is significantly higher in patients with biopsy-proven BKV nephropathy than in those without BKV nephropathy. A total of 78 renal transplant patients were followed for a median of 85 weeks after transplantation. BKV nephropathy was diagnosed in allograft biopsy specimens from five patients at a median of 28 weeks after transplantation. The diagnosis of infection on the basis of cytologic examination of urine specimens for the presence of decoy cells showed a sensitivity of 100% and specificity of 71% with a positive predictive value of 29% and a negative predictive value of 100%. The diagnosis of infection on the basis of cytologic examination of urine specimens for decoy cells was sensitive but had a low positive predictive value, suggesting that this approach could be used as a screening test. BKV viremia was detected in ten patients at a median of 23 weeks after transplant, with five having histologically proven BKV nephropathy. Interestingly, the mean viral DNA level in plasma was significantly higher in patients with histologically proven BKV nephropathy than in patients without histologic evidence of nephropathy (2×10^4 copies/ml vs 2×10^3 copies/ml, respectively; p<0.001). Furthermore, the plasma viral load increased to 7.7×10^3 copies/ml or more in all patients in whom BKV nephropathy developed, with three of the five patients reaching viral load levels of 1×10^7 copies/ml. For all patients with histologically proven BKV nephropathy, BKV viral load had a sensitivity of 100%, a specificity of 88%, a positive predictive value of 50%, and a negative predictive value of 100%. These findings offer a basis for identifying patients at risk for BKV nephropathy who may be candidates for preemptive reduction in immunosuppressive therapy or initiation of antiviral therapy.

BKV viral load testing of renal transplant patients has shown utility not only for diagnosing BKV nephropathy but also for monitoring the response to antiviral therapy or reduction of immunosuppressive therapy.[40–42] Limaye et al.[40] prospectively collected samples from four renal transplant patients with histologically diagnosed BKV nephropathy (cases) and 16 renal transplant patients who did not develop BKV nephropathy (controls). Serum samples were collected from all patients at the time of transplantation, during clinic visits, and during readmissions to the hospital. The case patients were more likely than the control patients to have BKV detected in serum samples (4 of 4 patients vs 0 of 16 patients). In all four patients, BKV DNA was detected in serum samples before histologic diagnosis of BKV nephropathy. Interestingly, prolonged viremia, in some cases over 50 weeks, was found in three case patients. Furthermore BKV DNA was detected in blood coincident with persistent unexplained inflammatory changes in biopsies weeks to months before characteristic histologic changes consistent with BKV nephropathy became evident. A reduction of the viral load was demonstrated after reduction in immunosuppression or transplant nephrectomy or both.[40]

BKV also is associated with the development of late-onset hemorrhagic cystitis (HC) in allogeneic BMT patients. HC is an important cause of morbidity and occasional mortality in BMT patients. The incidence of HC in this patient population varies from 5% to 35% and is characterized by lower abdominal pain, dysuria, frequent micturition, and hematuria. The manifestations vary from microscopic hematuria to severe hemorrhage, leading to clot retention and renal failure. HC had been ascribed solely to the toxic effects of drugs utilized during BMT, but recently BKV reactivation has been associated with HC. During BMT, intense immunosuppressive therapy leads to increased viral replication, which results in viruria. Since BKV can be detected in urine samples of 77% to 90% of all adult BMT patients, both with and without HC, it is apparent that BKV reactivation alone is not sufficient to cause HC.[43–45] Several studies have tried to identify other factors such as graft-vs-host disease, primary infection, or even specific types of BKV that might be involved in the development of HC, with little success.[34]

One of the biggest challenges in trying to evaluate the clinical utility of molecular tests for the diagnosis and monitoring of BKV-associated disease is the lack of standardized molecular assays. The performance of these assays can vary widely due to differences in specimen type used, methodology, and limit of detection. As a result, values obtained from different laboratory-developed assays may not be comparable, which makes it very difficult to establish interpretive guidelines that can be applied broadly in clinical practice. Further studies are needed to better define the role of BKV infection and the role of molecular qualitative and quantitative assays for diagnosis and monitoring BKV nephropathy.

HCV

End-stage liver disease secondary to HCV infection is the most common indication for liver transplantation in this country, accounting for one third of all liver transplants. A variety of molecular methods for detection and quantitation of HCV RNA genomes are used in the management of patients with HCV infection before and after liver transplantation. Three methods are used to detect and quantify HCV RNA: reverse transcription–PCR (RT-PCR), TMA, and the bDNA technique.[46] Refer to chapter 4 for a detailed discussion of these assays and their performance characteristics.

In patients transplanted for HCV cirrhosis, reinfection and recurrence of HCV disease occurs in most cases.[47–52] Reinfection refers to the presence of HCV in blood, while recurrence of disease refers to histologic evidence of liver damage. Therefore, the diagnosis of recurrent disease requires histologic changes in the presence of persistent HCV viremia. Detectable HCV RNA is present in nearly all HCV-related liver transplant recipients within 1 month after transplant, while histologic recurrence of HCV disease occurs in 50% within 2 years after transplant. The rate of histologic disease development is accelerated in liver transplant patients as compared to the general population, where chronic hepatitis develops in 80% of patients after a decade or more of infection. Moreover, development of cirrhosis also is accelerated in this patient population, with 10% to 20% of patients developing cirrhosis within 5 years of transplant, compared to the general population, in which 20% develop cirrhosis after 2 to 3 decades after infection. Many patients (20% to 40%) will have a benign course after transplant, while a few patients develop more severe disease with rapid progression to fibrosis and cirrhosis.[47–49] Although there is strong data supporting an accelerated disease process in transplanted patients, controversy remains regarding the impact of recurrent HCV on patient and graft survival. These findings underscore the need to identify prognostic factors that may predict the course of disease after transplant.

Prognostic factors for outcome after liver transplantation[53–56] include early recurrence of disease, viral load, and genotype. Early recurrence of HCV disease is associated with increased risk for cirrhosis, as well as decreased graft and patient survival. Liver transplant patients who developed recurrent HCV disease within 6 months of transplant are two to three times more likely to develop cirrhosis than recipients who developed histologic recurrence after 6 months. Patients who developed HCV recurrence within 1 year of transplantation are more likely to lose their graft.

The role of HCV viral load in predicting poor graft survival is controversial.[53] In an early study, using the National Institute of Diabetes and Digestive and Kidney Diseases Liver Transplantation Database, transplant patients with HCV RNA titers greater than 1×10^6 mEq/ml had worse patient and graft survival rates compared to patients with lower HCV RNA levels.[57] In a more recent study of 79 patients who underwent liver transplantation for chronic HCV infection, neither pretransplant nor posttransplant HCV RNA levels were significantly associated with the occurrence of graft hepatitis. However, there was a trend of more severe recurrent disease in patients with subtype 1b and high viral load soon after transplant.[54]

Another prognostic factor associated with a poor outcome after liver transplant is HCV genotype.[53,55] In nontransplant patients with HCV infection, patients with genotype 1 having a lower rate of sustained virologic response (SVR) to antiviral therapy compared to patients with genotypes 2 or 3 (see chapter 4). The association of genotype and outcome after liver transplantation has been controversial. Earlier studies showed no significant association with genotype 1b and disease severity or graft survival after transplant.[57,58] In contrast, more recent studies have shown that HCV genotype 1b is associated with a higher recurrence of HCV disease 3 years after transplant compared to genotype non-1b.[53] Although there is no uniform agreement regarding the prognostic factors associated with graft and patient survival, HCV RNA testing and genotyping will remain key parameters in future studies.

EBV

EBV-induced posttransplant lymphoproliferative disorders (PTLD) continue to be a rare but severe complication following transplantation. PTLD represents a heterogeneous group of abnormal lymphoid proliferations, generally of B-cell origin, that occur in an environment of ineffective T-cell function. The ineffective T-cell function is the result of pharmacologic immunosuppression after transplant. PTLD represents a spectrum of EBV-related clinical diseases, from benign mononucleosis-like illness to fulminate non-Hodgkin lymphoma.

The origin of the EBV in PTLD is varied. In SOT patients, the PTLD cells are usually of recipient origin, suggesting that the EBV infection represents reactivation of prior latent virus. Most cases of PTLD in BMT patients involve seropositive donors and recipients, and the PTLD cells are usually of donor origin because the host lymphoid tissue has been eradicated.

EBV-induced PTLD has an incidence of 0.8% to 20% depending on the type of organ transplant, patient age, and the type of immunosuppression.[59] Pretransplantation EBV seronegativity and the development of CMV disease, especially in the donor positive–recipient negative CMV serogroup, are significant risk factors. PTLD occurs more frequently in children than adults, probably because children are more likely to be EBV seronegative (49%) than adults (8%) at the time of transplant. Other risk factors for the development of PTLD include HLA-mismatched T-cell depletion, the use of antilymphocytic antibodies for conditioning, and treatment of graft-vs-host disease.[60–62]

PTLD has a variety of clinical presentations and may be related to viral infection, organ dysfunction, or lymphoma-related symptoms. Early diagnosis of PTLD requires diligent surveillance in appropriate patient populations. The median time to onset of PTLD in SOT patients is 6 months, whereas in BMT patients, signs and symptoms could appear within 70 to 90 days after transplant. Clinical features of PTLD are similar in both SOT and BMT patients, but there appears to be a greater incidence of fulminate, disseminated disease in BMT patients. Given the number of other diagnoses that PTLD can mimic, tissue biopsy is usually required for accurate diagnosis. A variety of special studies have been applied to the diagnosis of PTLD, such as immunophenotyping by flow cytometry, immunohistochemical staining, and molecular tests.[62–64]

Early detection of PTLD may allow for prompt therapy and potentially decreased mortality. Experience with monitoring patients for the development of PTLD is limited; however, several reports suggest that active surveillance for the presence of primary or reactivated EBV infection may be a useful approach to early detection of PTLD.[64–66]

Molecular tests, in particular quantitative PCR assays, are a promising advance that may allow for early diagnosis of PTLD. However, standardized methods and consensus on the appropriate clinical specimens are needed. Since EBV causes a latent infection, PCR assays for the detection of EBV in PBMC will have the same limitations as seen for CMV; that is, EBV DNA will be detected in patients regardless of PTLD status. Quantitative PCR assays have been used to distinguish asymptomatic EBV infection from PTLD. Furthermore, PTLD in SOT patients differs from that in BMT patients with regard to the source of EBV, the time of disease outbreak, and the course of the disease itself. For these reasons, not all patients should be grouped and analyzed together, and broad conclusions from different studies should be drawn cautiously.[64,66,67]

Several studies using quantitative PCR assays on a limited number of patients have shown that high levels of EBV DNA in lymphocytes are associated with the development of PTLD.[68–70] A recent study[68] described the use of a quantitative PCR assay to determine EBV viral load at the time of PTLD diagnosis in a group of allogeneic BMT recipients. The assay quantified between 20 and 10^6 copies of EBV DNA/µg of DNA from peripheral blood lymphocytes (PBL). The EBV viral loads in patients with PTLD were compared with the viral loads of transplant recipients without PTLD. EBV DNA was detected in 26 of the 59 patients, indicating primary infection or reactivation. The EBV viral load was significantly higher in patients with PTLD compared to those without PTLD. For the nine patients diagnosed with PTLD, the median EBV viral load was 1.6×10^6 copies/µg PBL DNA, compared to 4×10^3 copies/µg PBL DNA in patients without PTLD. Using the different median values in the two patient populations, a threshold value of 10^5 EBV copies/µg PBL DNA for the diagnosis of PTLD was selected, which resulted in both a sensitivity and specificity of approximately 90%. However, in transplant patients with fewer than three major risk factors for PTLD, the positive predictive value of this threshold was low. In addition, there were still a small number of patients with a high viral load that did not develop PTLD during the course of the study.

In an effort to simplify the method needed for EBV detection by PCR, Campe et al.[69] studied the utility of a quantitative PCR assay using sera and PBL in pediatric renal transplant patients. The advantage of using serum is that sample processing does not require the separation and quantitation of PBL from blood. In addition, the authors hypothesized that the detection of EBV DNA in serum would occur only for patients with a high EBV viral load, and might better distinguish patients with PTLD from transplant recipients that have low levels of EBV DNA secondary to immunosuppression, but not PTLD. This prospective study[69] evaluated 25 pediatric renal transplant recipients that were 1 to 8 years after transplant. PBL and serum were collected at each outpatient visit over a 6-month period. A mononucleosis-like syndrome with persistent symptoms of low-grade fever, cervical adenopathy, and hyperplastic adenoids was diagnosed in 11 patients. A total of 38.4% of PBL samples from asymptomatic patients were positive by PCR. PBL samples from two asymptomatic patients were continuously positive for EBV DNA over the period of the study. The mean viral load of positive samples was 480 copies/10,000 PBL. However, 100% of PBL samples from symptomatic patients were positive for EBV DNA with a mean viral load of 1500 copies/10,000 PBL. On the other hand, 14.3% of the serum samples from asymptomatic patients were positive by PCR, with a mean viral load of 13,250 copies/ml serum, while EBV DNA was detected in 81.9% of serum samples of symptomatic patients with a mean viral load of 22,500 copies/ml serum. Detection of EBV DNA in serum always was associated with EBV DNA in the corresponding sample of PBL in symptomatic patients. Thus, positive EBV PCR results in PBL and serum were more likely in symptomatic children. Therefore, patients who have EBV DNA detected simultaneously in PBL and serum may be at higher risk of developing PTLD.

There is some evidence that detection and quantitation of EBV DNA in peripheral blood can be utilized as prognostic markers for development of PTLD, with a correlation between high levels of EBV DNA in the blood and development of PTLD. A study by Kogan-Liberman et al.[70] addressed the value of EBV viral load monitoring and pre-

emptive reduction in immunosuppressive therapy in a group of pediatric liver transplant recipients. The authors prospectively followed monthly EBV viral load in 23 pediatric liver transplant recipients for 18 months after transplantation. A preemptive reduction in immunosuppressive therapy was instituted for significant EBV replication indicated by a positive PCR result. Patients were divided into two groups: group 1 was seropositive for EBV before transplant (13 patients), and group 2 was seronegative for EBV before transplant (10 patients). Nine of the 13 patients in the seropositive group 1 had positive PCR results at a mean time of 22.4 weeks after transplant. All but one of these patients was asymptomatic. In 7 of the 9 PCR-positive patients, preemptive reduction in immunosuppressive therapy was undertaken without development of PTLD or rejection. The two patients in whom immunosuppressive therapy could not be reduced experienced low-grade and medically responsive PTLD. On the other hand, in seronegative group 2 patients, no patient developed a positive EBV viral load, no intervention was necessary, and none of these patients developed PTLD. Since the number of patients enrolled in this study was small, further studies addressing this issue are warranted.

HHV-6

HHV-6 is another herpesvirus of emerging clinical significance. Although overt clinical disease is infrequent in healthy adults, HHV-6 reactivates in immunosuppressed individuals. HHV-6 infection is common in the first 2 years of life, and about 90% of adults are seropositive. HHV-6 can be reactivated following SOT, causing nonspecific febrile illness, bone marrow suppression, interstitial pneumonitis, rash, and hepatitis. The role of HHV-6 in this setting is difficult to determine, since the virus is latent and can be detected in asymptomatic patients, and CMV causes identical syndromes.[71] The reported incidence of HHV-6 infection after transplant varies according to the diagnostic method and ranges from 48% of BMT to 32% of SOT patients.

One of the most interesting features of HHV-6 is its interaction with other viruses. The indirect clinical sequelae of HHV-6 after transplant include altering the net state of immunosuppression with modification of the natural history of CMV disease. Interactions between HHV-6 and CMV have been well documented in liver transplant patients. HHV-6 infection is associated with severe clinical symptoms in SOT patients if concomitant CMV infection occurs. There is evidence that HHV-6 infection in liver or renal transplant patients is an independent risk factor for the development of CMV disease.[72–75]

Laboratory-developed PCR assays have been used to understand the significance of HHV-6 infection in SOT recipients.[74,76,77] One prospective study[74] followed 200 consecutive patients undergoing liver transplantation using a quantitative laboratory-developed PCR assay to detect

HHV-6 DNA in PBL obtained at baseline and weeks 1, 2, 3, 4, 6, 8, 10, and 12, or when clinically indicated. A positive HHV-6 PCR result was obtained in 51.1% of the patients at a median of 27 days after transplant. Peak viral load occurred by day 22 after transplant in 25% of the patients, by day 35 in 50% of the patients, by day 63 in 75% of the patients, and by day 90 in 90% of the patients. The median peak viral load was 200 copies/µg DNA (range 3 to 10,000 copies/µg DNA). To differentiate latent infection from active infection, patients were categorized into two groups, those with peak viral load under 100 copies/µg DNA and those with peak viral load greater than 100 copies/µg DNA. Using this cutoff value, 56 patients had HHV-6 infection. Interestingly, patients on GCV prophylaxis had a lower incidence of HHV-6 infection than those who did not receive prophylaxis (12.9% vs 30.8%, p = 0.042). HHV-6-associated disease was documented in only two patients (1%). Both patients had unexplained fever, leukopenia, and thrombocytopenia with negative CMV laboratory results and an HHV-6 viral load greater than 1,000 copies/µg DNA. CMV infection occurred in 40% of the patients, with symptomatic CMV disease in 16.6% of patients. HHV-6 infection was significantly associated with CMV disease. Furthermore, CMV viral load was significantly higher in patients with HHV-6 infection than those without HHV-6 infection (median viral load 1,560 copies/ml (0 to 181,000 copies/ml) vs median viral load undetectable [0 to 14,000 copies/ml], respectively; p < 0.001]). Risk factors for development of CMV disease were analyzed in a multivariate logistic regression model, and HHV-6 infection and anti-lymphocyte globulin administration were the only risk factors identified. In the same study, the association of HHV-6 infection with development of opportunistic infections was evaluated.[74] A total of 74 opportunistic infections, including CMV disease ($n = 32$), invasive fungal infection ($n = 17$), EBV-related PTLD ($n = 6$), disseminated zoster ($n = 11$), and other infections ($n = 8$), were diagnosed. An increase in HHV-6 viral load was significantly associated with the development of opportunistic infections. In addition, HHV-6 infection was associated with rejection in a subgroup of patients whose rejection occurred greater than 30 days after transplantation. Of the 41 patients in this subgroup, the median peak HHV-6 viral load was 40 copies/µg DNA compared to undetectable in those without rejection (p = 0.004).

Further studies are needed to better define HHV-6 pathogenesis and its interaction with CMV and other opportunistic pathogens. However, it is clear that molecular methods for the detection and quantitation of HHV-6 will play a crucial role in this area of research, as well as in routine clinical testing in the future.

References

1. Rubin RH. The direct and indirect effects of infection in liver transplantation: pathogenesis, impact, and clinical management. *Curr Clin Top Infect Dis.* 2002;22:125–154.

2. Ljungman P. Beta-herpesvirus challenges in the transplant recipient. *J Infect Dis.* 2002;186(suppl 1):S99–S109.

3. Sissons JG, Carmichael AJ. Clinical aspects and management of cytomegalovirus infection. *J Infect.* 2002;44:78–83.

4. Rubin RH. Cytomegalovirus in solid organ transplantation. *Transpl Infect Dis.* 2001;3(suppl 2):1–5.

5. Aitken C, Barrett-Muir W, Millar C, et al. Use of molecular assays in diagnosis and monitoring of cytomegalovirus disease following renal transplantation. *J Clin Microbiol.* 1999;37:2804–2807.

6. Caliendo AM, Schuurman R, Yen-Lieberman B, et al. Comparison of quantitative and qualitative PCR assays for cytomegalovirus DNA in plasma. *J Clin Microbiol.* 2001;39:1334–1338.

7. Caliendo AM, St George K, Allega J, et al. Distinguishing cytomegalovirus (CMV) infection and disease with CMV nucleic acid assays. *J Clin Microbiol.* 2002;40:1581–1586.

8. Mazzulli T, Drew LW, Yen-Lieberman B, et al. Multicenter comparison of the digene hybrid capture CMV DNA assay (version 2.0), the pp65 antigenemia assay, and cell culture for detection of cytomegalovirus viremia. *J Clin Microbiol.* 1999;37:958–963.

9. Gerna G, Baldanti F, Middeldorp JM, et al. Clinical significance of expression of human cytomegalovirus pp67 late transcript in heart, lung, and bone marrow transplant recipients as determined by nucleic acid sequence-based amplification. *J Clin Microbiol.* 1999;37:902–911.

10. Razonable RR, Brown RA, Wilson J, et al. The clinical use of various blood compartments for cytomegalovirus (CMV) DNA quantitation in transplant recipients with CMV disease. *Transplantation.* 2002;73:968–973.

11. Middeldorp J, Sillekens P, Lunenberg J. Diagnosis of active HCMV infection: the mRNA approach. *Organs and Tissue.* 2000;2:99–107.

12. Weinberg A, Hodges TN, Li S, et al. Comparison of PCR, antigenemia assay, and rapid blood culture for detection and prevention of cytomegalovirus disease after lung transplantation. *J Clin Microbiol.* 2000;38:768–772.

13. Caliendo AM, St George K, Kao SY, et al. Comparison of quantitative cytomegalovirus (CMV) PCR in plasma and CMV antigenemia assay: clinical utility of the prototype AMPLICOR CMV MONITOR test in transplant recipients. *J Clin Microbiol.* 2000;38:2122–2127.

14. Patel R, Smith TF, Espy M, et al. A prospective comparison of molecular diagnostic techniques for the early detection of cytomegalovirus in liver transplant recipients [comment]. *J Infect Dis.* 1995;171:1010–1014.

15. Humar A, Gregson D, Caliendo AM, et al. Clinical utility of quantitative cytomegalovirus viral load determination for predicting cytomegalovirus disease in liver transplant recipients. *Transplantation.* 1999;68:1305–1311.

16. Ferreira-Gonzalez A, Fisher RA, Weymouth LA, et al. Clinical utility of a quantitative polymerase chain reaction for diagnosis of cytomegalovirus disease in solid organ transplant patients. *Transplantation.* 1999;68:991–996.

17. Cope AV, Sabin C, Burroughs A, et al. Interrelationships among quantity of human cytomegalovirus (HCMV) DNA in blood, donor-recipient serostatus, and administration of methylprednisolone as risk factors for HCMV disease following liver transplantation. *J Infect Dis.* 1997;176:1484–1490.

18. Oldenburg N, Lam KM, Khan MA, et al. Evaluation of human cytomegalovirus gene expression in thoracic organ transplant recipients using nucleic acid sequence-based amplification. *Transplantation.* 2000;70:1209–1215.

19. Razonable RR, Brown RA, Espy MJ, et al. Comparative quantitation of cytomegalovirus (CMV) DNA in solid organ transplant recipients with CMV infection by using two high-throughput automated systems. *J Clin Microbiol.* 2001;39:4472–4476.

20. Norris S, Kosar Y, Donaldson N, et al. Cytomegalovirus infection after liver transplantation: viral load as a guide to treating clinical infection. *Transplantation.* 2002;74:527–531.

21. Razonable RR, van Cruijsen H, Brown RA, et al. Dynamics of cytomegalovirus replication during preemptive therapy with oral ganciclovir. *J Infect Dis.* 2003;187:1801–1808.

22. Hebart H, Rudolph T, Loeffler J, et al. Evaluation of the NucliSens CMV pp67 assay for detection and monitoring of human cytomegalovirus infection after allogeneic stem cell transplantation. *Bone Marrow Transplant.* 2002;30:181–187.

23. Li H, Dummer JS, Estes WR, et al. Measurement of human cytomegalovirus loads by quantitative real-time PCR for monitoring clinical intervention in transplant recipients. *J Clin Microbiol.* 2003;41:187–191.

24. Sia IG, Wilson JA, Groettum CM, et al. Cytomegalovirus (CMV) DNA load predicts relapsing CMV infection after solid organ transplantation. *J Infect Dis.* 2000;181:717–720.

25. Humar A, Kumar D, Boivin G, et al. Cytomegalovirus (CMV) virus load kinetics to predict recurrent disease in solid-organ transplant patients with CMV disease. *J Infect Dis.* 2002;186:829–833.

26. Fisher RA, Saggi BH, Ferreira-Gonzalez A, et al. Prospective validation of quantitative polymerase chain reaction for management of cytomegalovirus disease in solid-organ transplant patients. *Transplantation.* 2002;74:573–576.

27. Chou S. Antiviral drug resistance in human cytomegalovirus. *Transpl Infect Dis.* 1999;1:105–114.

28. Chou S, Erice A, Jordan MC, et al. Analysis of the UL97 phosphotransferase coding sequence in clinical cytomegalovirus isolates and identification of mutations conferring ganciclovir resistance. *J Infect Dis.* 1995;171:576–583.

29. Chou S, Guentzel S, Michels KR, et al. Frequency of UL97 phosphotransferase mutations related to ganciclovir resistance in clinical cytomegalovirus isolates. *J Infect Dis.* 1995;172:239–242.

30. Chou S, Lurain NS, Thompson KD, et al. Viral DNA polymerase mutations associated with drug resistance in human cytomegalovirus. *J Infect Dis.* 2003;188:32–39.

31. Chou S, Miner RC, Drew WL. A deletion mutation in region V of the cytomegalovirus DNA polymerase sequence confers multidrug resistance. *J Infect Dis.* 2000;182:1765–1768.

32. Chou S, Waldemer RH, Senters AE, et al. Cytomegalovirus UL97 phosphotransferase mutations that affect susceptibility to ganciclovir. *J Infect Dis.* 2002;185:162–169.

33. Hamprecht K, Eckle T, Prix L, et al. Ganciclovir-resistant cytomegalovirus disease after allogeneic stem cell transplantation: pitfalls of phenotypic diagnosis by in vitro selection of an UL97 mutant strain. *J Infect Dis.* 2003;187:139–143.

34. Kwak EJ, Vilchez RA, Randhawa P, et al. Pathogenesis and management of polyomavirus infection in transplant recipients. *Clin Infect Dis.* 2002;35:1081–1087.

35. Lin PL, Vats AN, Green M. BK virus infection in renal transplant recipients. *Pediatr Transplant.* 2001;5:398–405.

36. Boubenider S, Hiesse C, Marchand S, et al. Post-transplantation polyomavirus infections. *J Nephrol.* 1999;12:24–29.

37. Vats A, Shapiro R, Singh Randhawa P, et al. Quantitative viral load monitoring and cidofovir therapy for the management of BK virus-associated nephropathy in children and adults. *Transplantation.* 2003;75:105–112.

38. Randhawa PS, Finkelstein S, Scantlebury V, et al. Human polyoma virus-associated interstitial nephritis in the allograft kidney. *Transplantation.* 1999;67:103–109.

39. Hirsch HH, Knowles W, Dickenmann M, et al. Prospective study of polyomavirus type BK replication and nephropathy in renal-transplant recipients [comment]. *N Engl J Med.* 2002;347:488–496.

40. Limaye AP, Jerome KR, Kuhr CS, et al. Quantitation of BK virus load in serum for the diagnosis of BK virus-associated nephropathy in renal transplant recipients [comment]. *J Infect Dis.* 2001;183:1669–1672.

41. Ginevri F, De Santis R, Comoli P, et al. Polyomavirus BK infection in pediatric kidney-allograft recipients: a single-center analysis of incidence, risk factors, and novel therapeutic approaches. *Transplantation.* 2003;75:1266–1270.

42. Leung AY, Chan M, Tang SC, et al. Real-time quantitative analysis of polyoma BK viremia and viruria in renal allograft recipients. *J Virol Methods.* 2002;103:51–56.

43. Azzi A, Cesaro S, Laszlo D, et al. Human polyomavirus BK (BKV) load and haemorrhagic cystitis in bone marrow transplantation patients. *J Clin Virol.* 1999;14:79–86.

44. Iwamoto S, Azuma E, Hori H, et al. BK virus-associated fatal renal failure following late-onset hemorrhagic cystitis in an unrelated bone marrow transplantation. *Pediatr Hematol Oncol.* 2002;19:255–261.

45. Leung AY, Suen CK, Lie AK, et al. Quantification of polyoma BK viruria in hemorrhagic cystitis complicating bone marrow transplantation. *Blood.* 2001;98:1971–1978.

46. Gretch D. Standardization of hepatitis C virus—RNA quantification: advances and unfinished business [comment]. *Hepatology.* 2000; 31:788–789.

47. Chan SE, Rosen HR. Outcome and management of hepatitis C in liver transplant recipients. *Clin Infect Dis.* 2003;37:807–812.

48. Wali MH, Heydtmann M, Harrison RF, et al. Outcome of liver transplantation for patients infected by hepatitis C, including those infected by genotype 4. *Liver Transpl.* 2003;9:796–804.

49. Alonso O, Loinaz C, Abradelo M, et al. Changes in the incidence and severity of recurrent hepatitis C after liver transplantation over 1990–1999. *Transplant Proc.* 2003;35:1836–1847.

50. Berenguer M. Natural history of recurrent hepatitis C. *Liver Transpl.* 2002;8(suppl 1):S14–S18.

51. Firpi RJ, Abdelmalek MF, Soldevila-Pico C, et al. Combination of interferon alfa-2b and ribavirin in liver transplant recipients with histological recurrent hepatitis C. *Liver Transpl.* 2002;8:1000–1006.

52. McCaughan GW, Zekry A. Pathogenesis of hepatitis C virus recurrence in the liver allograft. *Liver Transpl.* 2002;8(suppl 1):S7–S13.

53. Costes V, Durand L, Pageaux GP, et al. Hepatitis C virus genotypes and quantification of serum hepatitis C RNA in liver transplant recipients. Relationship with histologic outcome of recurrent hepatitis C. *Am J Clin Pathol.* 1999;111:252–258.

54. Nuovo GJ, Holly A, Wakely P Jr, et al. Correlation of histology, viral load, and in situ viral detection in hepatic biopsies from patients with liver transplants secondary to hepatitis C infection. *Hum Pathol.* 2002;33:277–284.

55. Gigou M, Roque-Afonso AM, Falissard B, et al. Genetic clustering of hepatitis C virus strains and severity of recurrent hepatitis after liver transplantation. *J Virol.* 2001;75:11292–11297.

56. Feray C, Caccamo L, Alexander GJ, et al. European collaborative study on factors influencing outcome after liver transplantation for hepatitis C. European Concerted Action on Viral Hepatitis (EUROHEP) Group. *Gastroenterology.* 1999;117:619–625.

57. Charlton M, Seaberg E, Wiesner R, et al. Predictors of patient and graft survival following liver transplantation for hepatitis C. *Hepatology.* 1998;28:823–830.

58. Zhou S, Terrault NA, Ferrell L, et al. Severity of liver disease in liver transplantation recipients with hepatitis C virus infection: relationship to genotype and level of viremia. *Hepatology.* 1996;24:1041–1046.

59. Holmes RD, Sokol RJ. Epstein-Barr virus and post-transplant lymphoproliferative disease. *Pediatr Transplant.* 2002;6:456–464.

60. Muti G, Cantoni S, Oreste P, et al. Post-transplant lymphoproliferative disorders: improved outcome after clinico-pathologically tailored treatment. *Haematologica.* 2002;87:67–77.

61. Ho M. Risk factors and pathogenesis of posttransplant lymphoproliferative disorders. *Transplant Proc.* 1995;27(suppl 1):38–40.

62. Ho M, Miller G, Atchison RW, et al. Epstein-Barr virus infections and DNA hybridization studies in posttransplantation lymphoma and lymphoproliferative lesions: the role of primary infection. *J Infect Dis.* 1985;152:876–886.

63. Matsukura T, Yokoi A, Egawa H, et al. Significance of serial real-time PCR monitoring of EBV genome load in living donor liver transplantation. *Clin Transplant.* 2002;16:107–112.

64. Merlino C, Cavallo R, Bergallo M, et al. Epstein Barr viral load monitoring by quantitative PCR in renal transplant patients. *New Microbiol.* 2003;26:141–149.

65. Orentas RJ, Schauer DWJ, Ellis FW, et al. Monitoring and modulation of Epstein-Barr virus loads in pediatric transplant patients. *Pediatr Transplant.* 2003;7:305–314.

66. Limaye AP, Huang ML, Atienza EE, et al. Detection of Epstein-Barr virus DNA in sera from transplant recipients with lymphoproliferative disorders [comment]. *J Clin Microbiol.* 1999;37:1113–1116.

67. Riddler SA, Breinig MC, McKnight JL. Increased levels of circulating Epstein-Barr virus (EBV)-infected lymphocytes and decreased EBV nuclear antigen antibody responses are associated with the development of posttransplant lymphoproliferative disease in solid-organ transplant recipients. *Blood.* 1994;84:972–984.

68. Gartner BC, Schafer H, Marggraff K, et al. Evaluation of use of Epstein-Barr viral load in patients after allogeneic stem cell transplantation to diagnose and monitor posttransplant lymphoproliferative disease [erratum appears in *J Clin Microbiol.* 2002;40:2316]. *J Clin Microbiol.* 2002;40:351–358.

69. Campe H, Jaeger G, Abou-Ajram C, et al. Serial detection of Epstein-Barr virus DNA in sera and peripheral blood leukocyte samples of pediatric renal allograft recipients with persistent mononucleosis-like symptoms defines patients at risk to develop post-transplant lymphoproliferative disease. *Pediatr Transplant.* 2003;7:46–52.

70. Kogan-Liberman D, Burroughs M, Emre S, et al. The role of quantitative Epstein-Barr virus polymerase chain reaction and preemptive immunosuppression reduction in pediatric liver transplantation: a preliminary experience [comment]. *J Pediatr Gastroenterol Nutr.* 2001;33:445–449.

71. Griffiths PD, Clark DA, Emery VC. Betaherpesviruses in transplant recipients. *J Antimicrob Chemother.* 2000;45(suppl T3):29–34.

72. Boutolleau D, Fernandez C, Andre E, et al. Human herpesvirus (HHV)-6 and HHV-7: two closely related viruses with different infection profiles in stem cell transplantation recipients. *J Infect Dis.* 2003;187:179–186.

73. Kidd IM, Clark DA, Sabin CA, et al. Prospective study of human beta-herpesviruses after renal transplantation: association of human herpesvirus 7 and cytomegalovirus co-infection with cytomegalovirus disease and increased rejection. *Transplantation.* 2000;69:2400–2404.

74. Humar A, Kumar D, Caliendo AM, et al. Clinical impact of human herpesvirus 6 infection after liver transplantation. *Transplantation.* 2002;73:599–604.

75. Gautheret-Dejean A, Manichanh C, Thien-Ah-Koon F, et al. Development of a real-time polymerase chain reaction assay for the diagnosis of human herpesvirus-6 infection and application to bone marrow transplant patients. *J Virol Methods.* 2002;100:27–35.

76. Ljungman P, Wang FZ, Clark DA, et al. High levels of human herpesvirus 6 DNA in peripheral blood leucocytes are correlated to platelet engraftment and disease in allogeneic stem cell transplant patients. *Br J Haematol.* 2000;111:774–781.

77. Nitsche A, Muller CW, Radonic A, et al. Human herpesvirus 6A DNA Is detected frequently in plasma but rarely in peripheral blood leukocytes of patients after bone marrow transplantation. *J Infect Dis.* 2001;183:130–133.

Chapter 6

Viral Infections of the Central Nervous System

Christine C. Ginocchio

Introduction

Viral infections of the central nervous system (CNS) are relatively infrequent and usually result in a benign, self-limiting disease.[1-4] However, in a small percentage of cases, viral infection of the CNS can have extremely serious consequences that result in a spectrum of permanent neurologic damage or death. Viral agents gain access to the CNS by either neuronal or hematogenous spread, and infections can occur at a multitude of sites including the spinal cord, leptomeninges, dorsal nerve roots, nerves, and brain parenchyma. Viral CNS infections are classified clinically as either meningitis or encephalitis, although a close interrelationship occurs between the two disease states.[1-4] Host factors (age, sex, immune status, genetic differences) and viral factors (serotype, receptor preference, cell tropism, viral load) in concert with geographic and seasonal factors contribute to the potential for the development of CNS disease.[1-4]

Epidemiology

Viral meningitis, meningoencephalitis, and encephalitis frequently occur in epidemics and as seasonal outbreaks (late spring through autumn) and account for the majority of viral CNS infections.[1-4] The most common viral agents responsible for CNS disease are listed in Table 6-1. In the United States and in countries that immunize against mumps, enteroviruses account for approximately 80% to 92% of all cases of meningitis in which a causative agent is identified.[3,4] In countries that do not include mumps in their immunization programs, mumps account for as many as 30% of viral meningitis cases.[5] The arthropod-borne viruses (arboviruses) (Table 6-2) account for the majority of the remaining cases in the United States.[6-8]

Encephalitis occurs at a lower frequency, with arboviruses being the leading cause both worldwide and in the United States.[6-8] The flaviviruses and alphaviruses are the most important and are responsible for the majority of

mosquito and tick-borne encephalitis that cause epidemic and endemic disease in Asia, Europe, and the Americas.[6-8] Case fatality rates vary greatly, ranging from 5% to 70%. Human immunodeficiency virus (HIV) and rabies (genus *Lyssavirus*) are other important causes of encephalitis worldwide.[1,2] Herpes simplex virus (HSV) CNS infections affect all ages, occur at all times of the year, and have the highest mortality rate in the United States.[1-4] In a small number of cases, childhood viral diseases including rubella, measles, varicella-zoster virus (VZV), mumps, and human herpes virus 6 (HHV-6), can progress to neurologic disease during primary infection or with viral reactivation (VZV, HHV-6). Cytomegalovirus (CMV)[9-11] and JC polyomavirus (JCV)[12] are responsible for encephalitides in immunocompromised patients.

Overview of Diagnostic Testing for Viral CNS Disease

Traditionally, the diagnosis of viral CNS infection was based on laboratory findings in conjunction with patient history, clinical manifestations, and geographic and epidemiologic factors.[1-4,7,8] The diagnosis of viral encephalitis requires supplemental tests, including lumbar puncture, radiographic imaging such as computed tomography (CT) scans and magnetic resonance imaging (MRI) studies, and in some cases brain biopsy.

In general, patients with viral meningitis typically have a cerebrospinal fluid (CSF) pleocytosis with 10 to 500 leukocytes, a slightly elevated protein (<100 md/dL), and a glucose level greater than 40% of a simultaneously drawn serum sample.[1,2] However, there can be a tremendous range of values that often overlap with those indicative of bacterial meningitis. Patients with viral encephalitis or meningitis may or may not exhibit a CSF pleocytosis.[13] Therefore, normal CSF cell counts should not be used as a sole exclusion criterion for both diagnosis and determining which samples should be tested by molecular methods for viral pathogens. CSF glucose levels can be normal or low, as seen

Table 6-1. Primary Viral Agents Causing Central Nervous System Disease

Herpesviruses	Herpes simplex 1 and 2
	Varicella-zoster
	Epstein-Barr
	Cytomegalovirus
	Human herpesvirus 6
Enteroviruses	Poliovirus
	Coxsackievirus
	Echovirus
	Numbered enteroviruses
Arboviruses	See Table 6-2
Childhood illness associated	Measles
	Mumps
	Rubella
Rabies	
JC polyoma virus	
Human immunodeficiency virus type 1	

often takes weeks to demonstrate a diagnostic rise in IgG antibody titers between acute and convalescent serum samples.[3,4,12,14–16,18,19] Some patients with West Nile viral infections have detectable IgM antibodies for up to 500 days after infection, making the distinction between recent and past infection difficult.[19] In addition, immune status of the patient can affect the development of viral-specific antibodies.

Currently, molecular amplification methods that detect viral pathogens in CSF play a critical role in the rapid and accurate diagnosis of viral CNS infections.[14,15,17] This approach has largely abrogated the need for brain biopsy for the diagnosis of encephalitis and, in cases where biopsy is needed, can be used to detect viral pathogens in tissue specimens. In most cases, CSF is easily obtained, especially compared to brain biopsy. CSF should be stored frozen, preferably at −70°C, to maintain the stability of viral nucleic acids. Isolation of the nucleic acids is achieved using a variety of methods (described in chapter 2) that also remove amplification inhibitors and neutralize any DNases or RNases present in the sample. The volume of CSF required can vary significantly and is dependent on the viral target, relative levels of virus present in CSF, and sensitivity of the testing method.

Results can be available within 24 hours and as soon as 2 hours for applications utilizing real-time technologies that incorporate amplification and detection in one step. This is in contrast to viral culture and serology, which can require up to 28 days for a final result. The rapid identification of the correct viral agent directs the selection of appropriate antiviral therapy, decreases the number of patients unnecessarily placed on empiric antibiotic therapy, shortens length of hospitalization, and saves medical costs. Overall, molecular amplification assays are highly sensitive and, depending on the virus and amplification target, can detect as low as one viral particle per reaction. High assay specificity is obtained by gene-specific targeting and often is significantly better than serologic testing, which can demonstrate cross-reactivity among related viral agents. Multiplex assays offer the ver-

with bacterial meningitis. Encephalitis can lead to hemorrhagic necrosis with elevated protein levels and the presence of red blood cells.

Cultures for bacterial, fungal, and mycobacterial pathogens can aid in the diagnosis of viral CNS infections but can take several weeks for definitive results. Bacterial cultures may be falsely negative if patients have been treated with antibiotics prior to sample collection. Traditionally, the identification of the specific viral agent relied on viral culture, serologic detection of virus-specific IgM and IgG antibodies, either systemic or intrathecal, or both.[3,4,14–16] However, the ability to isolate the viral agent is highly dependent on the viral species, time of sample collection, sample handling and processing, and treatment of the patient with antiviral agents. In only approximately 10% to 16% of viral meningitis cases is the responsible agent identified using viral culture.[3–5,14–17] Serologic diagnosis can be made in certain cases as early as 5 days after infection with the development of specific IgM antibodies   but

Table 6-2. Arthropod-Borne Viruses (Arboviruses) and Endemic Areas

Family	Genus	Virus	Predominant Regions
Togaviridae	Alphavirus	Eastern equine	Eastern, southern United States; Canada; Central, South America
		Western equine	Western, central United States; Central, South America
		Venezuelan equine	Central, South America; eastern, western United States
Flaviviridae	Flavivirus	St Louis	United States; South America
		Powassan	Canada; United States; Russia
		Tick-borne	Central Europe; Russia
		Japanese	Asia; USSR; India; Sri Lanka
		Murray Valley	United States
		West Nile	North America; Europe; Middle East; Africa; Asia; Australia; Oceania
Bunyaviridae	Bunyavirus	California group*	California; upper Midwest; West Virginia; Virginia; Kentucky; Tennessee; North Carolina; Alabama
Reoviridae	Coltivirus	Colorado tick fever	Western mountain United States
Rhabdoviruses	Lyssavirus	Rabies	Worldwide
		Vesicular stomatitis virus	

*La Crosse, Cache Valley, James-town Canyon, and snowshoe hare.

satility of screening for several pathogens in one test. Quantitative assays are useful for differentiating active from latent infection and for monitoring response to antiviral therapy.

This chapter reviews the advances in the molecular diagnosis of the most common causes of viral meningitis and encephalitis, including the enteroviruses, herpesviruses, and arboviruses. Viral agents affecting persons with immune suppression are briefly discussed, including human immunodeficiency virus type 1 (HIV-1), JC polyomavirus (JCV), and CMV.

ENTEROVIRUSES

Epidemiology and Disease

Enteroviruses are small single-stranded RNA viruses that comprise 64 serotypes distributed into five species of the Picornaviridae family.[20,21] The nonpolio enteroviruses, including the coxsackieviruses, echoviruses, and numbered enteroviruses, are responsible for approximately 50 million infections per year in the United States and possibly more than a billion worldwide.[4,21,22] Enteroviruses cause a diverse array of illnesses in both adults and children, including respiratory, ocular, cardiac, gastrointestinal, and neurologic diseases and skin and oral eruptions.[21,22] In the neonate, enteroviruses can cause a sepsislike picture or meningoencephalitis, which can be severe. Outside of the neonatal period, children under 5 years of age appear to be the most susceptible to infection, partly due to a lack of acquired immunity and poor hygienic habits. Encephalitis is uncommon and meningitis is rarely associated with complicated disease and poor clinical outcome, although it may be more severe in adults than in children. Although enteroviral infections can occur year-round, the majority of the infections occur during the summer through autumn months.

Laboratory Diagnosis

Many enteroviruses can be cultured in human and primate cell lines.[21] No single cell line is optimal for all enteroviral types, and therefore several different susceptible culture cell lines are used. Viral CSF culture has a sensitivity of approximately 65% to 75%, in part because of the lability of the virus, possible low levels in the CSF, and the inability to grow all enteroviral serotypes in tissue culture, including several coxsackievirus A strains that require mouse inoculation for detection. The results of viral culture can take 3 to 8 days and therefore are generally not rapid enough to affect either treatment options or length of hospitalization. Patients are placed on unnecessary antibiotic therapy until bacterial CSF cultures are negative at 48 to 72 hours. A variety of serologic assays can be used to diagnose enteroviral infections, but they can be cross-reactive, nonspecific, and difficult to interpret due to the extended incubation and prodromal periods found with many enteroviral illnesses, and hence are not clinically useful.

Molecular Tests

To increase the sensitivity of enterovirus detection and to reduce the time to results, a variety of molecular tests have been developed.[17,23-35] The methods utilize either reverse transcription–polymerase chain reaction (RT-PCR) amplification combined with enzyme-linked immuno sorbent assay (ELISA),[23-28,31] real-time RT-PCR[30] or nucleic acid sequence–based amplification (NASBA) combined with either electrochemiluminescence (ECL) detection[29,32,34] or molecular beacon technology.[33,35] The assays utilize primer sequences selected from the conserved 5′ nontranslated region of the enteroviral genome. Sequence variations are present in this region, and the scope of detection of the various enteroviral serotypes is dependent on primer selection.[23-35] Since different serotypes circulate in distinct areas of the world, assays should be validated using local clinical isolates and reference strains known to be endemic in the region. Overall, enterovirus molecular tests are highly sensitive, some detecting as low as 0.1 tissue culture infectious dose 50 ($TCID_{50}$) and the majority of enteroviral isolates.[23-35] The tests also are highly specific, showing no cross-reactivity with other viral agents, with the exception of a rare rhinovirus.[30,31,34]

Currently, analyte-specific reagents (ASRs) are available for enteroviral detection from CSF. The Enterovirus Consensus assay (Argene Biosoft, Varilhes, France) utilizes RT-PCR and a stair primer technology that was designed to overcome the problems associated with sequence divergence in the primer binding regions, thus ensuring the detection of all 64 enteroviral serotypes.[31] The assay was shown to be more sensitive than assays using the original Rotbart[23] and Zolli[25] primers, and exhibited cross-reactivity with rhinovirus type 3 only. Studies have determined that the sensitivity of the assay is <0.4 $TCID_{50}$ and can detect approximately 6 RNA copies per input reaction. A NucliSens Basic Kit assay (bioMérieux, Boxtel, the Netherlands) that combines NASBA and ECL detection shows reactivity with all enteroviral isolates tested and a sensitivity in the range of 10 to 100 RNA copies.[29,32,34] Minimal low-level cross-reactivity has been detected for one rhinovirus isolate when tested at high titers. No cross-reactivity was demonstrated for other viral isolates. The assay is 18% to 32% more sensitive than CSF viral culture and 100% specific.[29,32,34] This assay has been modified for rapid real-time detection using molecular beacons and is currently available as an ASR (bioMérieux, Durham, NC).[33,35] This modification has reduced the time to results from 5.5 hours to as little as 3.5 hours, thus permitting multiple test runs per day. An additional enterovirus ASR real-time RT-PCR assay, developed for use on the SmartCycler and GeneXpert instruments (Cepheid, Sunnyvale, CA), is currently under evaluation.

HERPESVIRUSES

The herpesviruses, including herpes simplex virus types 1 and 2 (HSV-1, HSV-2), VZV, CMV, and HHV-6, cause a broad spectrum of viral CNS disease including meningitis, encephalitis, meningoencephalitis, myelitis, and polyradiculitis.[1,2] Epstein-Barr virus (EBV) DNA has been detected in virtually all AIDS-related cases of primary CNS lymphomas.[36] CMV is discussed briefly under diseases associated with immunosuppression and in detail in chapter 5.

HERPES SIMPLEX

Epidemiology and Disease

HSV-2 is the usual cause of HSV meningitis and accounts for approximately 1% to 5% of all cases of viral meningitis and 4% to 6% of cases of viral encephalitis.[1–4,37,38] The clinical course of the disease usually is self-limiting and generally not associated with permanent neurological damage. HSV-2 also causes Mollaret meningitis, a benign recurrent meningitis.[39] HSV-1 is responsible for the majority of HSV-associated encephalitis and for about 10% to 20% (approximately 1250 cases per year in the United States) of all viral encephalitis cases. Approximately 30% are primary HSV-1 infection, and the remaining cases are due to HSV reactivation. In contrast to HSV meningitis, HSV encephalitis can be a devastating disease, presenting with focal neurologic disease resulting from damage to one or both temporal lobes.[1–4,37,38] Encephalitis occurs in approximately 60% to 75% of babies with disseminated HSV disease, and without appropriate antiviral therapy the mortality rate can be as high as 80%.[40]

Diagnosis

CSF viral cultures are positive only in approximately 15% of the cases of HSV meningitis due to primary infection and, with the exception of neonatal infection, are rarely positive in cases of HSV encephalitis.[1–4,37,38,40] Traditionally, the diagnosis of HSV encephalitis was dependent on brain biopsy for obtaining tissue for viral culture, electron microscopy, immunohistochemical staining, and the demonstration of intrathecal production of HSV-specific antibodies.[1–3,14–16,38,40] Over the last decade, studies comparing HSV CSF PCR with brain biopsy, intrathecal HSV-specific antibody production for the diagnosis of HSV CNS infections, or both demonstrated sensitivities and specificities for PCR ranging from 96% to 98% and 96% to 99%, respectively.[14,40–42] HSV PCR can identify infected persons who fail to either seroconvert in primary infection or demonstrate significant rises in antibody titers after

reactivation. Finally, HSV PCR can aid in differentiating HSV antibody increases due to active HSV CNS infection and reactivation in persons with concomitant CNS disease not related to HSV. Another advantage of PCR assays for diagnosis of HSV encephalitis is that the assay sensitivity remains high (95%) up to approximately 1 week after initiating therapy.[42] Since DNA can be slow to clear from the CSF (as many as 21% of CSF specimens can remain PCR positive for more than 15 days after completion of therapy), PCR should not be used as a test of cure.[42]

VARICELLA-ZOSTER

Epidemiology and Disease

The most common manifestation of VZV resulting from primary infection is chickenpox and generally occurs in early childhood.[43] VZV-associated neurologic syndromes include acute cerebella ataxia, diffuse or focal encephalitis, meningitis, transverse myelitis, and Reye syndrome.[1,2,43] Herpes zoster, resulting from the reactivation of latent VZV infection, occurs in approximately 20% of immunocompetent persons, generally 45 years or older, and the incidence is approximately 15% higher in persons with immunosuppression.[43,44] In a small percentage of these cases, severe complications, including meningitis, encephalitis, myelitis, Ramsay Hunt syndrome, Guillian-Barré syndrome, and contralateral hemiplegia can occur.[43–45]

Diagnosis

The recovery of VZV in culture is poor (20% positive), as is serologic diagnosis (48% positive).[46] Antigen detection by immunofluorescence improves detection (82% positive), and PCR is the most sensitive, with a detection rate of approximately 95%.[46] Based on improved detection with PCR assays, VZV accounts for 6% to 30% of all herpesviruses isolated from CSF.[46–54] However, results need to be interpreted cautiously since VZV DNA has been detected in CSF without overt disease, particularly in patients with immunosuppression.

HUMAN HERPES VIRUS 6

Epidemiology and Disease

HHV-6 is generally acquired early in life and is manifested as exanthem subitum, more commonly known as roseola or as a nonexanthemous febrile illness, sometimes accompanied by severe neurologic manifestations, including febrile seizures, meningitis, meningoencephalitis, and encephalitis.[55] Detection of HHV-6 in children with a febrile seizure is important for identifying children with a potential for the recurrence of seizure episodes due to ongoing HHV-6 infection. Immunocompromised patients can manifest severe postprimary infections, including encephalitis due to HHV-6 reactivation.[55]

Diagnosis

Culture confirmation of HHV-6 infection is not routinely performed in clinical virology laboratories since it requires purification and culture of patient lymphocytes or cocultivation of activated patient lymphocytes and activated human umbilical cord blood lymphocytes.[55] Serologic confirmation of the disease depends on the detection of IgM in primary infection or conversion from either a negative to a positive IgG antibody response or a four-fold or greater rise in IgG antibody titer.[55] Antibody titers can be difficult to interpret for several reasons. IgM antibodies may not develop in some children, can be positive with HHV-6 reactivation, and can remain positive for extended periods of time. Significant rises in HHV-6-specific IgG antibody titers can be found during infections with other herpesviruses. The detection of HHV-6 DNA in the CNS by PCR can support the diagnosis; however, in a percentage of cases, HHV-6 DNA can be found in normal brain tissue and in the CSF of children without evidence of CNS disease.[55] Quantitative methods may be more accurate for correlating the presence of HHV-6 with active disease.[56,57]

Molecular Tests for Herpesviruses

Comparisons of the sensitivity of HSV PCR to viral culture, antibody detection, and direct immunofluorescence assays have clearly established the utility of PCR as a first-line diagnostic test in the clinical laboratory.[5,14,15,17] Most PCR assays are applicable to the majority of conventional or real-time PCR instruments. The assays for herpesviruses use a variety of primer sets targeting a number of genes including: DNA polymerase gene (HSV-1, HSV-2, CMV, EBV, VZV, HHV-6); UL42, glycoprotein B (gB), glycoprotein D (gD), or thymidine kinase (TK) genes (HSV); genes 28 and 29 (VZV); and major capsid protein, U89/U90 (HHV-6). Identification of the specific herpesvirus is achieved using either traditional methods, including the use of species-specific primers, hybridization with species-specific probes, agarose gel electrophoresis, restriction enzyme analysis, and ELISA-based colorimetric detection methods,[46-49,51,52] or fluorescent probe technologies that permit real-time detection.[50,53,54] Currently, no test kits are approved or cleared by Food and Drug Administration (FDA) for the detection of herpesviruses; however, several commercial kits or ASRs are available for the detection of herpesviruses in CSF. Roche Diagnostics (Indianapolis, IN) has developed ASRs for HSV-1, HSV-2, VZV, and EBV identification using the LightCycler instrument.[50,53,54] A single-tube amplification and detection step allows the identification of both HSV-1 and HSV-2 and the differentiation of subtype by melting-curve analysis.[50] The manufacturer's claim of sensitivity is approximately 12.5 copies

or 2.5 to 6.3 genome equivalents per reaction. Artus Biotech (Artus GmbH, Hamburg, Germany) has real-time PCR assays (Real/Art LC PCR) for the detection of HSV-1, HSV-2, EBV, and VZV, for individual analytes (EBV, VZV) or as multiplex tests (HSV-1 and HSV-2, VZV and EBV, and HSV-1, HSV-2, VZV, and EBV). Each kit includes all PCR reagents, primers, probes, internal amplification control, and, for HSV, external calibration controls for quantitation. According to the manufacturer, the detection limits (95% probability) of the assays are 1 copy/mL for HSV, 0.7 copies/mL for VZV, and 0.2 copies/mL for EBV.

Multiplex assays that can screen simultaneously for the six major herpesviruses (HSV-1, HSV-2, CMV, VZV, EBV, HHV-6) offer some distinct advantages, including the detection of coinfections in the CNS and the identification of a herpesvirus that may not have been considered in the original diagnosis.[58] Several laboratory-developed assays have been validated for this purpose using either traditional or real-time PCR methods,[14,47-54] and currently two commercial ASR multiplex systems that use standard platform PCR and screen for all six herpesvirus are available.[48] The Herpes Mplex (Prodesse Inc, Waukesha, WI) includes primers, probes, internal and external controls, and all PCR reagents, with the exception of amplification enzyme. The Herpes Generic Consensus kit (Argene Biosoft, Varilhes, France) uses stair primers to compensate for sequence divergence in the primer binding regions of the six herpesviruses.[48] After PCR amplification and generic colorimetric detection of the herpesvirus, the Herpes Identification Hybridomawell kit (Argene Biosoft, Varilhes, France) is used to identify the specific herpesvirus present. All primers, probes, an internal control, external controls, and all PCR reagents, with the exception of amplification enzyme, are provided. Assay sensitivity varies between 5 and 50 copies per PCR reaction, with EBV being the least sensitive. Another Argene Biosoft kit (Herpes Simplex Consensus 1/2) is available to screen for just HSV-1 and HSV-2.

ARBOVIRUSES

Epidemiology and Disease

Alphaviruses, flaviviruses, and bunyaviruses are responsible for the majority of the arboviral encephalopathies (Table 6-2) and are found throughout the world.[1,2,6] The encephalitides are zoonotic, and transmission of the viruses occurs between susceptible amplifier vertebrate hosts, such as birds, squirrels, and chipmunks, via blood-feeding arthropods, including mosquitoes, psychodids, ticks, and ceratopogonids. Peak incidence occurs in summer and continues through the fall months, when arthropods are most active. In warmer regions cases can occur into the winter months. Humans, horses, and domestic animals can develop a clinical illness. The majority of human arboviral infections are either asymptomatic or manifest as a flulike self-limiting illness. Occasionally viruses enter the brain by mechanisms not clearly understood, and productive infection of brain cells occurs, resulting in encephalitis, often with a fatal outcome or permanent neurologic damage.[1,2,6]

The mosquito-borne viruses were first discovered in the 1930s.[6] Until 1999 and the emergence of West Nile virus (WNV) in Queens, New York,[59] the most important cause of epidemic and endemic encephalitis in the United States was St Louis encephalitis virus (SLE), which is found throughout the lower 48 states. Confirmed cases of SLE average approximately 193 per year, and 4437 cases have been reported to the Centers for Disease Control and Prevention (CDC; Atlanta, GA), since 1964.[7] Less than 1% of the cases are clinically apparent, with a case fatality rate of 5% to 25% for symptomatic persons.[7] Since the initial outbreak in 1999, WNV has migrated across the United States, and by August 2005 all but three states (Alaska, Hawaii, and Washington) have reported bird, mosquito, vertebrate, or human cases.[7,8] WNV is responsible for neuroinvasive disease (encephalitis and meningitis) and what is termed West Nile fever, which is typically less severe and does not show signs of neuroinvasion.[59] As of August 2005, 17,039 WNV cases with 674 deaths have been reported to the CDC.[7,8] Approximately one in 150 WNV cases progresses to meningitis or encephalitis, the most common neurological manifestation. Case fatality rates remain constant at approximately 12%, with advanced age being the most important risk factor for death.[6,7,8] In addition, WNV has been transmitted to persons receiving either transfusions or transplanted organs from asymptomatic donors infected with WNV.[8,59,60] La Crosse virus (LAC) is found in several midwestern and mid-Atlantic states, and an average of 70 cases are reported per year, usually in children under the age of 16. Since 1964, eastern equine encephalitis (EEE) virus and western equine encephalitis (WEE) virus have been responsible for 200 and 639 cases, respectively.[7] In the northern United States, Powassan virus is a minor cause of encephalitis and is transmitted by ticks.[7]

Japanese encephalitis (JE) virus, found mainly in Asia and the Pacific, is the leading cause of encephalitis worldwide, with more than 45,000 cases reported annually.[1,2,6] Venezuelan encephalitis virus remains the third most common cause of equine encephalitides and the most common cause of epidemic encephalitis in Central and South America.[1,2,6]

Diagnosis

By the time persons present with encephalitic symptoms, the viremic phase of the disease often has ceased and infected persons have developed serum and intrathecal IgM or IgG antibodies or both.[6,59] Since IgM antibodies do not cross the blood-brain barrier, the identification of virus-specific IgM antibodies in the CSF is strongly suggestive of CNS infection. A variety of assays including hemagglutination inhibition, complement fixation, plaque reduction neutralization test (PRNT), IgM antibody

capture ELISA (MAC-ELISA) and IgG antibody ELISA, indirect immunofluorescence (IFA), and antigen capture ELISA have been useful in the identification of arboviral infections.[6,59,61,62] Confirmation of the virus-specific IgM antibodies or the demonstration of a four-fold or greater rise in neutralizing IgG antibodies in either CSF or serum is achieved by performing PRNT with multiple arboviruses. Older serologic assays were technically demanding, lacked reproducibility, and were often poor measures of early IgM production. Recently developed MAC-ELISAs are more reliable, rapid and reproducible.[59,61,62] In persons with immunosuppressive disorders or who are very early in the course of the infection, antibody titers can be negative and the diagnosis is dependent on isolation of the virus. However, due to the transient nature of the viremic stage and probably low levels of virus in the CSF and serum, virus isolation using cell culture generally has been unsuccessful and not practical for most clinical laboratories.

Although serological confirmation of disease remains the gold standard, molecular tests are important for identifying early infection prior to seroconversion, infected transplant tissues and blood,[59,60] and infection in immunocompromised patients, and for diagnosis confirmation.[59,63-66] A positive result with a nucleic acid amplification assay is diagnostic of an arboviral infection; however, a negative result does not preclude the possibility of an arboviral infection. For example, up to 55% of CSF samples and only approximately 10% of serum samples are positive in patients with serologically confirmed cases of WNV disease.[59] The molecular detection of arboviral nucleic acids is standard for vector-borne disease surveillance studies and control programs[59,63,64,66,67] and for monitoring both the blood supply and transplantation tissues.[59,60]

Molecular Tests

Several assays using traditional RT-PCR, nested RT-PCR, Taqman-based RT-PCR, and NASBA combined with either ECL or molecular beacon detection have been developed for the identification of arboviral infections.[59,63-67] Assay methods are highly sensitive, specific, and rapid, with results available in as little as 2 hours for real-time RT-PCR and NASBA molecular beacon assays. Primers usually target the NS1, NS3, NS5, and 3' NC regions of the genomes of the flaviviruses. Primer probe sets may be virus specific,[63,64,66] or universal primers can be used for the detection of all flaviviruses.[65] Studies by Lanciotti et al., Division of Vector-Borne Infectious Diseases, CDC (Fort Collins, Colorado), have clearly defined the status of molecular testing for arboviral infections in both humans and surveillance populations, including mosquito pools, dead birds, horses, and other vertebrates.[63,64,66] The results of Lanciotti and colleagues' evaluations of laboratory-developed RT-PCR, Taqman RT-PCR, and NASBA-based assays for the detection of WNV, EEE, SLE, and WEE viruses are summarized

Table 6-3. Sensitivities of the RT-PCR, Taqman, NASBA ECL, and NASBA Molecular Beacon Assays for the Detection of WN, SLE, EEE, and WEE Viral Culture Isolates (PFU detected*)

Assay	WNV	SLE	EEE	WEE
RT-PCR	1.00	0.15	0.77	35
Taqman	0.10	0.15	0.77	0.35
NASBA-ECL	0.01	0.15	0.77	3.5
NASBA-MB	0.10	0.15	ND	ND

Sources: References 62 and 64.
*Number of plaque-forming units (PFU) detected by assay. NASBA, nucleic acid sequence–based amplification; ECL, electrochemiluminescence; MB, molecular beacon; WNV, West Nile virus; SLE, St Louis encephalitis virus; EEE, eastern equine encephalitis virus; WEE, western equine encephalitis virus; ND, not done; PFU, plaque-forming units.

in Tables 6-3 and 6-4. The Taqman and NASBA assays are currently used by the US Public Health Laboratories for both human diagnosis and surveillance studies. ASR for performing real-time RT-PCR (Real/Art WNV RT-PCR) are available from Artus Biotech with a manufacturer's claim of detection sensitivity of 5 to 20 nucleic acid copies per reaction. Prodesse has two ASR reagents available, one using standard RT-PCR and one using real-time RT-PCR, with limits of detection of 50 and 500 copies/mL, respectively, as per the manufacturer. Full assessment of the Artus Biotech and Prodesse assays is currently limited by the lack of sufficient clinical data.

VIRAL AGENTS ASSOCIATED WITH IMMUNOSUPPRESSION

CYTOMEGALOVIRUS

Epidemiology and Disease

CMV disease may be due to primary infection but generally is related to CMV reactivation in association with progressive immune deficiency.[9–11] Neurological syndromes associated with CMV include peripheral neuropathy, ventriculoencephalitis, myelitis/polyradiculopathy, and diffuse micronodular encephalitis with dementia.[9–11]

Diagnosis

The presumptive diagnosis of CMV CNS disease has been based primarily on clinical presentation, serologic testing, neuroradiologic studies including CT and MRI, CSF chemistries, and the magnitude and types of CSF pleocytosis.[9–11] CSF viral culture is positive in only approximately 50% of patients with CMV CNS disease, and culture is relatively slow, requiring between 1 and 4 weeks for detection.[9–11]

Molecular Tests

Various molecular methods have been used to more accurately and rapidly detect CMV in patients with active CMV CNS disease.[68] Several studies have determined that the detection of CMV DNA by PCR in CSF of aquired immunodeficiency syndrome (AIDS) patients was highly sensitive (100% negative predictive value for CNS disease) but did not always correlate with active CMV CNS disease (68.4% positive predictive value for CNS disease).[68] Sensitive qualitative PCR may detect nonreplicating virus, which could clearly limit the use of these tests in the differentiation of asymptomatic infection from active CNS disease. Quantitative PCR assays with established cut-off values for differentiating infection from active disease may provide an alternative superior to qualitative PCR. For example, CSF from AIDS patients with autopsy-proven CMV encephalitis had a median value of 3333 CMV genomes/10^5 cells compared to a median value of 125/10^5 cells for AIDS patients with neurologic symptoms not related to CMV, and a median value of 19/10^5 cells for HIV-1 seronegative controls.[68] High levels of cellular CMV correlated with marked histopathologic changes in AIDS patients.

Table 6-4. Sensitivities of Vero Cell Culture, Taqman Assay, NASBA-ECL Assay, and RT-PCR Assay for the Detection of EEE, WEE, and WNV from Mosquito Pools and WNV from Human CSF Specimens

Mosquito Pools

	Number Tested	Viral Culture Pos	Taqman Pos/Equiv	NASBA-ECL Pos/Equiv	RT-PCR Pos/Equiv
EEE	20	4	9	7	4
WEE	20	0	3	2	3
WNV	68	32	31/2	34	24/7

CSF Samples

	Number Tested	Serology Pos	Taqman Pos/Equiv	NASBA ECL Pos/Equiv	RT-PCR Pos/Equiv
WNV	10	10	4/3	7/0	0/0
WNV	10	0	0	0	0

Sources: References 62 and 64.
NASBA, nucleic acid sequence-based amplification; ECL, electrochemiluminescence; WNV, West Nile virus; SLE, St Louis Encephalitis virus; EEE, eastern equine encephalitis virus; WEE, western equine encephalitis virus; ND, not done; Pos, positive; Equiv, equivocal.

Additional studies are necessary to determine the level of CMV DNA that would be considered indicative of active CNS disease.

Several PCR-based commercial test kits, including the Amplicor Cytomegalovirus test (Roche Molecular Systems, Branchburg, NJ), PrimeCapture CMV DNA Detection Plate System (Synthetic Genetics, San Diego, CA), Herpes Mplex (Prodesse, Inc), and Herpes Generic Consensus kit (Argene, Inc), have been used to detect human CMV in CSF.[64] In addition, the Amplicor CMV Monitor test, the Digene CMV Hybrid Capture assay (Digene Corp, Gaithersburg, MD), and quantitative CMV real-time DNA-based PCR assays developed for use with the LightCycler instrument are available to quantify CMV DNA from a variety of clinical specimens.

A different approach, used in both transplantation recipients and HIV-1-infected persons for diagnosing active disease versus asymptomatic CMV infection, is based on detection of CMV mRNA transcripts (immediate-early and early, UL83, pp150, pp67).[68,69] The NucliSens pp67 assay (bioMérieux, Boxtel, the Netherlands) detects the presence of mRNA encoding for the phosphorylated matrix tegument protein pp67, one of the most abundant late gene transcripts that is detectable when viral replication is occurring. The detection of pp67 mRNA in CSF was found to be the most accurate in diagnosing active CMV CNS disease (100% positive predictive value [PPV], 97% negative predictive value [NPV]), when compared to viral culture (100% PPV, 82.7% NPV) and qualitative DNA PCR (68.4 % PPV, 100% NPV).[69] In addition to diagnostic utility, quantitative PCR and the NucliSens pp67 assay have been effective for monitoring response to therapy for CMV infections.[68]

HUMAN JC POLYOMAVIRUS

Epidemiology and Disease

Primary infection with human JCV generally occurs early in life, is usually asymptomatic, and results in a latent infection of both renal tissues and B lymphocytes.[12] Reactivation occurs during cell-mediated immune deficiency and can lead to the rapidly evolving severe demyelinating disease of the CNS, progressive multifocal leukoencephalopathy (PML). This disease is primarily seen in patients with AIDS and, prior to the era of highly active antiretroviral therapy (HAART), was a serious cause of infection in 2% to 10% of AIDS patients.

Diagnosis

The diagnosis of PML can be difficult, was generally presumptive, and was based on imaging techniques (CT and MRI) in combination with serologic studies, virus isolation by cell culture, and electron microscopy.[12] Often confir-

mation required histopathological analysis of brain biopsy materials.

Molecular Tests

Several PCR-based strategies to detect JCV in CSF have been established for the diagnosis of PML and to monitor patients with AIDS who achieved a PML remission as a result of HAART.[12,70-72] Testing has included unique or sequential CSF samples, with assays developed using single or nested PCR combined with conventional or real-time detection technologies. Primers have targeted different noncoding and coding (VP1, VP2, small T-antigen, large T-antigen) regions, often with variable results, presumably due to the large amount of sequence variation within the various subtypes of JCV.[12] Using a variety of PCR assays, the rate of detection of JCV in CSF from patients with PML ranged from 30% to 89.5%.[70-72] Specificity of PCR for identifying viral isolates of JCV was 100%, while specificity for the diagnosis of confirmed PML was generally about 95%.[70-72] In summary, CSF examination for JCV DNA was shown to be useful for confirming the diagnosis of PML. However, a negative test does not preclude the possibility of PML and brain biopsy is necessary to confirm such cases.

HUMAN IMMUNODEFICIENCY VIRUS

Early in the course of infection, HIV-1 enters the CNS.[73,74] A complex interaction between the virus and host immune responses leads to neurological damage that is manifested by a variety of syndromes including meningitis, encephalitis, peripheral neuropathies, and AIDS dementia complex (ADC).[73,74]

Molecular Tests

High HIV-1 RNA levels in CSF correlate with an increased incidence of ADC and with the presence of cerebral atrophy.[73] Most persons with high CSF viral load have concomitant high plasma viral load. However, there are patients on HAART with either very-low-level or undetectable plasma viral load (<50 copies/ml) who have signs of neurologic disease and high CSF viral load (>50,000 copies/ml). Studies have indicated that suppression of plasma viral load does not always correspond with HIV-1 suppression in other body compartments, and the monitoring of such compartments may be indicated in certain clinical situations. Therefore, when neurological symptoms are evident, it is important to measure HIV-1 levels in the CSF. Detectable viral load in the CSF can affect the selection of HAART, since not all drugs penetrate the CSF to the same degree. In addition, due to the large overlap of neurological symptoms associated with the various AIDS-related neurological disorders, such as CMV encephalopathies and PML, CSF viral load can aid in the differential diagnosis of ADC.[69] The measurement of CSF viral load can be achieved using a variety of commercially available methods described in chapter 3.

Conclusions and Future Considerations

Currently, the application of molecular testing for the detection of clinically relevant viral CNS infections is considered the standard of care. For certain viral pathogens, such as HSV, molecular tests are considered the new gold standard, whereas for arboviral infections, serology remains the gold standard for human disease, yet molecular assays are useful for mosquito, bird, and vertebrate surveillance studies. Molecular tests are rapid, accurate and significantly impact patient management and outcome. The selection of the best method or target must be carefully considered, as variations in both can affect the overall performance of the assays. In certain cases, where latent viruses may be detected, quantitative assays or assays that target mRNA rather than DNA may provide more useful clinical correlation for CNS disease. Laboratories must thoroughly evaluate and validate the tests, continue to monitor technical performance, and maintain strict environmental precautions to prevent cross-contamination of samples. Standardization of test methods and cooperative participation in proficiency programs will improve performance and correlation of intra- and interlaboratory results.

References

1. Cassady KA, Whitley RJ. Pathogenesis and pathophysiology of viral central nervous system diseases. In: Scheld WM, Whitey RJ, Durack DT, eds. *Infections of the Central Nervous System*. Philadelphia, Lippincott-Raven; 1997:7–22.
2. Cassady KA, Whitley RJ. Viral central nervous system infections. In: Richman DD, Whitley RJ, Hayden FG, eds. *Clinical Virology*. Washington, DC. ASM Press; 2002:27–44.
3. Hammer SM, Connolly KJ. Viral aseptic meningitis in the United States: clinical features, viral etiologies, and differential diagnosis. *Curr Clin Top Infect Dis*. 1992;12:1–25.
4. Rotbart HA. Viral meningitis. *Semin Neurol*. 2000;20:277–292.
5. Hosoya M, Honzumi K, Sato M, et al. Application of PCR for various neurotropic viruses on the diagnosis of viral meningitis. *J Clin Virol*. 1998;11:117–124.
6. Gubler DJ, Roehrig JT. Arboviruses (*Togaviridae* and *Flaviviridae*). In: Collier L, ed. *Topley and Wilson's Microbiology and Microbial Infections*. ASM Press, London; 1996.
7. Centers for Disease Control and Prevention. Division of Vector-Borne Infectious Diseases. Arboviral encephalitides. August 2005. Available at: http://www.cdc.gov/ncidod/dvbid/index.htm.
8. Centers for Disease Control and Prevention. Division of Vector-Borne Infectious Diseases. West Nile virus. August 2005. Available at: http://www.cdc.gov/ncidod/dvbid/westnile/index.htm.
9. Hibberd PL, Snydman DR. Cytomegalovirus infection in organ transplant recipients. *Infect Dis Clin North Am*. 1995;9:863–877.
10. Ives DV. Cytomegalovirus disease in AIDS. *AIDS*. 1997;11:1791–1797.
11. Cinque P, Marenzi R, Ceresa D. Cytomegalovirus infections of the nervous system. *Intervirology*. 1997;40:85–97.
12. Safak M, Khalili K. An overview: human polyomavirus JC virus and its associated disorders. *J Neurovirol*. 2003;9(suppl 1):3–9.
13. Landry ML. Frequency of normal cerebrospinal fluid protein level and leukocyte count in enterovirus meningitis. *J Clin Virol*. 2005;32:73–74.
14. Cinque P, Cleator GM, Weber T, et al. The role of laboratory investigation in the diagnosis and management of patients with suspected herpes simplex encephalitis: a consensus report. *J Neurol Neurosurg Psychiatry* 1996;61:339–345.
15. Thomson R, Bertram H. Laboratory diagnosis of central nervous system infections. *Infect Dis Clin North Am*. 2001;15:1047–1071.
16. Reiber H, Lange P. Quantitation of virus specific antibodies in cerebrospinal fluid and serum; sensitive and specific detection of antibody synthesis in the brain. *Clin Chem*. 1991;37:1153–1160.
17. Cinque P, Bossolasco S, Lundkvist A. Molecular analysis of cerebrospinal fluid in viral diseases of the central nervous system. *J Clin Virol*. 2003;26:1–28.
18. Johnson A, Martin D, Karabatsos N, et al. Detection of anti-arboviral immunoglobulin G by using a monoclonal antibody-based capture enzyme-linked immunosorbent assay. *J Clin Microbiol*. 2000;38:1827–1831.
19. Roehrig JT, Nash D, Maldin B, et al. Persistence of virus-reactive serum immunoglobulin M antibody in confirmed West Nile virus encephalitis cases. *Emerg Infect Dis*. 2003;9:376–379.
20. van Regenmortel MHG, Fauquet CM, Bishop EB, et al. *Virus Taxonomy. Seventh Report of the International Committee on Taxonomy of Viruses*. New York: Academic Press; 2000.
21. Pallansch MA, Roos RP. Enteroviruses: polioviruses, coxsackieviruses, echoviruses, and newer enteroviruses. In: Knipe DM, Howley PM, Griffin DE, et al., eds. *Fields Virology*. Philadelphia: Lippincott Williams and Wilkins; 2001:723–775.
22. Rotbart HA. Enteroviral infections of the central nervous system. *Clin Infect Dis*. 1995;20:971–981.
23. Rotbart HA. 1990. Enzymatic RNA amplification of the enteroviruses. *J Clin Microbiol*. 1990;28:438–442.
24. Rotbart HA. Diagnosis of enteroviral meningitis with the polymerase chain reaction. *J Pediatr*. 1990;117:85–89.
25. Zoll GJ, Melchers JG, Kopecka H, et al. General primer-mediated polymerase chain reaction detection of enteroviruses; application for diagnostic routine and persistent infections. *J Clin Microbiol*. 1992;30:160–165.
26. Oberste MS, Maher K, Flemister MR, et al. Comparison of classic and molecular approaches for the identification of untypeable enteroviruses. *J Clin Microbiol*. 2000;38:1170–1174.
27. Ramers C, Billman G, Hartin M, et al. Impact of a diagnostic cerebrospinal fluid enterovirus polymerase chain reaction test on patient management. *JAMA*. 2000;283:2680–2685.
28. Stellrecht KA, Harding I, Hussain FM, et al. A one-step RT-PCR assay using an enzyme-linked detection system for the diagnosis of enterovirus meningitis. *J Clin Virol*. 2000;17:143–149.
29. Fox JD, Han S, Samuelson A, et al. Development and evaluation of nucleic acid sequence based amplification (NASBA) for diagnosis of enterovirus infections using the NucliSens Basic Kit. *J Clin Virol*. 2002;24:117–130.
30. Verstrepen WA, Bruynseels P, Mertens AH. Evaluation of a rapid real-time RT-PCR assay for detection of enterovirus RNA in cerebrospinal fluid specimens. *J Clin Virol*. 2002;25:S39-S43.
31. Bourlet T, Caro V, Minjolle S, et al. New PCR test that recognizes all human prototypes if enterovirus: application for clinical diagnosis. *J Clin Microbiol*. 2003;41:1750–1752.
32. Landry ML, Garner R, Ferguson D. Rapid enterovirus RNA detection in clinical specimens by using nucleic acid sequence-based amplification. *J Clin Microbiol*. 2003;41:346–350.
33. Sillekens P, Foolen H, Overdijk M, et al. Development of a real-time NASBA application for the diagnosis of enteroviral meningitis

[abstract T4]. University of South Florida Clinical Virology Symposium, Pan American Society for Clinical Virology, Clearwater, Florida; April, 2003.

34. Ginocchio CC, Zhang F, Malhotra A, et al. Development, technical performance, and clinical evaluation of a NucliSens Basic Kit application for detection of enterovirus RNA in cerebrospinal fluid. *J Clin Microbiol.* 2005;43:2616–2623.

35. Landry ML, Garner R, Ferguson D. Real-time Rapid nucleic acid sequence-based amplification using molecular beacons for detection of enterovirus RNA in clinical specimens. *J Clin Microbiol.* 2005;43:3136–3139.

36. International Agency for Research on Cancer. Epstein-Barr virus and Kaposi's sarcoma herpesvirus/human herpes virus 8. *IARC Monogr Eval Carcinog Risk Chem Hum.* 1997;70:101–373.

37. Jackson AC. Acute viral infections [review]. *Curr Opin Neurol.* 1995;8:170–174.

38. Whitley RJ. Herpes simplex viruses. In: Knipe DM, Howley PM, Griffin DE, et al., eds. *Fields Virology.* Philadelphia: Lippincott Williams and Wilkins; 2001:2461–2509.

39. Tedder DG, Ashley R, Tyler R, et al. Herpes simplex virus infection as a cause of benign recurrent lymphocytic meningitis. *Ann Intern Med.* 1994;121:334–338.

40. Kimberlin DW, Whitley RJ. Neonatal herpes: what have we learned? *Semin Pediatr Infect Dis.* 2005;16:7–16.

41. Sauerbrei A, Eichorn U, Hottenrott G, et al. Virologic diagnosis of herpes simplex encephalitis. *J Clin Virol.* 2000;17:31–36.

42. Lakeman F, Whitley R, and the National Institute of Allergy and Infectious Diseases Collaborative Antiviral Study Group. Diagnosis of herpes simplex encephalitis: application of polymerase chain reaction to cerebrospinal fluid from brain-biopsied patients and correlation with disease. *J Infect Dis.* 1995;171:857–863.

43. Arvin AM. Varicella zoster virus. In: Knipe DM, Howley PM, Griffin DE, et al., eds. *Fields Virology.* Philadelphia: Lippincott Williams and Wilkins; 2001:2731–2768.

44. Gnann J, Whitley R. Herpes zoster. *N Engl J Med.* 2002;347:340–346.

45. Gilden DH, Kleinschmidt-DeMaster BK, LaGuardia JJ, et al. Neurologic complications of the reactivation of varicella-zoster virus. *N Engl J Med.* 2000;342:635–645.

46. Sauerbrei A, Eichorn U, Schacke M, et al. Laboratory diagnosis of herpes zoster. *J Clin Virol.* 1999;14:31–36.

47. Rowley A, Whitley R, Lakeman F, et al. Rapid detection of herpes simplex virus DNA in cerebrospinal fluid of patients with herpes simplex encephalitis. *Lancet.* 1990;335:440–441.

48. Minjolle S, Michelet C, Jusselin I, et al. Amplification of the six major human herpesviruses from cerebrospinal fluid in a single PCR. *J Clin Microbiol.* 1999;37:950–953.

49. Read SJ, Kurtz JB. Laboratory diagnosis of common viral infections of the central nervous system by using a single multiplex PCR screening assay. *J Clin Microbiol.* 1999;37:1352–1355.

50. Espy M, Uhl J, Mitchell P, et al. Diagnosis of herpes simplex virus infections in the clinical laboratory by LightCycler PCR. *J Clin Microbiol.* 2000;38:759–799.

51. Johnson G, Nelson S, Petric M, et al. Comprehensive PCR-based assay for detection and species identification of human herpesviruses. *J Clin Microbiol.* 2000;38:3274–3279.

52. Quereda C, Corral I, Laguna F, et al. Diagnostic utility of a multiplex herpesvirus PCR assay performed with cerebrospinal fluid from human immunodeficiency virus-infected patients with neurological disorders. *J Clin Microbiol.* 2000;38:3061–3067.

53. Read S, Mitchell J, Fink C. LightCycler multiplex PCR for the laboratory diagnosis of common viral infections of the central nervous system. *J Clin Microbiol.* 2001;39:3056–3059.

54. Weidmann M, Meyer-Konig U, Hufert F. Rapid detection of herpes simplex virus and varicella-zoster virus infections by real-time PCR. *J Clin Microbiol.* 2003;41:1565–1568.

55. Braun DK, Dominguez G, Pellett PE. Human herpesvirus 6. *Clin Microbiol Rev.* 1997;10:521–567.

56. Secchiero P, Zella D, Crowley R, et al. Quantitative PCR for human herpesviruses 6 and 7. *J Clin Microbiol.* 1995;33:2124–2130.

57. Van den Bosch G, Locatelli G, Geerts L, et al. Development of reverse transcriptase PCR assays for detection of active human herpesvirus 6 infection. *J Clin Microbiol.* 2001;39:2308–2310.

58. Tang Y, Espy M, Persing D, et al. Molecular evidence and clinical significance of herpesvirus coinfection in the central nervous system. *J Clin Microbiol.* 1997;35:2869–2872.

59. Campbell GL, Marfin AA, Lanciotti RS, et al. West Nile virus. *Lancet Infect Dis.* 2002;2:519–529.

60. Harrington T, Kuehnert MJ, Kamel H, et al. West Nile virus infection transmitted by blood transfusion. *Transfusion.* 2003;43:1018–1022.

61. Johnson A, Martin D, Karabatsos N, et al. Detection of anti-arboviral immunoglobulin G by using a monoclonal antibody-based capture enzyme-linked immunosorbent assay. *J Clin Microbiol.* 2000;38:1827–1831.

62. Martin D, Muth D, Brown T, et al. Standardization of immunoglobulin M capture enzyme-linked immunosorbent assay for routine diagnosis of arboviral infections. *J Clin Microbiol.* 2000;38:1823–1826.

63. Lanciotti R, Kerst A, Nasci R, et al. Rapid detection of West Nile virus from human clinical specimens, field-collected mosquitoes, and avian samples by a TaqMan reverse transcriptase-PCR assay. *J Clin Microbiol.* 2000;38:4066–4071.

64. Lanciotti R, Kerst A. Nucleic acid sequence-based amplification assays for rapid detection of West Nile and St. Louis Encephalitis viruses. *J Clin Microbiol.* 2001;39:4506–4513.

65. Scaramozzino N, Crance J, Jouan A, et al. Comparison of flavivirus universal primer pairs and development of a rapid, highly sensitive hemi-nested reverse transcription-PCR assay for detection of flaviviruses targeted to a conserved region of the NS5 gene sequences. *J Clin Microbiol.* 2001;39:1922–1927.

66. Lambert A, Martin D, Lanciotti R. Detection of North American eastern and western equine encephalitis viruses by nucleic acid amplification assays. *J Clin Microbiol.* 2003;41:379–385.

67. White D, Kramer L, Backenson P, et al. Mosquito surveillance and polymerase chain reaction detection of West Nile virus, New York State. *Emerg Infect Dis.* 2001;7:643–649.

68. Ginocchio CC. Laboratory diagnosis of human cytomegalovirus (HCMV) central nervous system disease in AIDS patients. *Int J Antimicrob Agents.* 2000;16:447–453.

69. Zhang F, Tetali S, Wang XP, et al. Detection of human cytomegalovirus pp67 late gene transcripts in cerebrospinal fluid of human immunodeficiency virus type 1 infected patients by nucleic acid sequence based amplification. *J Clin Microbiol.* 2000;38:1920–1925.

70. Hammarin A, Bogdanovic G, Svenhem V, et al. Analysis of PCR as a tool for detection of JC virus DNA in cerebrospinal fluid for diagnosis of progressive multifocal leukoencephalopathy. *J Clin Microbiol.* 1996;34:2929–2932.

71. De Viedma D, Alonson R, Miralles P, et al. Dual qualitative-quantitative nested PCR for detection of JC virus in cerebrospinal fluid: high potential for evaluation and monitoring of progressive multifocal leukoencephalopathy in AIDS patients receiving highly active antiretroviral therapy. *J Clin Microbiol.* 1999;37:724–728.

72. Whiley D, Mackay I, Sloots T. Detection and differentiation of Human polyomaviruses JC and BK by LightCycler PCR. *J Clin Microbiol.* 2001;39:4357–4361.

73. Albright AV, Soldan SS, Gonzalez-Scarano F. Pathogenesis of human immunodeficiency virus-induced neurological disease. *J Neurovirol.* 2003;9:222–227.

74. McArthur JC, Haughey N, Gartner S, et al. Human immunodeficiency virus-associated dementia: An evolving disease. *J Neurovirol.* 2003;9:205–221.

Chapter 7

Sexually Transmitted Diseases

Jeanne A. Jordan

CHLAMYDIA TRACHOMATIS AND NEISSERIA GONORRHEAE

Clinical Utility

Chlamydia trachomatis (CT) and *Neisseria gonorrheae* (GC) are presented together, not because of their similarities in disease presentation, but because of the current trend in screening samples for both simultaneously. Historically, these organisms were identified using very different laboratory methods: CT by tissue culture and GC by growth in specialized bacterial medium. However, over the past decade a revolutionary change has taken place in the approach used to detect these two sexually transmitted infections (STIs). In many instances, molecular testing, either nucleic acid hybridization or nucleic acid amplification, has replaced culture and immunoassays.

Chlamydia Trachomatis

Chlamydia trachomatis is a gram-negative, obligate intracellular bacterium of global public health significance. Infection with CT is associated with three different disease presentations; trachoma (serovars A, B, B$_1$, and C), genital infection (serovars D-K), and lymphogranuloma venereum (LV) (serovars L$_1$, L$_2$, and L$_3$).[1] This chapter focuses on the diagnosis of those serovars causing genital infections.

Genital CT infections represent a major reproductive health problem. The World Health Organization (WHO) estimates that annually there are 89 million new cases of genital CT globally, with more than 4 million cases occurring annually in North America. In the developed world, CT is the likely cause of secondary infertility in females, due to its association with cervicitis, endometritis, and urethritis. Between 10% and 40% of CT infections in females will result in pelvic inflammatory disease (PID), whose sequelae include ectopic pregnancy, tubal factor infertility, and chronic pelvic pain.[2] The risk of developing any one of these sequelae increases with the number of PID episodes that an individual experiences. Additionally, pregnant women infected with CT are at risk of transmitting the infection to their newborn infant in the form of conjunctivitis or pneumonia. In males, genital CT infection is associated with nongonococcal urethritis (NGU), epididymitis, urethritis, prostatitis, proctitis, and Reiter syndrome.[1,3]

The individuals at greatest risk of genital CT infections are adolescents and young adults, ages 14 to 24 years, which is similar to the age of prevalence for human papillomavirus (HPV). Intervention based on selective screening for genital CT infection has reduced its prevalence, as well as the incidence of PID and ectopic pregnancy. These improved outcomes have occurred with the implementation of nucleic acid amplification testing (NAT), use of less-invasive and better-tolerated collection techniques, and development of more stable specimen transport systems. Molecular testing for sexually transmitted diseases (STDs) is an advantageous approach, especially in the high prevalence or high-risk patient populations.

CT infection often is silent, with up to 70% of infected females and 50% of infected males being asymptomatic; therefore, a significant number of individuals do not seek treatment and are at risk of developing complications from the infection. Mass screening programs in Europe have led to a significant reduction in CT prevalence. However, to be successful, these programs must be practical and acceptable to the targeted patient populations. Acceptable screening programs might include the use of self-collected vaginal specimens or first-void urines that could be stably shipped at ambient temperatures. This strategy has the advantage of limiting the number of physician office visits for individuals, thereby increasing compliance.

Neisseria Gonorrhoeae

Neisseria gonorrhoeae is a gram-positive, oxidase-positive, intracellular diplococcus. Microscopically, the microorganism has a characteristic kidney or coffee bean

Table 7-1. Summary of Selected NAT Platforms for *Chlamydia trachomatis* and *Neisseria Gonorrheae*

Manufacturer	Assay Method	Sample Preparation	Amplification Strategy	Detection Strategy	Contamination Controls	IAC
Becton Dickinson	SDA	Crude cell lysate	Target	Fluorescence	Closed System Postamplification Bleach	Yes
Digene Corporation	hc2	Hybrid capture	Signal	Chemiluminescence	No recommendations	No
Gen-Probe, Inc	TMA	Target capture	Target	Chemiluminescence Dual Kinetics Assay	Postamplification Bleach	No
Roche Diagnostics	PCR	Crude cell lysate	Target	Colorimetric	Preamplification dUTP, UNG	Yes

SDA, strand displacement amplification; IAC, internal amplification control; NASBA, nucleic acid sequence–based amplification; hc2, Hybrid Capture 2; TMA, transcription-mediated amplification; PCR, polymerase chain reaction; NAT, nucleic acid amplification testing.

appearance. GC is a fastidious organism, being highly susceptible to temperature extremes and desiccation, which results in less-than-satisfactory isolation by culture, especially when off-site specimen transportation is required before culture.[4]

The fastidious nature of GC has led to a trend from culture toward molecular testing.[5] Interestingly, experiences in GC testing have led some investigators to conclude that NAT for GC does not appreciably increase the number of positive specimens compared to culture methods, if optimal transport conditions have been maintained. However, NAT allows for the use of alternative, less-invasive specimens such as urine and self-collected vaginal swabs for GC detection. This strategy avoids the need to collect urethral or endocervical specimens, which should increase compliance with testing.

Like CT, the incidence of GC is highest among young adults under the age of 24 years. GC remains second only to CT infection in the number of cases of a reportable STD. Worldwide, approximately 62 million new cases of GC occur annually. GC-associated urogenital tract infections can lack symptoms altogether, or present with mild to severe symptoms. In men, symptoms include acute urethritis and discharge, which if left untreated can lead to epididymitis, prostatitis, or urethral strictures. In women, symptoms can include endocervical inflammation and discharge, which if not treated can lead to abscess formation, salpingitis, or PID. Disseminated GC infection, although not common, can occur in a small percentage of infected individuals and is usually has a poor outcome.

Available Tests

Prior to the introduction of molecular testing, CT and GC were detected from clinical specimens primarily by culture. For CT, more rapid tests were developed to facilitate shorter turnaround times and included enzyme immunoassays (EIA) to detect either the LPS or MOMP antigen and direct fluorescence assays (DFA) that used genus-specific or species-specific monoclonal antibodies.[1] For GC, direct gram stain and culture have been used. Guidelines for CT and GC testing now include molecular testing as a recommended test method.

More molecular testing platforms for detection of CT and GC have been cleared or approved by the Food and Drug Administration (FDA) than for any other infectious pathogen. These platforms include both nonamplified (e.g., the PACE DNA probe assay, GenProbe, San Diego, CA) and amplified testing methods (Table 7-1). The nonamplified probe-based assays are not discussed further in this chapter.

The popularity of using NAT for CT and GC can be partially explained by market pressures; the sheer volume of STD testing performed annually drives commercial interests. In addition, there are a wide variety of validated specimen types that have been approved for use with these testing platforms, which help to facilitate compliance in high-risk groups for this ever-growing public health concern.

Table 7-1 lists four of the most commonly used, commercially available NAT platforms for CT and GC; three use target amplification and one uses signal amplification methods.[6-10] The table summarizes the test methods, purification strategies, amplification and detection schemes, and types of contamination controls and internal amplification controls included in each kit. The sample preparation protocols vary widely for these kits and range from using crude cell lysates to using purified nucleic acid as the input specimen. The different sample types used and the extent of sample purification affect the rates of inhibition and thus the need to include an internal amplification control.

Interpretation of Test Results

Tables 7-2 through 7-4 describe in detail the three most commonly used NAT platforms for CT and GC, specifically, ProbeTec ET (Becton, Dickinson and Co, Franklin Lakes, NJ), Aptima Combo 2 (Gen-Probe, Inc, San Diego, CA), and Amplicor CT/NG Assays (Roche Diagnostics, Indianapolis, IN). The tables provide the gene targeted for CT and GC detection, the recommended clinical specimens, optimal transport and storage conditions, processing deadlines, test interpretations, workflow issues, and other features of these test methods. Many investigators have published performance data using these platforms.[6,7,9-16]

Table 7-2. BD ProbeTec™ ET CT/GC SDA Assays: Parameters and Test Interpretation for CT/GC Detection

Target	CT: Cryptic plasmid
	GC: Piv_{Ng} gene
Specimens	Female and male urine
	Endocervical and urethral swabs
Specimen handling	Urines: Adding a UPP to urine sample at specimen collection site permits 15°C to 27°C transport; process within 2 days of collection. Unpreserved urines should be transported at 2°C to 8°C; process within 7 days of collection. See package insert for all approved variations for urine specimens.
	Swabs: Transport swabs at 2°C to 27°C; process within 4 days.

Test interpretations

IAC	CT/GC MOTA Score	AC MOTA Score	Result	Interpretation
No	<2,000	NA	Negative	CT and/or GC not detected
	2,000 to 9,999	NA	Low positive	CT and/or GC likely, supplemental testing
	≥10,000	NA	Positive	CT and/or GC detected
Yes	<2,000	<1,000	Indeterminate	Inhibition
	<2,000	≥1,000	Negative	CT and/or GC not detected
	2,000 to 9,999	Any	Low positive	CT and/or GC likely, supplemental testing
	≥10,000	Any	Positive	CT and/or GC detected

Workflow issues	Individual amplification and detection reactions required for CT and GC, or CT, GC, and IAC.
Other features	CT: IAC consists of 1,000 copies of a linearized GC DNA containing plasmid.
	GC: Cross-reactivity to some nongonococcal *Neisseria* species.

Complete package insert is available at: http://www.bd.com.
IAC, Internal amplification control; MOTA, method other than acceleration; NA, not applicable; UPP, urine processing pouch.

Table 7-3. Gen-Probe Aptima Combo 2 Assays: Parameters and Test Interpretation for CT/GC Detection Using TMA and DKA Technologies

Target	23S rRNA/16S rRNA
Specimens	Female and male urine
	Endocervical and male urethral swabs
Specimen handling	Urines and Swabs: Transport at 2°C to 30°C and process within 60 days of collection.
	Transport both specimen types in the proper collection devices.

Test interpretation
Signals in relative light units (RLU)

		Negative	Equivocal	Positive
For CT	CT only	1 to <25	25 to <100	100 to <3000
	CT and GC	1 to <85	85 to <250	250 to <3000
For GC	CT indeterminate	1 to <85	85 to <3000	NA
	Rapid "flasher" kinetics			
	Slower "glower" kinetics	Negative	Equivocal	Positive
	CT only	1 to <60	60 to <150	150 to <4500
	CT and GC	1 to <85	85 to <250	250 to <4500
	CT indeterminate	1 to <85	85 to <4500	NA

Workflow issues	Simultaneous amplification and detection of CT and GC.
	Options include manual assay or Tecan-assisted assay.
Other features	No known cross-reactivity with nongonococcal *Neisseria* species.

Complete package insert is available at: http://www.gen-probe.com.
TMA, transcription-mediated amplification; DKA, dual kinetic assay; NA, not applicable.

Table 7-4. Roche Amplicor and Cobas Amplicor CT/NG PCR Assay: Parameters and Test Interpretation for CT/NG Detection

Targets	Cryptic plasmid/*M·Ngo* PII (*Cytosine DNA methyltransferase*)				
Specimens	Female and male urine (CT only)				
	Endocervical and male urethral swabs (CT/NG)				
Specimen handling	Transport swabs and urines at 2° to 8°C				
	Store swabs and urines at 2° to 8°C; process within 7 days of collection; –20°C: process within 30 to 60 days of collection.				
Test interpretation					
For CT	IC	A_{660}	CT Result	IC Result	Interpretation
	Without	<0.2	NA	NA	Negative
		≥0.2 to <2.0	NA	NA	Equivocal
		≥2.0	NA	NA	Positive
	With	<0.2	Negative	Positive	CT not detected
		<0.2	Negative	Negative	Inhibition
		≥0.2 to <2.0	Equivocal	Any	Equivocal
For NG	IC	A_{660}	NG Result	IC Result	Interpretation
	Without	<0.2	NA	NA	Negative
		≥0.2 to <3.5	NA	NA	Equivocal
		≥2.0	NA	NA	Positive
	With	<0.2	Negative	Positive	GC not detected
		<0.2	Negative	Negative	Inhibition
		≥0.2 to <3.5	Equivocal	Any	Equivocal
		≥2.0	Positive	Any	GC detected
Workflow issues	Simultaneous amplification of CT/NG/IC with separate detection reactions.				
Other issues	IC is a plasmid-containing CT primer binding sites and randomized internal sequence.				
	Cross-reactivity with certain nongonococcal *Neisseria* species.				

PCR, polymerase chain reaction; A_{660}, Absorbance$_{660}$; IC, internal control.
More information is available at: http://www.roche-diagnostics.us.

Laboratory Issues

The following laboratory issues are noteworthy when NAT platforms for CT and GC testing are selected.[17–21]

Inhibitors and Internal Controls

Amplification inhibition is common within urogenital specimens, with consequent negative effects on test results.[22] The percentage of specimens containing amplification inhibitors ranges from 1% to 5% for urines and as much as 20% for cervical swabs. Initial studies found that inhibition could be reduced or eliminated if specimens were first refrigerated overnight or frozen and thawed before testing, pointing to the labile nature of some inhibitors. However, other inhibitors are quite stable and thus more difficult to neutralize. Some of the commercially available platforms include an internal amplification control (IAC) to identify specimens containing inhibitors. Alternatively, inhibitors can be removed if nucleic acid purification steps are included in the sample preparation protocol. For testing platforms that include an IAC, the testing algorithm states that when the internal control fails, the results of a specimen without detectable CT and/or GC cannot be reported as negative due to the likelihood that amplification inhibitors are present in the specimen.

Cross-Reactivity with Nongonnococcal Neisseria Species

The specificity for some GC NAT platforms has been problematic due to cross-reactivity with certain nongonococcal species of *Neisseria*.[23,24] This problem is thought to arise from the intraspecies and interspecies genetic recombination that occurs between *Neisseria* species, which can result in false-positive NAT results with certain of the commensal *Neisseria* species.[16] Of eight nongonococcal species tested, five species demonstrated cross-reactivity: *N. cinerea*, *N. flavescens*, *N. lactamica*, *N. subflava*, and *N. sicca*. False-positive results were seen with *N. flavescens*, *N. lactamica*, *N. subflava*, and *N. cinerea* using the BD ProbeTec assay, and with *N. flavescens*, *N. lactamica*, and *N. sicca* using the Roche Amplicor assay. Since *N. cinerea*, *N. lactamica*, *N. subflava*, and *N. sicca* isolates have been recovered from genital mucosa, it is possible to generate false-positive results from genital specimens as well as pharyngeal specimens. Therefore, confirmatory testing using a different gene target may be useful.

Confirmatory Testing

When a testing platform is being selected, the prevalence of infection in the population being tested is of significance. The analytical performance of any test is dependent on the prevalence of infection, with the risk of generating false-positive results being inversely related to the prevalence. These issues have fueled the debate over the need for confirmatory testing for CT and GC. Both are reportable infections, with the potential for psychosocial and/or medico-legal consequences for a false-positive or a true-positive result.[17,18,25] FDA-cleared confirmatory tests for CT and GC are now available.

The most recent CDC Guidelines for STD testing have addressed the issue of confirmatory testing, providing a variety of options.[26] These guidelines are especially critical for confirmatory testing in low-prevalence populations where the positive predictive value (PPV) of the assay is known to be less than 90%. In fact, the manufacturers' package inserts illustrate this point, with a PPV of 32% to 60% for any of these tests when the GC prevalence is 1%. This also is true for CT testing, with a PPV range from 56% and 74% when the prevalence is 5%. The most recent options recommended by the CDC for confirmatory testing are summarized as follows:

- Test another specimen with a different assay that has a different target.
- Test the original specimen with a different assay that has a different target.
- Test the original specimen using the original test, incorporating a blocking antibody or competitive probe.
- Test the original specimen again using the original test.

To this end, many laboratories have developed algorithms to incorporate confirmatory testing in their workflow. Some laboratories establish an equivocal range for specimens with an initial low-level positive or high-level negative result. Although laboratory personnel feel more confident in reporting positive results that are confirmed by repeat testing, this has cost implications. Questions remain about the proper reporting strategy for specimens that do not reconfirm as positive on repeat testing.

Amplification Contamination Control

The advent of NAT, with its exquisite sensitivity, has given birth to a whole new mind-set for cleanliness in the molecular testing laboratory. No longer is disinfection of the benchtop after a day's work adequate. New standards strive to "nuclease" the laboratory environment to remove or prevent amplicon contamination. Strategies includes daily cleaning of laboratory surfaces with a bleach solution, and frequently replacing disposable gloves and gowns while working in the pre- and postamplification area(s). A regular schedule for performing wipe testing to monitor for amplicon contamination should be enforced. For many of the current NAT platforms, pre- and postamplification steps should be performed, if possible, in separate rooms with positive and negative airflow, respectively. In the future, much of the monumental efforts currently taken to minimize amplicon contamination may be reduced or eliminated altogether with the introduction of fully auto-

mated, closed real-time NAT systems that incorporate sample preparation, nucleic acid amplification, and detection in a single closed reaction.

Future Directions

Testing Noninvasive Specimen Types

One of the more recent changes to STD testing has been the use of noninvasively collected samples, including self-collected vaginal swabs and first-void urines.[20,27–32] The greatest impact of this change will be seen in the young adult patient population, age range from 14 to 24 years, where the prevalence of CT and GC infections is highest and the willingness to undergo a pelvic examination or urethral swab collection is lowest.

Out-of-the-Vial Testing

Another concept currently being marketed is out-of-the-vial testing for STDs.[11] This testing approach would use the remainder of liquid-based cytology fluid collected for Pap testing not only for HPV testing but also for CT and GC testing. Many critical issues must be addressed before this approach can be implemented; these include technical issues (cross contamination), ethical issues (waiting to perform the infectious disease testing until after the cytology screening is completed), and legal issues (cancer diagnosis takes precedence over STD diagnosis). Successful implementation of this strategy will require the cooperation of many interested groups. The ability to use a pre-aliquot of the sample from the liquid-based cytology specimen for STD testing prior to the Pap analysis may provide a workable solution.

Automated NAT

Fully automated instrumentation (including specimen processing, amplification, detection, and reporting) will facilitate testing. Gen-Probe launched the Tigris, a fully automated high-throughput system, while Cepheid has introduced the GeneXpert System. Other manufacturers have similar systems in development.

TRICHOMONAS VAGINALIS

Clinical Utility

Trichomonas vaginalis (TV) is a flagellated protozoan and the only species within its genus that can infect squamous epithelial cells of the human urogenital tract.[33] TV infection is considered to be a nonulcerative STD but is associated with severe local inflammation. In women, symptoms may include vulvar irritation and vaginal discharge, which appears frothy, mucopurulent, and yellow-green in color. During a TV infection, the vaginal pH is often abnormally elevated (pH > 4.5). Complications of TV infection in untreated women include endometritis, infertility, and cervical erosion. In men infected with TV, symptoms may include profuse purulent urethritis and a form of NGU, with complications including chronic prostatitis, urethral strictures, epididymitis, and/or infertility if the infection is untreated.[34,35]

Detection of TV infections in males has received much less attention than detection in females. However, with the advent of NAT, this understudied infection in men has become more appreciated, and thus research studies have provided important information on its prevalence, clinical symptoms, sequelae, and the most appropriate specimen to collect for proper diagnosis. TV has a greater role in NGU than previously thought.[36] As in females, direct microscopic examination of urethral discharge in males has poor sensitivity for detection of TV.

Worldwide, TV infection accounts for more than 167 million to 200 million cases annually. WHO estimates that TV infection accounts for close to half of all treatable STIs worldwide. In the United States, the annual incidence of TV infection is estimated between 5 million and 8 million cases. However, because TV infection is not a reportable disease, this number may be an underestimate. Unlike CT and GC, where prevalence is higher in adolescents and young adults, TV is more equally distributed among all age groups.

The detection of TV in an individual is considered by healthcare providers to be a red flag for high-risk sexual behavior and is frequently present along with other STIs in the same individual. Diagnosing TV is difficult, because 50% to 70% of all infected individuals are asymptomatic. Without a sensitive assay, infected individuals left untreated continue to act as a reservoir for ongoing disease transmission.

TV infection is associated with two important sequelae: (1) an increased risk of acquiring human immunodeficiency virus (HIV) and (2) an increased risk of perinatal morbidity and mortality.[37–40] HIV transmission is enhanced by the local inflammation reaction within the genital tract that is present with TV infections. In women, TV infection is strongly associated with an abnormal vaginal ecology. Harboring TV may contribute to the change in vaginal flora, which is associated with decreased lactic acid production and subsequent increase in vaginal pH. Lactic acid production and the normally low pH of the genital tract environment help to inactivate HIV. Therefore, a change in the vaginal environment to a less-hostile environment promotes an increased survival of HIV. If this hypothesis is correct, then controlling TV infections could lower HIV acquisition.

The increased risk of perinatal morbidity and mortality with TV infection is associated with premature rupture of membranes (PROM), preterm delivery, and low-birth-weight infants in pregnant women infected with TV.[41] Although controversial, these associations suggest a

Table 7-5. Summary of the Commonly Used *Trichomonas Vaginalis* Specific Targets for NAT

Primer Pair	DNA Target	Amplicon (bp)
TVK3, TVK7	Repetitive DNA	312
TVK3, TVK4	Repetitive DNA	350
BTUB2, BTUB9	*Beta Tubulin*	112
TV1, TV2	*18S rRNA* gene	312
TV-E650	E650	650
TVA5, TVA6	*Ferredoxin* gene	102

need for increased efforts to detect and treat this infection in pregnant women.[42]

Screening for TV infection is usually done only in public health STD clinics and some obstetrical practices. Successful control of this STI would be aided greatly by performing contact follow-ups with sexual partners and using a more sensitive diagnostic assay. Improved detection of TV by using NAT, as was the case for CT, would be predicted to reduce the incidence of TV infection and assist in reducing HIV transmission and possibly even poor pregnancy outcomes.[43]

Available Tests

Historically, the most common means of diagnosing TV in urogenital discharge was direct microscopic examination, broth culturing, or both. Direct microscopic examination of genital discharge material on a slide is certainly the most rapid and inexpensive method to use, but it lacks adequate sensitivity, which is reported to be approximately 40% to 70%.[44] The low level of sensitivity with microscopic examination may be due to the rapid loss of the characteristic protozoan motility once TV has been removed from a 37°C environment, and to the fact that nonmotile TV organisms are difficult to differentiate from leukocytes, being similar in size.

Currently, broth culturing is the gold standard for detection of TV.[45] Successful growth in culture can be achieved with as few as 300 to 500 TV organisms per milliliter of vaginal fluid, but this approach requires 2 to 7 days of incubation and daily microscopic examination. Culture methods have sensitivities that range between 50% and 80% but require specialized medium such as Diamond's broth, Tricosel medium, or the In-Pouch system. These specialized media may not be available in the physician's office. In addition, some TV isolates do not grow in culture due to strain requirements, low numbers of organisms, or damaged/nonviable organisms.

These limitations have led some laboratories to develop NAT for TV DNA. Although none of the NAT are commercially available, numerous assays have been described that are specific for TV.[46–53] A range of testing platforms has been developed, including conventional and real-time NAT assays. The most commonly cited TV targets used for NAT are listed in Table 7-5. The repetitive DNA sequences have a higher copy number per organism and therefore may result in a more sensitive assay.

Interpretation of Test Results

Currently, no FDA-approved test kits or analyte-specific reagents for TV are commercially available. Therefore, the individual laboratories performing NAT for TV DNA need to establish the interpretation criteria. The following issues should be included in the development and validation of NAT for TV:

- Rule out cross-reactivity of primers and probes with non-TV targets that could be present within the specimens.
- Validate the different specimen types to be tested, and the handling conditions to be used.
- Establish a protocol for specimen preparation.
- Establish the limit of detection for TV DNA.
- Establish analytical performance of the assay including sensitivity and specificity, and positive and negative predictive values.
- If applicable, include the rationale for establishing positive and negative cutoff values and whether an equivocal zone is used.
- Establish a protocol for repeat testing and reporting of indeterminate results.
- Address resolution of culture-negative, NAT-positive discrepancies.
- Assess the presence of interfering substances by including an internal amplification control.
- Ensure specimen adequacy by testing for an endogenous housekeeping gene such as beta globin.
- Develop an alternative proficiency testing program for TV NAT because an external program is not available.

Laboratory Issues

Target Selection

Validation of the primers and probes is necessary for laboratory-developed NAT to rule out cross-reactivity with other *Trichomonas* species, such as *T. tena*, as well as to other organisms that may be present within the urogenital tract specimen, including human genomic DNA. The TV-specific primer pairs and probes described in the literature recognize different gene targets that vary in their copy number. In general, choosing a gene target that is present in multiple copies per genome is usually preferable to choosing a single-copy gene target.

Internal Control

Both vaginal swabs and urine specimens can contain inhibitors that interfere with the nucleic acid amplification reaction. For interpreting negative results, it is important to include an internal control in the assay, especially if a crude cell lysate is used as the input material for testing.

More details on inhibitors can be found within the CT and GC section of this chapter.

Specimen Collection

The optimal specimen to collect differs for women and men. For women, the specimen of choice is vaginal discharge collected using a Dacron-tipped, plastic-shaft swab, while for men, the sediment from the first-void urine is superior to a urethral swab specimen. For increased analytical sensitivity, only the first 20 ml to 30 ml of the first-void urine should be collected.

Specimen Transport

TV expresses and secretes numerous proteases. Therefore, for greatest target stability, specimens should be transported at temperatures below room temperature ($\leq 2°C$ to $8°C$).

Future Directions

Multiplex Testing for CT, GC, and TV

Multiplex testing for CT and GC has been available for years. Recently, there has been increased attention given to including TV as a target. With the prevalence of TV being greater than that of CT and GC combined in many regions, along with the association of TV infection with increased risk of HIV acquisition, inclusion of TV in a multiplex STD panel is a reasonable idea. Depending on the prevalence of other STIs within a patient population or geographic area, additional targets may be considered applicable for a multiplex STD panel.

Greater Use of Noninvasive Specimens

As with CT and GC detection, collection of first-void urines or self-collected vaginal swab-based specimens may improve patient compliance for TV testing.[32] This approach may in turn help to identify the asymptomatic, infected individuals and reduce transmission to sexual partners.

HUMAN PAPILLOMAVIRUS

Clinical Utility

Human papillomaviruses (HPV) are small, nonenveloped, double-stranded, circular DNA (~8 kilobases [kb]) viruses with a very limited cell tropism. To date, more than 100 different types of HPV have been identified.[54] HPV can infect and replicate in the nuclei of only certain squamous epithelial cells, which are classified as either cutaneous or mucosal in nature. In general, the cutaneous types of HPV infect keratinizing epithelium, while mucosal types infect nonkeratinizing epithelium. This section focuses on the approximately 30 types of anogenital HPV, which can be spread through sexual contact.

The sexually transmitted HPV types can be further classified by their risk of disease progression. Infection with a low-risk HPV is commonly associated with condyloma accuminata or genital warts, and is considered benign or low-risk for progression to malignancy.[55] In contrast, infection with a high-risk HPV can be associated with cervical cancer in women and penile cancer in men.[56-58] High-risk HPV types play a major role in the pathogenesis of epithelial cell cancers of the anogenital tract, as they induce epithelial cell proliferation.[59,60]

HPV is one of the most common sexually transmitted infections. It is estimated that more than 5 million new cases are contracted annually in the United States, with more than 20 million men and women currently infected. The prevalence of HPV is highest among sexually active young women ages 15 through 25 years.

While most men and women infected with anogenital HPV types will not develop cancer, a subset will; a process that may take decades to occur.[61,62] Certain cofactors may be important in disease progression as well, including the individual's immune status, certain HLA types, smoking, nutritional status, or possibly coinfection with HIV-1, herpes simplex virus, or *Chlamydia trachomatis*.[63-67] Women ages 30 years or older who are persistently infected within the cervix with a high-risk HPV type are at an increased risk for developing cervical cancer. Thus, HPV acquisition during adolescence may have long-term consequences for health later in adulthood.[68,69]

Worldwide, cervical cancer is the second most common female cancer, with approximately 493,000 women developing cervical cancer each year. In the United States, approximately 13,000 new cases of cervical cancer are diagnosed annually. Cervical cancer is a highly preventable disease if detected and treated early. Infection with high-risk HPV types is associated with the appearance of clinical lesions. In fact, HPV now is considered to be a necessary cause of invasive cervical cancer.[70] Abnormal cell growth or cervical dysplasia is an early manifestation of HPV infection. The characteristic cellular changes caused by HPV infection can be detected on Pap smear evaluations or in cervical biopsies. The morphologic changes of dysplasia are classified as atypical squamous cells of undetermined significance (ASCUS), low-grade squamous intraepithelial lesion (LSIL), or high-grade squamous intraepithelial lesion (HSIL).[71,72]

Annually, approximately 2 million Pap tests performed in the United States are interpreted as an ASCUS-grade result. ASCUS rates typically fall within the range of 5% to 10% but can be as high as 20% in younger women. Current recommendations include reflex testing (triage) for high-risk HPV for patients with an ASCUS-grade Pap smear result; patients testing negative for HPV DNA can be followed according to routine practice, while those testing positive for high-risk HPV should be referred to col-poscopy, as progression to high-grade disease is probable.[73,74] Patients with abnormal Pap smears whose specimens contain high-risk HPV DNA require immediate medical attention.[75-78]

In 2003, the FDA approved the Digene Hybrid Capture 2 (hc2) assay for use with a Pap test for adjunct screening of women ages 30 years and older for high-risk HPV infection. This recommendation was based on the theory that in this age group, the combined negative predictive value of Pap and hc2 would improve the sensitivity of cervical screening. Women who have both a normal Pap test and a negative high-risk HPV screen can be screened once every 3 years instead of annually.

Available Tests

Molecular testing platforms have been particularly helpful in detecting and classifying the HPV DNA within clinical specimens, as viral culturing is not easily accomplished and cytological examinations cannot differentiate between low-risk and high-risk types of HPV. Several nucleic acid–based tests have been developed for the detection and typing of HPV strains. These tests include signal amplification assays, polymerase chain reaction (PCR), and in situ hybridization.

Digene Hybrid Capture 2 Assay

Currently, the Hybrid Capture 2 (hc2) HPV Assay (Digene Corp, Gaithersburg, MD) is the only FDA-approved test kit for detecting low-risk or high-risk HPV types from cervical specimens.[79] This test is a signal amplification assay, with separate tests for high-risk and low-risk HPV types. The indicated uses for both the high-risk and the low-risk HPV hc2 assay include aiding in the diagnosis of sexually transmitted HPV infections. In contrast, the indicated uses for the high-risk assay include (1) screening specimens from patients with an ASCUS-grade Pap test result to determine the need for colposcopy[73,78] and (2) as a primary screening tool in conjunction with a Pap test for women 30 years and older.[76] Recommended specimen types for this assay include cervical swabs and liquid-based cytology specimens. The recommended collection devices and transport media include cervical brushes and cervical biopsies transported in specimen transport medium (STM), or a cervical broom transported in Cytyc Preserv-Cyt (PC) solution.

The principle of the hc2 HPV assay is as follows: Target DNA, liberated from the virus, is denatured and allowed to hybridize with a specific cocktail of RNA probes. The high-risk cocktail contains 13 RNA probes recognizing HPV types 16, 18, 31, 33, 35, 39, 45, 51, 52, 56, 58, 59, and 68. The low-risk cocktail contains five RNA probes recognizing HPV types 6, 11, 42, 43, and 44. The resulting DNA-RNA hybrids are captured onto the surface of a microtiter well coated with polyclonal antibodies specific for RNA-DNA hybrids. Alkaline phosphatase (AP) conjugated antibodies recognizing the immobilized hybrids bind several molecules per target to provide signal amplification. Finally, the chemiluminescent substrate CDP-Star with Emerald II is added to the wells and cleaved by the AP enzyme. The resulting light emission is measured as relative light units (RLUs) using a luminometer.

Interpretation of Test Results

Prior to interpreting the patient specimen results of the hc2 HPV test, assay calibration verification must meet the following criteria:

- Mean value of the negative control must be <250 RLU with a %CV ≤ 25% for at least 2 of the 3 values.
- %CV of the calibrator mean value must be <15% for at least 2 of the 3 values.
- Ratio of the calibrator mean over the negative control mean must be ≥2.0.

If the above criteria are met, then the cutoff value can be calculated for determining positive specimens. The calibrator mean value serves as the cutoff value. A ratio of specimen RLU/cutoff value (CO) is generated, and, according to the package insert:

- Specimens with RLU/CO ratios ≥1.0 are interpreted as positive.
- Specimens with RLU/CO ratios <1.0 are interpreted as negative, or nondetected for the 13 high-risk HPV types tested.
- When testing PC solution specimens, if the RLU/CO ratio of a specimen is ≥1.0 and <2.5, the specimen must be retested. If the initial retest result is positive (≥1.0 RLU/CO), the specimen can be reported as positive. If the first retest is negative (<1.0), then a second retest should be performed. The result of the second retest is considered the final result and is to be reported.

Laboratory Issues

Specimen Expiration Date

Routinely, the liquid-based cytological evaluation (Pap test) is performed before the HPV DNA testing is done. Therefore, the DNA testing laboratory must carefully monitor the specimen-collection and testing dates to assure that the specimens have not exceeded their expiration date as stated in the package insert for the hc2 HPV assay.

Low-Volume Specimens Received for HPV DNA Testing

Inadequately collected specimens may contain fewer cells than normal, which results in a greater volume of the spec-

imen being used for the Pap test, leaving fewer than normal cell numbers for the HPV DNA testing. Lower than usual cell numbers may still occur even if the specimen contains the required 4.0 ml volume. Technologists need to be aware of this issue when visually inspecting the pelleted material during HPV sample preparation to ensure quality results.

Assay Reproducibility

As with any test, reproducibility is most problematic at the assay's limit of detection. Therefore, specimens containing a limited number of HPV also will be the least reproducible specimens. In contrast, specimens containing a high level of HPV will have the greatest reproducibility. It is important to remember that the positive predictive value of any assay will decrease when the test is used in populations with low prevalence.

False-Positive Results

False-positive results are known to occur with the hc2 HPV assay due to the following conditions:

- Contamination of specimen with exogenous alkaline phosphatase.
- Inadequate denaturation of initial specimen.
- Inadequate washing during the assay.
- Cross-reactivity with HPV types 40, 53 and 66.
- Cross-reactivity with low-risk HPV types. Hybridization exists between low-risk HPV types 6 and 42 with the high-risk probe set. Specimens containing high levels (≥4 ng/ml) of HPV 6 or 42 DNA may be falsely positive in the hc2 high-risk HPV assay.

HPV PCR

There are numerous PCR assays in the literature describing HPV DNA amplification.[80–82] A common strategy utilizes the L1 consensus primer pair MY09 and MY11 to amplify HPV DNA, followed by hybridization with specific probes for amplicon detection and confirmation. Recent modifications to the MY09/11 assay have been described using the PGMY primers, which amplify a smaller region internal to the MY09/11 sequence and have improved detection of HPV DNA in genital samples.[83] HPV genotyping can be performed using line blot or line probe assays or DNA sequencing.[84] Currently there are no FDA-cleared PCR assays for HPV detection or typing. However, outside of the United States, Roche Diagnostics offers the Amplicor HPV test, which detects 13 high-risk HPV types, and the Linear Array HPV Genotyping test, which detects 37 high- and low-risk HVP types.

Inform HPV Assay

The Inform HPV assay (Ventana Medical Systems, Inc, Tucson, AZ) is an in situ hybridization (ISH) test used in conjunction with the company's Benchmark IHC and ISH staining system.[85] The Inform HPV assay is not an FDA-approved test kit. The automated ISH technology is a slide-based HPV assay that provides HPV DNA detection in the context of cervical cell morphology. The assay does not detect cell-free HPV DNA. The company offers both high-risk and low-risk HPV genomic fluorescently labeled probe cocktails for ISH testing.

Invader HPV Reagents

Third Wave Technologies (Madison, WI) offers analyte-specific reagents (ASR) for detecting the DNA of 13 HPV types, including types 16, 18, 31, 33, 35, 39, 45, 51, 52, 56, 58, 59, and 68, along with the human histone gene. The HPV ASR are packaged as four separate mixtures based on phylogenic relatedness, and include A5/A6, A7, A9 and human histone. Analytical and performance characteristics are established by individual laboratories.

Summary

In summary, the limits of detection for the various assays are between 50 and 100 genome copies for PCR, approximately 500 to 1000 genome copies for signal amplification assays, and approximately 100,000 genome copies for DNA in situ hybridization assays.

Future Directions

A number of possible applications are on the horizon for HPV testing.

- Several manufacturers are marketing out-of-the-vial testing for HPV detection from liquid-based cytology specimens. More comments can be found on this topic in the CT/GC section of this chapter.[86]
- There is potential prognostic value in determining quantitative HPV viral load measurements. Further studies will be needed before any conclusions can be made on this topic including addressing variations in the cell numbers present within specimens and the viral copy number present per cell.
- In light of the recent findings of an elevated risk of cervical precancer and cancer in women with HPV type 16 or 18 compared to the other high-risk HPV types, HPV viral typing may prove informative in differentiating between viral persistence and reinfection.[87]
- Virus persistence and disease progression will be assessed relative to HPV E6 and E7 mRNA gene expression.
- The level of CpG methylation of high-risk HPV DNA may be explored.

References

1. Moss T, ed. *International Handbook of Chlamydia*. Exeter, UK: Polestar Wheatons Ltd; 2001.
2. Scholes D, Stergachis A, Heidrich FE, et al. Prevention of pelvic inflammatory disease by screening for cervical chlamydial infection. *N Engl J Med*. 1996;334:1362–1366.
3. Burstein GR, Zenilman JM. Nongonococcal urethritis—a new paradigm. *Clin Infect Dis*. 1999;28(suppl 1):S66–S73.
4. Judson FN. Gonorrhea. *Med Clin North Am*. 1990;74:1353–1366.
5. Koumans EH, Johnson RE, Knapp JS, et al. Laboratory testing for *Neisseria gonorrhoeae* by recently introduced nonculture tests: a performance review with clinical and public health considerations. *Clin Infect Dis*. 1998;27:1171–1180.
6. Chernesky MA, Martin DH, Hook EW, et al. Ability of new APTIMA CT and APTIMA GC assays to detect *Chlamydia trachomatis* and *Neisseria gonorrhoeae* in male urine and urethral swabs. *J Clin Microbiol*. 2005;43:127–131.
7. Gaydos CA, Quinn TC, Willis D, et al. Performance of the APTIMA combo 2 assay for detection of *Chlamydia trachomatis* and *Neisseria gonorrhoeae* in female urine and endocervical swab specimens. *J Clin Microbiol*. 2003;41:304–309.
8. Modarress KJ, Cullen AP, Jaffurs WJ Sr, et al. Detection of *Chlamydia trachomatis* and *Neisseria gonorrhoeae* in swab specimens by the Hybrid Capture II and PACE 2 nucleic acid probe tests. *Sex Transm Dis*. 1999;26:303–308.
9. Van der Pol B. COBAS Amplicor: an automated PCR system for detection of *C. trachomatis* and *N. gonorrhoeae*. *Expert Rev Mol Diagn*. 2002;2:379–389.
10. Van Der Pol B, Ferrero DV, Buck-Barrington L, et al. Multicenter evaluation of the BDProbeTec ET System for detection of *Chlamydia trachomatis* and *Neisseria gonorrhoeae* in urine specimens, female endocervical swabs, and male urethral swabs. *J Clin Microbiol*. 2001;39:1008–1016.
11. Bianchi A, Moret F, Desrues JM, et al. PreservCyt transport medium used for the ThinPrep Pap test is a suitable medium for detection of *Chlamydia trachomatis* by the COBAS Amplicor CT/NG test: results of a preliminary study and future implications. *J Clin Microbiol*. 2002;40:1749–1754.
12. Chong S, Jang D, Song X, et al. Specimen processing and concentration of *Chlamydia trachomatis* added can influence false-negative rates in the LCx assay but not in the APTIMA Combo 2 assay when testing for inhibitors. *J Clin Microbiol*. 2003;41:778–782.
13. Diemert DJ, Libman MD, Lebel P. Confirmation by 16S rRNA PCR of the COBAS AMPLICOR CT/NG test for diagnosis of *Neisseria gonorrhoeae* infection in a low-prevalence population. *J Clin Microbiol*. 2002;40:4056–4059.
14. Farrell DJ. Evaluation of AMPLICOR *Neisseria gonorrhoeae* PCR using *cppB* nested PCR and 16S rRNA PCR. *J Clin Microbiol*. 1999;37:386–390.
15. Livengood CH 3rd, Wrenn JW. Evaluation of COBAS AMPLICOR (Roche): accuracy in detection of *Chlamydia trachomatis* and *Neisseria gonorrhoeae* by coamplification of endocervical specimens. *J Clin Microbiol*. 2001;39:2928–2932.
16. Palmer HM, Mallinson H, Wood RL, et al. Evaluation of the specificities of five DNA amplification methods for the detection of *Neisseria gonorrhoeae*. *J Clin Microbiol*. 2003;41:835–837.
17. McAdam AJ. Discrepant analysis: how can we test a test? *J Clin Microbiol*. 2000;38:2027–2029.
18. Schachter J, Hook EW, Martin DH, et al. Confirming positive results of nucleic acid amplification tests (NAATs) for *Chlamydia trachomatis*: All NAATs are not created equal. *J Clin Microbiol*. 2005;43:1372–1373.
19. Schachter J, Hook EW 3rd, McCormack WM, et al. Ability of the Digene hybrid capture II test to identify *Chlamydia trachomatis* and *Neisseria gonorrhoeae* in cervical specimens. *J Clin Microbiol*. 1999;37:3668–3671.

20. Stary A. Correct samples for diagnostic tests in sexually transmitted diseases: which sample for which test? *FEMS Immunol Med Microbiol.* 1999;24:455–459.

21. Watson EJ, Templeton A, Russell I, et al. The accuracy and efficacy of screening tests for *Chlamydia trachomatis*: a systematic review. *J Med Microbiol.* 2002;51:1021–1031.

22. Rosenstraus M, Wang Z, Chang SY, et al. An internal control for routine diagnostic PCR: design, properties, and effect on clinical performance. *J Clin Microbiol.* 1998;36:191–197.

23. Hagblom P, Korch C, Jonsson AB, et al. Intragenic variation by site-specific recombination in the cryptic plasmid of *Neisseria gonorrhoeae. J Bacteriol.* 1986;167:231–237.

24. Miyada CG, Born TL. A DNA sequence for the discrimination of *Neisseria gonorrhoeae* from other Neisseria species. *Mol Cell Probes.* 1991;5:327–335.

25. Van Der Pol B, Martin DH, Schachter J, et al. Enhancing the specificity of the COBAS AMPLICOR CT/NG test for *Neisseria gonorrhoeae* by retesting specimens with equivocal results. *J Clin Microbiol.* 2001;39:3092–3098.

26. Centers for Disease Control. Sexually transmitted diseases treatment guidelines 2002. *MMWR Recomm Rep.* 2002;51:1–78.

27. Gaydos CA, Crotchfelt KA, Shah N, et al. Evaluation of dry and wet transported intravaginal swabs in detection of *Chlamydia trachomatis* and *Neisseria gonorrhoeae* infections in female soldiers by PCR. *J Clin Microbiol.* 2002;40:758–761.

28. Hardy PH, Hardy JB, Nell EE, et al. Prevalence of six sexually transmitted disease agents among pregnant inner-city adolescents and pregnancy outcome. *Lancet.* 1984;2:333–337.

29. Mahony JB, Jang D, Chong S, et al. Detection of *Chlamydia trachomatis, Neisseria gonorrhoeae, Ureaplasma urealyticum,* and *Mycoplasma genitalium* in first-void urine specimens by multiplex polymerase chain reaction. *Mol Diagn.* 1997;2:161–168.

30. Ostergaard L, Moller JK, Andersen B, et al. Diagnosis of urogenital *Chlamydia trachomatis* infection in women based on mailed samples obtained at home: multipractice comparative study. *BMJ.* 1996;313:1186–1189.

31. Sugunendran H, Birley HD, Mallinson H, et al. Comparison of urine, first and second endourethral swabs for PCR based detection of genital *Chlamydia trachomatis* infection in male patients. *Sex Transm Infect.* 2001;77:423–426.

32. Wiesenfeld HC, Lowry DL, Heine RP, et al. Self-collection of vaginal swabs for the detection of chlamydia, gonorrhea, and trichomoniasis: opportunity to encourage sexually transmitted disease testing among adolescents. *Sex Transm Dis.* 2001;28:321–325.

33. Petrin D, Delgaty K, Bhatt R, et al. Clinical and microbiological aspects of *Trichomonas vaginalis. Clin Microbiol Rev.* 1998;11:300–317.

34. Graves A, Gardner WA Jr. Pathogenicity of *Trichomonas vaginalis. Clin Obstet Gynecol.* 1993;36:145–152.

35. Schwebke JR. Update of trichomoniasis. *Sex Transm Infect.* 2002;78:378–379.

36. Krieger JN. Trichomoniasis in men: old issues and new data. *Sex Transm Dis.* 1995;22:83–96.

37. Laga M, Manoka A, Kivuvu M, et al. Non-ulcerative sexually transmitted diseases as risk factors for HIV-1 transmission in women: results from a cohort study. *AIDS.* 1993;7:95–102.

38. Moodley P, Connolly C, Sturm AW. Interrelationships among human immunodeficiency virus type 1 infection, bacterial vaginosis, trichomoniasis, and the presence of yeasts. *J Infect Dis.* 2002;185:69–73.

39. Rendon-Maldonado J, Espinosa-Cantellano M, Soler C, et al. Trichomonas vaginalis: in vitro attachment and internalization of HIV-1 and HIV-1-infected lymphocytes. *J Eukaryot Microbiol.* 2003;50:43–48.

40. Sorvillo F, Kerndt P. *Trichomonas vaginalis* and amplification of HIV-1 transmission. *Lancet.* 1998;351:213–214.

41. Cotch MF, Pastorek JG 2nd, Nugent RP, et al. *Trichomonas vaginalis* associated with low birth weight and preterm delivery. The Vaginal Infections and Prematurity Study Group. *Sex Transm Dis.* 1997;24:353–360.

42. Klebanoff MA, Carey JC, Hauth JC, et al. Failure of metronidazole to prevent preterm delivery among pregnant women with asymptomatic Trichomonas vaginalis infection. *N Engl J Med.* 2001;345:487–493.

43. Sutton MY, Sternberg M, Nsuami M, et al. Trichomoniasis in pregnant human immunodeficiency virus-infected and human immunodeficiency virus-uninfected Congolese women: prevalence, risk factors, and association with low birth weight. *Am J Obstet Gynecol.* 1999;181:656–662.

44. McCann JS. Comparison of direct microscopy and culture in the diagnosis of trichomoniasis. *Br J Vener Dis.* 1974;50:450–452.

45. Garber GE, Sibau L, Ma R, et al. Cell culture compared with broth for detection of *Trichomonas vaginalis. J Clin Microbiol.* 1987;25:1275–1279.

46. Caliendo AM, Jordan JA, Green AM, et al. Real-time PCR improves detection of Trichomonas vaginalis infection compared with culture using self-collected vaginal swabs. *Infect Dis Obstet Gynecol.* 2005;13:145–150.

47. Heine RP, Wiesenfeld HC, Sweet RL, et al. Polymerase chain reaction analysis of distal vaginal specimens: a less invasive strategy for detection of Trichomonas vaginalis. *Clin Infect Dis.* 1997;24:985–987.

48. Jordan JA, Lowery D, Trucco M. TaqMan-based detection of *Trichomonas vaginalis* DNA from female genital specimens. *J Clin Microbiol.* 2001;39:3819–3822.

49. Kengne P, Veas N, Vidal J, et al. *Trichomonas vaginalis*: repeated DNA target for highly sensitive and specific polymerase chain reaction diagnosis. *Cell Mol Biol.* 1994;40:819–831.

50. Madico G, Quinn TC, Rompalo A, et al. Diagnosis of *Trichomonas vaginalis* infection by PCR using vaginal swab samples. *J Clin Microbiol.* 1998;36:3205–3210.

51. Mayta H, Gilman RH, Calderon MM, et al. 18S ribosomal DNA-based PCR for diagnosis of *Trichomonas vaginalis. J Clin Microbiol.* 2000;38:2683–2687.

52. Paces J, Urbankova V, Urbanek P. Cloning and characterization of a repetitive DNA sequence specific for Trichomonas vaginalis. *Mol Biochem Parasitol.* 1992;54:247–255.

53. Riley DE, Roberts MC, Takayama T, et al. Development of a polymerase chain reaction-based diagnosis of *Trichomonas vaginalis. J Clin Microbiol.* 1992;30:465–472.

54. Reid R, Greenberg M, Jenson AB, et al. Sexually transmitted papillomaviral infections. I. The anatomic distribution and pathologic grade of neoplastic lesions associated with different viral types. *Am J Obstet Gynecol.* 1987;156:212–222.

55. Gissmann L, Wolnik L, Ikenberg H, et al. Human papillomavirus types 6 and 11 DNA sequences in genital and laryngeal papillomas and in some cervical cancers. *Proc Natl Acad Sci USA.* 1983;80:560–563.

56. Bosch FX, Manos MM, Munoz N, et al. Prevalence of human papillomavirus in cervical cancer: a worldwide perspective. International biological study on cervical cancer (IBSCC) Study Group. *J Natl Cancer Inst.* 1995;87:796–802.

57. McCance DJ, Walker PG, Dyson JL, et al. Presence of human papillomavirus DNA sequences in cervical intraepithelial neoplasia. *Br Med J (Clin Res Ed).* 1983;287:784–788.

58. Zbar AP, Fenger C, Efron J, et al. The pathology and molecular biology of anal intraepithelial neoplasia: comparisons with cervical and vulvar intraepithelial carcinoma. *Int J Colorectal Dis.* 2002;17:203–215.

59. Crum CP, Ikenberg H, Richart RM, et al. Human papillomavirus type 16 and early cervical neoplasia. *N Engl J Med.* 1984;310:880–883.

60. Herrero R. Epidemiology of cervical cancer. *J Natl Cancer Inst Monogr.* 1996;21:1–6.

61. Ellerbrock TV, Chiasson MA, Bush TJ, et al. Incidence of cervical squamous intraepithelial lesions in HIV-infected women. *JAMA.* 2000;283:1031–1037.

62. Svare EI, Kjaer SK, Worm AM, et al. Risk factors for genital HPV DNA in men resemble those found in women: a study of male attendees at a Danish STD clinic. *Sex Transm Infect.* 2002;78:215–218.

63. Behbakht K, Friedman J, Heimler I, et al. Role of the vaginal micro-biological ecosystem and cytokine profile in the promotion of cervical dysplasia: a case-control study. *Infect Dis Obstet Gynecol.* 2002;10:181–186.

64. Chin-Hong PV, Palefsky JM. Natural history and clinical management of anal human papillomavirus disease in men and women infected with human immunodeficiency virus. *Clin Infect Dis.* 2002;35:1127–1134.

65. Goedert JJ, Cote TR, Virgo P, et al. Spectrum of AIDS-associated malignant disorders. *Lancet.* 1998;351:1833–1839.

66. Smith JS, Herrero R, Bosetti C, et al. Herpes simplex virus-2 as a human papillomavirus cofactor in the etiology of invasive cervical cancer. *J Natl Cancer Inst.* 2002;94:1604–1613.

67. Wallin KL, Wiklund F, Luostarinen T, et al. A population-based prospective study of *Chlamydia trachomatis* infection and cervical carcinoma. *Int J Cancer.* 2002;101:371–374.

68. Cothran MM, White JP. Adolescent behavior and sexually transmitted diseases: the dilemma of human papillomavirus. *Health Care Women Int.* 2002;23:306–319.

69. Ressel GW. CDC releases 2002 guidelines for treating STDs: part II. Human papillomavirus and hepatitis. *Am Fam Physician.* 2002;66: 1996, 1999.

70. Walboomers JM, Jacobs MV, Manos MM, et al. Human papillomavirus is a necessary cause of invasive cervical cancer worldwide. *J Pathol.* 1999;189:12–19.

71. Ronnett BM, Manos MM, Ransley JE, et al. Atypical glandular cells of undetermined significance (AGUS): cytopathologic features, histopathologic results, and human papillomavirus DNA detection. *Hum Pathol.* 1999;30:816–825.

72. Schenck U, Herbert A, Solomon D, et al. Terminology. International Academy of Cytology Task Force summary. Diagnostic cytology towards the 21st century: an international expert conference and tutorial. *Acta Cytol.* 1998;42:5–15.

73. Cox JT, Lorincz AT, Schiffman MH, et al. Human papillomavirus testing by hybrid capture appears to be useful in triaging women with a cytologic diagnosis of atypical squamous cells of undetermined significance. *Am J Obstet Gynecol.* 1995;172:946–954.

74. Solomon D, Schiffman M, Tarone R. Comparison of three management strategies for patients with atypical squamous cells of undetermined significance: baseline results from a randomized trial. *J Natl Cancer Inst.* 2001;93:293–299.

75. Berkova Z, Kaufmann RH, Unger ER, et al. The effect of time interval between referral and colposcopy on detection of human papillomavirus DNA and on outcome of biopsy. *Am J Obstet Gynecol.* 2003;188:932–937.

76. Kulasingam SL, Hughes JP, Kiviat NB, et al. Evaluation of human papillomavirus testing in primary screening for cervical abnormalities: comparison of sensitivity, specificity, and frequency of referral. *JAMA.* 2002;288:1749–1757.

77. Nobbenhuis MA, Walboomers JM, Helmerhorst TJ, et al. Relation of human papillomavirus status to cervical lesions and consequences for cervical-cancer screening: a prospective study. *Lancet.* 1999;354: 20–25.

78. Wang SS, Walker JL, Schiffman M, et al. Evaluating the risk of cervical precancer with a combination of cytologic, virologic, and visual methods. *Cancer Epidemiol Biomarkers Prev.* 2005;14:2665–2668.

79. Peyton CL, Schiffman M, Lorincz AT, et al. Comparison of PCR- and hybrid capture-based human papillomavirus detection systems using multiple cervical specimen collection strategies. *J Clin Microbiol.* 1998;36:3248–3254.

80. Gravitt PE, Peyton CL, Alessi TQ, et al. Improved amplification of genital human papillomaviruses. *J Clin Microbiol.* 2000;38:357–361.

81. Kornegay JR, Shepard AP, Hankins C, et al. Nonisotopic detection of human papillomavirus DNA in clinical specimens using a consensus PCR and a generic probe mix in an enzyme-linked immunosorbent assay format. *J Clin Microbiol.* 2001;39:3530–3536.

82. Manos MM, Ting Y, Wright DK, et al. The use of polymerase chain reaction amplification for the detection of genital human papillomaviruses. *Cancer Cells.* 1989;7:209–214.

83. Coutlee F, Gravitt P, Kornegay J, et al. Use of PGMY primers in L1 consensus PCR improves detection of human papillomavirus DNA in genital samples. *J Clin Microbiol.* 2002;40:902–907.

84. van Doorn LJ, Quint W, Kleter B, et al. Genotyping of human papillomavirus in liquid cytology cervical specimens by the PGMY line blot assay and the SPF(10) line probe assay. *J Clin Microbiol.* 2002;40:979–983.

85. Menezes G, Euscher E, Schwartz B, et al. Utility of the in situ detection of HPV in Pap smears diagnosed as within normal limits. *Acta Cytol.* 2001;45:919–926.

86. Castle PE, Solomon D, Hildesheim A, et al. Stability of archived liquid-based cervical cytologic specimens. *Cancer.* 2003;99:89–96.

87. Khan MJ, Castle PE, Lorincz AT, et al. The elevated 10-year risk of cervical precancer and cancer in women with human papillomavirus (HPV) type 16 or 18 and the possible utility of type-specific HPV testing in clinical practice. *J Nat Cancer Inst.* 2005;97:1072–1079.

Chapter 8

Respiratory Pathogens

Julie D. Fox and Peter A. Tilley

Introduction

Respiratory tract infections are among the most common presenting complaints of patients in both hospital and community settings. They are a considerable burden in terms of both patient morbidity and public health interventions. Laboratory diagnosis of respiratory tract infections should provide guidance in therapy and prognosis, as well as useful epidemiological information reflecting trends in the community. Understanding and monitoring such trends facilitates early recognition of new infectious agents in a population. A summary of the common viruses and bacteria causing respiratory tract infections and their clinical relevance is given in Tables 8-1 and 8-2, respectively.

Even with a significant clinical effort and analysis of multiple specimens, current laboratory methods fail to diagnose approximately half of lower respiratory tract infections. In fact, laboratory diagnosis of community-acquired pneumonia (CAP) is so poor that current clinical practice guidelines do not recommend testing for all but the most severely affected patients and advise use of empiric therapy.[1] This pragmatic approach fails to address issues of antimicrobial overuse and resistance, public health surveillance, and advancement of medical knowledge.

Many "atypical" bacteria are known to cause severe respiratory symptoms, but lack of good diagnostic procedures has hampered the measurement of the real impact of such infections in the community. Despite vaccination policies, *Bordetella pertussis* infection remains relatively common in children and adults and is associated with chronic cough in adults.[2] *Mycoplasma pneumoniae, Legionella pneumophila,* and *Chlamydophilia* (previously *Chlamydia) pneumoniae* are all recognized causes of lower respiratory tract infections, but again, their impact has not been studied in detail. In addition, despite the well-recognized association of viral infections with upper and lower respiratory tract infections, the current diagnostic virology procedures do not provide an answer rapidly enough to

prevent inappropriate antibiotic use or to consider use of antiviral therapy.[3,4]

Molecular techniques have the potential to enhance our diagnostic approaches to respiratory pathogen identification and enable more detailed analysis of outbreaks. Use of nucleic acid detection methods has demonstrated that some organisms are more common and important causes of respiratory infection and disease than previously appreciated. Molecular methods are applied to the diagnostic detection and analysis of the viral and some of the atypical bacterial causes of respiratory infections.

Clinical Utility

Limitations of Conventional Diagnostic Procedures

Conventional diagnostic techniques (culture, antigen, and antibody detection) have been widely utilized for the diagnosis of individual infections and for the identification of respiratory outbreak pathogens with varying success. Culture-based methods are the mainstay for the diagnosis of more typical bacterial infections, such as *Streptococcus pneumoniae* and *Staphylococcus aureus,* and provide isolates for antimicrobial susceptibility testing. For many agents of CAP, however, culture methods have significant drawbacks. In particular, such diagnostic approaches have very low sensitivity for atypical bacteria, due to the fastidious nature of the organisms (e.g., *M. pneumoniae, C. pneumoniae, Bordetella pertussis*), and are too slow to influence patient management. In other cases, culture methods are hazardous and require enhanced containment laboratories (e.g., *Chlamydophilia psittaci, Coxiella burnetii, Francisella tularensis, Yersinia pestis*), which is a costly and not widely available option.

Cell culture for respiratory viruses is cumbersome, expensive, and available only in major medical centers. For many viral infections, suitable culture techniques and antibodies for isolate identification are not available. Thus, infections

J.D. Fox and P.A. Tilley

Table 8-1. Respiratory Viruses in Acute and Public Health Settings

Viruses	Acute Infection	Public Health Significance and Community Impact	Conventional Diagnostics	Molecular Diagnostics and Typing
Influenza viruses (A and B)	Mild to severe URT and LRT infection	Responsible for outbreaks in the community and in immunocompromised individuals	DFA or culture can be utilized, but sensitivity depends on sample quality	Utilized for subtype and strain identification, particularly when culture is inefficient or impractical
Parainfluenza viruses (HPIV1-4)	Mild to severe URT and LRT infection	Impact of parainfluenza 4 not clear; others associated with outbreaks in the community and in immunocompromised individuals	DFA or culture can be utilized, but sensitivity depends on sample quality; HPIV4 is not usually identified	Some outbreaks investigated by sequencing to confirm relationship among viruses
Coronaviruses (and SARS-CoV)	Thought to be mild for most coronaviruses; SARS-CoV has a high morbidity and mortality	SARS-CoV spread by close contact and responsible for outbreaks in multiple countries; other coronaviruses not well studied	Not readily available and lack sensitivity; antibody responses slow to develop	Used to confirm SARS-CoV as a new introduction to man; sequencing used to differentiate among coronaviruses
Rhinoviruses	Usually mild in healthy individuals; exacerbations in asthmatic individuals reported	Common cause of mild URT symptoms with significant economic impact	Not readily available and lack sensitivity	Of only academic interest to date but potentially useful for studying the impact of this common virus in the community
Enteroviruses	Recognized as a cause of wide-ranging respiratory symptoms	Not well established for respiratory symptoms but recognized for other clinical manifestations	Only a proportion is culturable; DFA not established for all serotypes	Range of methods used to mirror serotyping procedures; molecular methods likely to replace typing methods that depend on culture
Respiratory syncytial virus (RSV)	Cause of mild to severe infection, particularly in infants and elderly	Responsible for outbreaks in the community and in immunocompromised individuals	DFA or culture can be utilized, but sensitivity depends on sample quality	Differentiated into subtypes RSVA and B based on sequence differences, but clinical relevance unproven
Metapneumovirus	Studies to date indicate clinical presentation similar to that of RSV	Common infection; likely responsible for outbreaks in the community and in immunocompromised individuals; common copathogen	Culture thought to be insensitive; DFA not yet available	Differentiated into two lineages based on sequence differences, but clinical relevance unproven
Respiratory adenoviruses	Mild to severe respiratory infection (URT and LRT)	Responsible for outbreaks in the community and in immunocompromised individuals	DFA or culture can be utilized, but sensitivity depends on sample quality	Differentiated into types and subtypes with recognized clinical relevance; persistence may create problems in interpretation

DFA, direct fluorescent antibody; HPIV, human parainfluenza virus; LRT, lower respiratory tract; RSV, respiratory syncytial virus; SARS-CoV, severe acute respiratory syndrome coronavirus; URT, upper respiratory tract.

Table 8-2. Respiratory Bacteria in Acute and Public Health Settings

Organism	Acute Infection	Public Health Significance and Community Impact	Conventional Diagnostics	Molecular Diagnostics and Typing
Bordetella pertussis	Mild to severe infection, especially in infants	Large community outbreaks are common	Culture and DFA have low sensitivity; latter also compromised by artifacts	PCR superior to culture but requires standardization; gradual evolution of strains reported
Legionella species	Mild to fatal infection	Frequent outbreaks, water or soil related	Culture performs well, but is slow; Urine antigen detection useful for *L. pneumophila* serogroup 1 in high-prevalence areas	PCR similar to culture for *L. pneumophila*; likely better for non-*pneumophila* species; typing may be useful for outbreaks, but available data are limited
Mycoplasma pneumonia	Common cause of CAP, usually mild	Endemic with occasional epidemics	IgM test useful for primary infection	PCR useful for rapid, sensitive detection
Chlamydophila pneumoniae	Common cause of CAP requiring hospitalization	Community outbreaks described	Limited; serology by MIF most accurate, but slow	PCR useful for rapid, sensitive detection; role of *C. pneumoniae* prolonged infection or colonization needs to be determined

DFA, direct fluorescent antibody; CAP, community acquired pneumonia; MIF, microimmunofluorescence; PCR, polymerase chain reaction.

with parainfluenza virus type 4, human coronaviruses, rhinoviruses, and some enteroviruses would not ordinarily be identified without RNA detection methods. The impact of such infections is only just being realized, and there is probably an underestimation of their clinical importance, particularly for immunocompromised individuals, the elderly, or those with underlying conditions such as asthma.[5,6]

Human metapneumovirus has been confirmed as an important cause of severe lower respiratory tract infection. The virus has been circulating for more than 50 years, and studies using molecular assays have confirmed its wide distribution,[7,8] but many laboratories have not been successful in isolating this virus. The recent identification of the agent causing severe acute respiratory syndrome (SARS), known as SARS-CoV, has illustrated the need for expansion of diagnostic testing to encompass new emerging viruses and the limitations of conventional virological laboratory approaches to respiratory pathogen diagnosis.[9,10]

Even if it is possible to culture viruses efficiently, isolation and confirmation of the cause of a cytopathic effect can take days to weeks, depending on the pathogen. Waiting for a culture-positive result can take many days, during which time the patient may be inappropriately treated and, if hospitalized, infection control measures may not be initiated. Also, the use of primary primate cells in culture (which gives the best yields of influenza and parainfluenza viruses) is unlikely to be sustainable in the long term.

When available, monoclonal antibodies are useful in direct virus-specific antigen detection tests, and these can be used for rapid diagnosis. Many laboratories are able to provide diagnostic testing for influenza, parainfluenza (types 1–3), respiratory syncytial virus (RSV), and respiratory adenoviruses. A respiratory specimen containing cells is necessary for sensitive detection of viruses by immunofluorescence or other antigen-detection methods.

Good-quality diagnostic samples (often lavage or aspirate samples) can usually be obtained from young, immunocompetent, hospitalized individuals, but in other circumstances the ideal sample may not be available. Delays in transportation may reduce specimen quality and compromise assay results. The most-difficult (and least-efficient) specimens for diagnostic testing are swab samples containing minimal cellular material taken from largely asymptomatic individuals in the community. Smears from these samples can be difficult to interpret in a direct antigen test and thus culture of the sample is usually required for pathogen identification. Bacterial antigen detection by a direct fluorescent antibody (DFA) test is similarly compromised by poor sensitivity and has the added concern of artifacts leading to false-positive results, particularly for *B. pertussis* and *L. pneumophila*.

Serological assays of an antibody response to infection are available for some respiratory pathogens. Although useful for retrospective evidence of infection in a community, the results are not timely enough for patient management. For some cell-associated or intracellular bacteria and viruses, antibody responses develop slowly, if they develop at all, and convalescent sera taken many weeks after disease onset are required to make a definitive diagnosis (e.g., for *C. pneumoniae*, *Legionella* species, RSV). For other infections such as influenza, antibody responses are brisk, but frequent reinfection reduces the IgM response and convalescent sera are required to demonstrate changing titers.

Application of Molecular Assays to Respiratory Pathogen Diagnosis

The limitations of conventional testing are well recognized for viral[11,12] and bacterial[13,14] pathogens, and some of the

Table 8-3. Comparison of Nucleic Acid and Culture/Antigen Detection Methods for Respiratory Pathogen Diagnosis

	Nucleic Acid Methods	Culture/Antigen Methods
Cost	Tests tend to be expensive (but getting cheaper)	Relatively inexpensive in laboratories already set up for these procedures, but "real" cost of maintaining cultures often underestimated
Speed	Rapid diagnostic methods	Speed very variable depending on the pathogen and method used
Infrastructure	Specialized laboratory set-up required	Specialized laboratory set-up required
Spectrum	Specific sequence information required for design; triage of testing can be difficult; generic primers may be used to identify novel pathogens	"Catch-all" approach, which may be advantageous when novel pathogens need to be identified
Sensitivity	Exquisite sensitivity but can be prone to cross-contamination problems	Generally less sensitive than nucleic acid detection methods
Specificity	Careful handling required to avoid contamination (common problem); primer/probe design crucial	Careful handling required to avoid contamination, but less-common problem than for molecular methods; DFA subject to over interpretation
Strain typing	Most definitive method	Limited serotyping (e.g., influenza, *Legionella*)
Automation	Automated extraction equipment becoming available; automated detection commonplace	Difficult to automate
Safety	Inactivated before analysis, but antimicrobial sensitivity information requires knowledge of genotypic mutation	Isolates useful for antimicrobial sensitivity testing and phenotyping, but specialized safety requirements needed for culture of category 3/4 pathogens
Quality assurance	Proficiency and validation of methods not well established	Culture depends critically on cell line or medium quality; maintaining quality can be difficult

key differences between nucleic acid and culture or direct antigen testing methods are summarized in Table 8-3. Utilization of rapid viral diagnostic procedures, such as may be provided by molecular amplification methods, could help to reduce the emergence of antibiotic-resistant bacteria. One study demonstrated that a 52% reduction in antibiotic use was possible using molecular methods for viral diagnosis.[15]

Despite the obvious economic burden of CAP, we do not have accurate data on how many of these infections are viral in origin or caused by the atypical bacteria for which routine diagnostic testing is not readily available. The identification of emerging human viral infections (such as H5N1 influenza and SARS-CoV) has heightened awareness of the gaps in respiratory pathogen diagnosis. Nucleic acid detection assays are likely to be utilized more widely to identify novel emerging pathogens that could result in worldwide outbreaks. Molecular amplification assays are being used successfully for the identification of organisms associated with pneumonia.[16]

The potential for nosocomial spread of respiratory pathogens is well recognized for patients admitted to the hospital with RSV, parainfluenza, or other infections, serving as a reservoir for transmission to vulnerable patients and leading to possible outbreaks.[17] Previously, available diagnostic methods were not sensitive enough to identify sources of outbreaks, but the advent of molecular amplification methods has allowed even environmental sampling to be helpful in confirming outbreak sources and linking clustered cases of infection.[18]

Molecular Tests for Respiratory Pathogens

Samples and Nucleic Acid Extraction

Samples used for detection of respiratory pathogens include swabs (usually nasopharyngeal or throat), aspirates (nasopharyngeal or tracheal), sputum (usually from individuals presenting with pneumonia), or bronchoalveolar lavage specimens. For infections involving the entire respiratory tract, nasopharyngeal specimens are practical for diagnosis. For other infections, which are more focal,

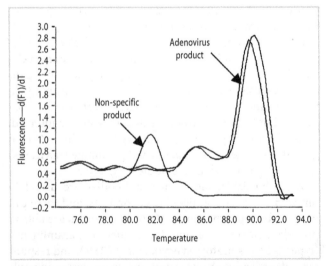

Figure 8-1. Melting-curve analysis of PCR products using the intercalating dye SYBR Green differentiates between specific and nonspecific products without further manipulation of the PCR products.

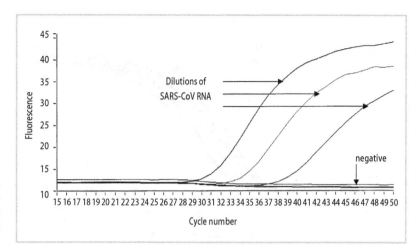

Figure 8-2. Detection of RT-PCR products for severe acute respiratory syndrome coronavirus (SARS-CoV) by a real-time PCR assay utilizing a hydrolysis (TaqMan) probe. The fluorescence signal is produced by measurement of the amount of fluorescent dye released each cycle.

lower respiratory tract specimens are required (e.g., for *Legionella*).

Sample preparation is a critical step for the detection and analysis of organisms. Numerous methods, from simple boiling to sophisticated automated protocols, are available for disruption of the organism and purification of the nucleic acids. Many studies have demonstrated inhibitors in respiratory specimens, making some form of extraction (with or without freezing) necessary to avoid frequent false negative results. Commercial kits for preparation of samples are available and should reduce interlaboratory variation in results. Simultaneous extraction of RNA and DNA facilitates assays for both viruses and bacteria.

Diagnostic Detection of Nucleic Acid

Molecular techniques for the detection and analysis of pathogens associated with respiratory infection provide specific diagnoses for individual cases and for outbreaks. Currently, FDA-cleared molecular tests are not available

for the detection of respiratory pathogens, with the exception of *Mycobacterium tuberculosis* (see chapter 10). Molecular tests are performed using either validated laboratory-developed procedures or commercial testing reagents. Published diagnostic methods for detection of respiratory pathogen DNA or RNA directly from clinical specimens utilize target amplification procedures such as polymerase chain reaction (PCR) or nucleic acid sequence-based amplification (NASBA). Although direct detection methods based on nucleic acid hybridization would be theoretically possible, the amount of target nucleic acid in specimens may be minimal and such methods would lack sensitivity compared to amplification methods, unless the organism was propagated before analysis. Thus, the molecular amplification procedures reported for direct detection of respiratory pathogens in clinical samples include PCR (e.g., Reference 19 and Figure 8-1), reverse transcription-polymerase chain reaction (RT-PCR) (e.g., Reference 20 and Figures 8-2 and 8-3), and NASBA (e.g., References 21–23 and Figures 8-4 and 8-5). Target nucleic acid for amplification assays usually is a pathogen-specific gene or genes from the pathogen genomic DNA or RNA, but some

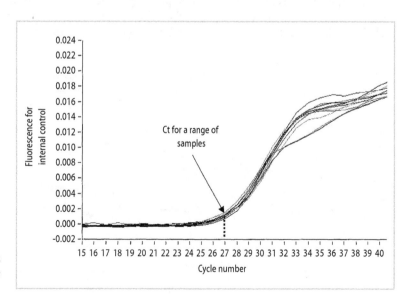

Figure 8-3. Analysis of internal control reactions for clinical samples in a real-time RT-PCR assay ensures that nucleic acid extraction of the sample was efficient and no residual inhibitors are present.

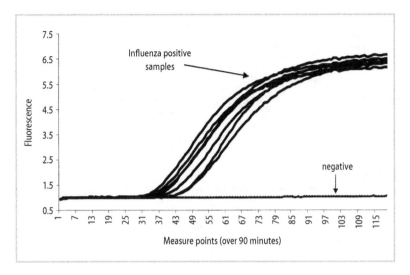

Figure 8-4. Real-time NASBA assay for influenza with detection of amplified products using a molecular beacon probe. Differentiation of positive from negative results is straightforward in this example.

assays have utilized bacterial ribosomal RNA (rRNA; e.g., Reference 22). For cellular samples tested for respiratory pathogens, targeting messenger RNA (mRNA) or genomic antisense RNA may enhance diagnostic sensitivity.

A variety of formats have been utilized for the detection of amplified products. Procedures that separate target amplification from the detection phase (agarose gel analysis or endpoint hybridization) are well established[24,25] and may allow multiple targets to be analyzed in a single reaction, providing added typing information.

For ease of use and incorporation into diagnostic laboratories, most laboratory-developed assays for detection of respiratory pathogens utilize real-time amplification methods in which the amplification and detection steps are combined. Some methods use intercalating dyes with the analysis of PCR product melting temperatures (e.g., as described previously[26] and illustrated in Figure 8-1), whereas others use fluorogenic primers or probes (e.g., TaqMan, hybridization format, and molecular beacons[19,21–23,27]) to ensure the specificity of the reaction. Figure 8-2 illustrates a real-time RT-PCR assay for SARS-CoV using probe-specific detection of amplified products (one fluorescence measurement per cycle). The range of real-time PCR or RT-PCR and NASBA methodologies used

for respiratory targets is diverse given the fact that assays are laboratory developed.[28,29]

The difficulty with diagnosis of respiratory infections is the wide range of pathogens with similar presentations. The nucleic acid technologies utilized currently in the majority of diagnostic laboratories are real-time PCR single-target assays. In some cases, generic primers can be designed to pick up several related pathogens. Such generic primers may be based on conserved protein coding sequences (such as those essential for enzyme function) or noncoding regions for which variation is limited because of the need for maintenance of secondary structure. The use of primer sets to pick up genera or even families of organisms has shown promise in limited studies, including analysis of *Legionella* and *Mycobacteria*. Generic assays have the ability to detect many related organisms and may be used to characterize previously undescribed species in respiratory infection.

Limited multiplex procedures have been reported for detection of related organisms using real-time PCR or NASBA procedures, but such assays are difficult to set up and control. For many respiratory pathogens, there is sufficient variation that multiplex approaches have been developed to detect, for example, all possible respiratory

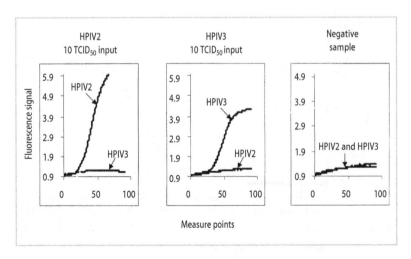

Figure 8-5. Multiplex real-time NASBA assay for human parainfluenza virus (HPIV) with simultaneous detection and differentiation of two target types using two sets of primers and specific molecular beacons labeled with FAM and ROX, respectively. TCID$_{50}$, 50% Tissue Culture Infecting Dose.

adenovirus,[19] influenza,[20] or parainfluenza[21] types. A simple, dual-labeled multiplex NASBA assay is shown in Figure 8-5 that uses separate primer sets and specific molecular beacon probes for parainfluenza types 2 and 3 (HPIV2 and HPIV3) in the same reaction mix. Each probe is labeled with a different fluorophore, allowing detection and differentiation of both viruses in a single reaction. An ambitious multiplex nested RT-PCR procedure with gel analysis of the amplicons detects influenza A, B, and C viruses, RSV (A and B subtypes), and adenoviruses in a single assay.[30] The procedure, while complex to set up and validate, was reported to have good specificity and better sensitivity than antigen/culture procedures.

Interpretation and validation of a negative result are important parts of diagnostic tests based on nucleic acid amplification. Some assays incorporate an internal control system to distinguish true-negative from false-negative results. The internal control may amplify with the pathogen-specific primers but result in an amplicon with a different size or internal sequence from the pathogen amplicon. Alternatively, the internal control may be an external sequence spiked into the reaction (heterologous control) and amplified with a primer set different from the pathogen primers. In the example shown in Figure 8-3, amplification of the RNA heterologous control is consistent across many clinical samples and ensures that there are no gross inhibitors present in the reactions. For cellular samples obtained for detection of respiratory pathogens, the internal control reaction can utilize human DNA, rRNA, or mRNA detection. Such approaches have the added value of assessing for sample collection and integrity, as well as amplification inhibitors.

The relative merits of commercial versus laboratory-developed tests depend on the laboratory facilities, the technical expertise available, and the clinical need for expanded diagnosis. Commercial testing reagents provide quality controls and procedure standardization that facilitate clinical studies.[24,32] Many companies are focusing on providing analyte-specific reagents (ASRs) for respiratory pathogen assays. ASRs will provide the laboratory with quality-controlled primers and probes, while allowing

them the flexibility to test for currently known circulating pathogens or according to a local testing algorithm. Microarray-based detection of multiplexed PCR products also has been reported.[31]

Microbial Typing and Respiratory Outbreak Investigation

Classically, typing of bacteria or viruses has used serological techniques that rely on antibody-antigen interactions. One benefit of approaches based on DNA or RNA detection is the more-detailed, quantitative assessment of the relationship between organisms, providing valuable data relevant to outbreak investigations and community health. Variation at the nucleic acid sequence level is not necessarily reflected in altered protein sequence or function; thus, additional sequence variation information may not correlate with conventional typing methods.

Restriction fragment length polymorphism (RFLP) analysis by pulsed field gel electrophoresis (PFGE), either with or without blot hybridization, has been utilized for analysis of complex DNA genomes from a variety of respiratory pathogens. RFLP analysis also has been applied to PCR or RT-PCR products from respiratory bacteria and viruses. In general, such methods can provide resolution down to the subtype level and have proven useful in outbreak investigation, as illustrated in Figure 8-6 for *B. pertussis* isolates. The difficulty with gel-based typing assays, such as PFGE, is standardizing results and sharing data between laboratories. Amplified fragment length polymorphism (AFLP) analysis represents an alternative method with better discriminatory power and portability, but this approach has not been used extensively for respiratory isolates to date.

For respiratory viruses, other methods have been used for typing, including heteroduplex mobility assay (HMA), single-strand conformation polymorphism (SSCP), and RFLP analysis of amplified PCR products. In general, HMA is considered technically complex but has the capacity to distinguish viral quasispecies with >3% nucleotide

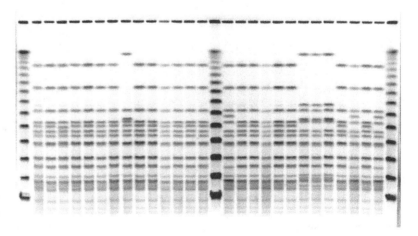

Figure 8-6. Pulsed field gel electrophoresis for analysis of *Bordetella pertussis* isolates. (Figure kindly provided by Dr, M. Peppler, University of Alberta.)

differences. SSCP and RFLP, while technically easier, generally can resolve viruses only to the subtype level, and RFLP has the added constraint of assessing only sequence differences in restriction sites.

The use of sequencing to assess the relationship among viruses is well established, and molecular phylogenetic knowledge is expanding, allowing modeling of viral populations and prediction of new outbreaks.[33] The level of resolution using primary sequence is at one genome, and point mutations can be identified. Sometimes this provides more information than originally sought and creates problems in interpretation; while in other circumstances even small sequence variations can confer important changes in viral transmissibility and disease outcome. Identification of emerging viruses, which may have been recently introduced into the human population (e.g., SARS-CoV and influenza A H5N1 types), is critical to public health. Analysis of such novel viruses has relied heavily on sequencing of isolates or amplicons.[9,10,34]

Human influenza A viruses are associated with enhanced morbidity and mortality compared with influenza B or influenza C viruses. Differences in pathogenicity for subtypes of influenza A also have been reported; for example, H3N2 is associated with more severe infection than H1N1. Such types and subtypes of

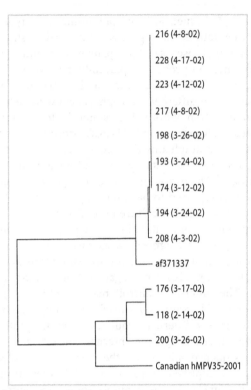

Figure 8-8. Phylogenetic tree illustrating the relationships among fusion gene sequences for 12 human metapneumovirus strains (from 2002). af371337 is the GenBank accession number for the prototype human metapneumovirus strain, and HMPV 35 is a Canadian strain isolated in 2001. (Reprinted from Boivin G, De Serres G, Cote S, et al. Human metapneumovirus infections in hospitalized children. *Emerg Infect Dis.* 2003;9:634–640.)

influenza A can circulate independently, and their identification is important for assessment of current vaccine efficacy. Reassortment of the two predominant influenza subtypes infecting humans in recent times has been reported, and analysis of main hemagglutinin (HA) types has been undertaken by a range of molecular and nonmolecular methods.[35,36] Detailed sequence comparison for HA of H1N1 and H1N2 viruses circulating in the United Kingdom in 2001–2002 (Figure 8-7 and Reference 37) illustrates the utility of sequence analysis in understanding viral divergence and relationship to current vaccine use. Reports of avian H5N1 viruses infecting humans (1997–1998 and 2003–2004[34,38]) emphasize the need for detailed surveillance of influenza viruses and vigilance in identification of emerging viruses of importance to public health. Detailed analysis of avian H5N1 viruses that have infected humans to date have confirmed that all genes are of avian origin and are associated with minimal or very inefficient human-to-human spread. The potential for reassorted viruses that could more easily spread among humans is clear, and molecular methods are now an important part of influenza surveillance.

Recent studies of human metapneumovirus have identified two main lineages, with sequence diversity within each group (Figure 8-8[40]), thus displaying a similar pattern to RSV isolates that are classified into two major

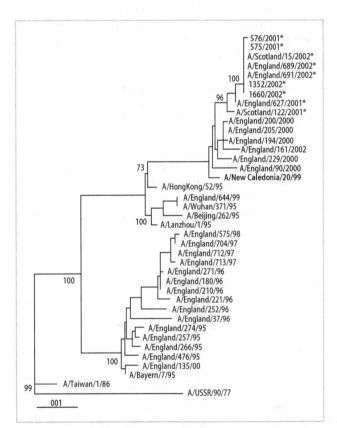

Figure 8-7. Sequence comparison of hemagglutinin (HA) for H1N1 and H1N2 viruses circulating in the United Kingdom in 2001 to 2002. The H1N1 vaccine strain is in bold typeface. H1N2 strains are indicated with asterisks. (Reproduced from Ellis JS, Alvarez-Aguero A, Gregory V, et al. Influenza AH1N2 viruses, United Kingdom, 2001–02 influenza season. *Emerg Infect Dis.* 2003;9:304–310.)

groups, A and B.[39] Further studies will confirm whether this distinction is associated with differences in virulence.

Sequence analysis for typing of bacteria has been slower to develop than that for viruses but has been utilized for investigation of some atypical bacteria associated with outbreaks of respiratory infection (e.g., *Legionella*[41]). Due to the problem of recombination, characterization of a single bacterial gene often does not reflect the organism as a whole. Multilocus sequence typing is a strategy that addresses this and appears useful for analysis of *B. pertussis*.[42]

Microarray hybridization methods have been used to identify and differentiate related pathogens.[31] Such an approach was useful in first identifying the agent of SARS as a coronavirus.[43] Molecular methods provide additional information about the virulence and type of infectious organism, as illustrated by recent experience with SARS-CoV and influenza types.

Interpretation of Test Results

Molecular tests have advantages over conventional procedures, but the sensitivity of molecular amplification methods can lead to problems with interpretation of results. For many organisms, a gold standard method is not available that accurately reflects the enhanced sensitivity of molecular methods, as has been seen with PCR testing for *B. pertussis* or *C. pneumoniae* in clinical samples. Studies confirm that PCR tests are very sensitive, and PCR-positive individuals may be culture negative or asymptomatic, so that results must always be interpreted in the clinical context.

Inhibitors of amplification are common in respiratory specimens, so a negative result must be interpreted in the context of the nucleic acid extraction method and the control results to monitor for nucleic acid degradation and amplification inhibition. When assays for the detection of respiratory pathogens are designed, primers and probes should not cross-react with normal respiratory flora or other respiratory pathogens.

Laboratory Issues

The triage of molecular testing for respiratory infection diagnosis is difficult. Currently, a single respiratory pathogen test detects only one or a few related pathogens. Also, bacterial testing and viral testing are not combined. Thus, many molecular tests must be used to screen for all appropriate pathogens, which increases testing costs. Thus, a laboratory that embarks on using molecular methods for the diagnosis of respiratory infections may require a complex testing algorithm. One approach is use a multiplex amplification procedure to identify multiple pathogens in a single assay, with certain assays now commercially available.[24,32] Unfortunately, such tests tend to be expensive

and, if developed by the laboratory, are very difficult to control and ensure equal sensitivity and specificity for all pathogens. Thus, despite the potential for replacement of many culture and antigen procedures with nucleic acid amplification assays, such a molecular diagnostic revolution has not yet happened. The exception is for new pathogens when nucleic acid amplification and detection methods are clearly far superior to alternatives (e.g., metapneumovirus, SARS-CoV) or for testing of samples that are suboptimal for routine procedures (e.g., in surveillance situations).

Future Directions

Respiratory infections are currently underdiagnosed, despite the fact that accurate pathogen identification is important to ensure appropriate patient management and monitor infectious trends in the community. The major stumbling blocks in the diagnosis and investigation of respiratory infections are the complexity of testing algorithms and the number of potential targets that cause both upper and lower respiratory tract symptoms. Real-time PCR methods have vastly improved the sensitivity for detection and recognition of some difficult-to-culture organisms, and will likely become standard practice in the clinical laboratory in the next few years. There is, however, a limit to how many organisms can be "multiplexed" in a single test.

Microarray hybridization of randomly amplified PCR products from respiratory cultures and clinical samples has shown some success.[31] If the promise of early experiments is maintained when applied to large-scale clinical studies, this could answer some of the technical problems surrounding the use of multiplex systems. Microarray hybridization, while not currently as convenient as real-time PCR detection methods, potentially has the benefit of being able to resolve complex product mixtures and provide clinically valuable information.

The use of molecular methods for typing and outbreak investigation of respiratory pathogens of public health importance is well established and is likely to expand. Future directions will incorporate the use of microarray systems for respiratory pathogen detection and analysis to allow crossing of the barriers between conventional virology and bacteriology (and mycology/parasitology). Once microarray systems have been developed and validated, the costs of this enhanced technology may be reduced and justifiable.

Identification of novel viruses, which have presumably only recently been introduced to humans, has reinforced the need for careful surveillance of emerging respiratory pathogens and institution of appropriate infection control measures. Lessons should be learned from the continuous sensitive surveillance and typing of organisms such as influenza and *B. pertussis* to direct the use and efficacy of available vaccines.

Molecular techniques developed for detection and analysis of the microbes responsible for respiratory infections will be vital to our understanding of pathogenic mechanisms, appropriate management, and prevention of outbreaks in the future. Gel-based typing procedures (PFGE, HMA, SSCP) slowly will be replaced by sequence-based alternatives (e.g., multilocus sequence typing or MLST), which are more amenable to standardization and sharing of data among laboratories.

References

1. Mandell LA, Marrie TJ, Grossman RF, et al. Canadian guidelines for the initial management of community-acquired pneumonia: an evidence-based update by the Canadian Infectious Diseases Society and the Canadian Thoracic Society. The Canadian Community-Acquired Pneumonia Working Group. *Clin Infect Dis.* 2000;31:383–421.
2. Birkebaek NH. Bordetella pertussis in the aetiology of chronic cough in adults. Diagnostic methods and clinic. *Dan Med Bull.* 2001;48: 77–80.
3. Barenfanger J, Drake C, Leon N, et al. Clinical and financial benefits of rapid detection of respiratory viruses: An outcomes study. *J Clin Microbiol.* 2000;38:2824–2828.
4. Zambon MC, Stockton JD, Clewley JP, et al. Contribution of influenza and respiratory syncytial virus to community cases of influenza-like illness: an observational study. *Lancet.* 2001;358:1410–1416.
5. Atmar RL, Guy E, Guntupalli KK, et al. Respiratory tract viral infections in inner-city asthmatic adults. *Arch Intern Med.* 1998;158:2453–2459.
6. van Elden LJ, van Kraaij MG, Nijhuis M, et al. Polymerase chain reaction is more sensitive than viral culture and antigen testing for the detection of respiratory viruses in adults with hematological cancer and pneumonia. *Clin Infect Dis.* 2002;34:177–183.
7. Falsey AR, Erdman D, Anderson LJ, et al. Human metapneumovirus infections in young and elderly adults. *J Infect Dis.* 2003;187:785–790.
8. Stockton J, Stephenson I, Fleming D, et al. Human metapneumovirus as a cause of community-acquired respiratory illness. *Emerg Infect Dis.* 2002;8:897–901.
9. Poutanen SM, Low DE, Henry B, et al. Identification of severe acute respiratory syndrome in Canada. *N Engl J Med.* 2003;348:1967–1976.
10. Drosten C, Gunther S, Preiser W, et al. Identification of a novel coronavirus in patients with severe acute respiratory syndrome. *N Engl J Med.* 2003;348:1995–2005.
11. Mitchell S, O'Neill HJ, Ong GM, et al. Clinical assessment of a generic DNA amplification assay for the identification of respiratory adenovirus infections. *J Clin Virol.* 2003;26:331–338.
12. Ong GM, Wyatt DE, O'Neill HJ, et al. A comparison of nested polymerase chain reaction and immunofluorescence for the diagnosis of respiratory infections in children with bronchiolitis, and the implications for a cohorting strategy. *J Hosp Infect.* 2001;49: 122–128.
13. Tilley PA, Kanchana MV, Knight I, et al. Detection of Bordetella pertussis in a clinical laboratory by culture, polymerase chain reaction, and direct fluorescent antibody staining; accuracy, and cost. *Diagn Microbiol Infect Dis.* 2000;37:17–23.
14. Qasem JA, Khan ZU, Shiji G, et al. Polymerase chain reaction as a sensitive and rapid method for specific detection of Mycoplasma pneumoniae in clinical samples. *Microbiol Res.* 2002;157:77–82.
15. Woo PCY, Chiu SS, Seto W-H, et al. Cost-effectiveness of rapid diagnosis of viral respiratory tract infections in pediatric patients. *J Clin Microbiol.* 1997;35:1579–1581.
16. Murdoch DR. Nucleic acid amplification tests for the diagnosis of pneumonia. *Clin Infect Dis.* 2003;36:1162–1170.
17. Zambon M, Bull T, Sadler CJ, et al. Molecular epidemiology of two consecutive outbreaks of parainfluenza 3 in a bone marrow transplant unit. *J Clin Microbiol.* 1998;36:2289–2293.
18. Echavarria M, Kolavic SA, Cersovsky S, et al. Detection of adenoviruses (AdV) in culture-negative environmental samples by PCR during an AdV-associated respiratory disease outbreak. *J Clin Microbiol.* 2000;38:2982–2984.
19. Gu Z, Belzer SW, Gibson CS, et al. Multiplexed, real-time PCR for quantitative detection of human adenovirus. *J Clin Microbiol.* 2003;41:4636–4641.
20. Smith AB, Mock V, Melear R, et al. Rapid detection of influenza A and B viruses in clinical specimens by Light Cycler real time RT-PCR. *J Clin Virol.* 2003;28:51–58.
21. Hibbitts S, Rahman A, John R, et al. Development and evaluation of NucliSens basic kit NASBA for diagnosis of parainfluenza virus infection with "end-point" and "real-time" detection. *J Virol Methods.* 2003;108:145–155.
22. Loens K, Ieven M, Ursi D, et al. Detection of Mycoplasma pneumoniae by real-time nucleic acid sequence-based amplification. *J Clin Microbiol.* 2003;41:4448–4450.
23. Fox JD, Han S, Samuelson A, et al. Development and evaluation of nucleic acid sequence based amplification (NASBA) for diagnosis of enterovirus infections using the NucliSens Basic Kit. *J Clin Virol.* 2002;24:117–130.
24. Fan J, Henrickson KJ, Savatski LL, et al. Rapid simultaneous diagnosis of infections with respiratory syncytial viruses A and B, influenza viruses A and B, and human parainfluenza virus types 1, 2, and 3 by multiplex quantitative reverse transcription-polymerase chain reaction-enzyme hybridization assay (Hexaplex). *Clin Infect Dis.* 1998;26:1397–1402.
25. Stockton J, Ellis JS, Saville M, et al. Multiplex PCR for typing and subtyping influenza and respiratory syncytial viruses. *J Clin Microbiol.* 1998;36:2990–2995.
26. Boivin G, Cote S, Dery P, et al. Multiplex real-time PCR assay for detection of influenza and human respiratory syncytial viruses. *J Clin Microbiol.* 2004;42:45–51.
27. Templeton KE, Scheltinga SA, Sillekens P, et al. Development and clinical evaluation of an internally controlled, single-tube multiplex real-time PCR assay for detection of Legionella pneumophila and other Legionella species. *J Clin Microbiol.* 2003;41:4016–4021.
28. Mackay IM, Arden KE, Nitsche A. Real-time PCR in virology. *Nucleic Acids Res.* 2002;30:1292–1305.
29. Chan AB, Fox JD. NASBA and other transcription-based amplification methods for research and diagnostic microbiology. *Rev Med Microbiol.* 1999;10:185–196.
30. Coiras MT, Perez-Brena P, Garcia ML, et al. Simultaneous detection of influenza A, B, and C viruses, respiratory syncytial virus, and adenoviruses in clinical samples by multiplex reverse transcription nested-PCR assay. *J Med Virol.* 2003;69:132–144.
31. Wang D, Coscoy L, Zylberberg M, et al. Microarray-based detection and genotyping of viral pathogens. *Proc Natl Acad Sci U S A.* 2002;99:15687–15692.
32. Hindiyeh M, Hillyard DR, Carroll KC, et al. Evaluation of the Prodesse Hexaplex multiplex PCR assay for direct detection of seven respiratory viruses in clinical specimens. *Am J Clin Pathol.* 2001;116: 218–224.
33. McCormack GP, Clewley JP. The application of molecular phylogenetics to the analysis of viral genome diversity and evolution. *Rev Med Virol.* 2002;12:221–238.
34. Subbarao K, Shaw MW. Molecular aspects of avian influenza (H5N1) viruses isolated from humans. *Rev Med Virol.* 2000;10:337–348.
35. Ellis JS, Zambon MC. Molecular diagnosis of influenza. *Rev Med Virol.* 2002;12:375–389.
36. Poddar SK. Influenza virus types and subtypes detection by single step single tube multiplex reverse transcription-polymerase chain reaction (RT-PCR) and agarose gel electrophoresis. *J Virol Methods.* 2002;99:63–70.
37. Ellis JS, Alvarez-Aguero A, Gregory V, et al. Influenza AH1N2 viruses, United Kingdom, 2001–02 influenza season. *Emerg Infect Dis.* 2003;9: 304–310.

38. Shaw M, Cooper L, Xu X, et al. Molecular changes associated with the transmission of avian influenza A H5N1 and H9N2 viruses to humans. *J Med Virol.* 2002;66:107–114.

39. Peret TC, Hall CB, Schnabel KC, et al. Circulation patterns of genetically distinct group A and B strains of human respiratory syncytial virus in a community. *J Gen Virol.* 1998;79:2221–2229.

40. Boivin G, De Serres G, Cote S, et al. Human metapneumovirus infections in hospitalized children. *Emerg Infect Dis.* 2003;9:634–640.

41. Cloud JL, Carroll KC, Pixton P, et al. Detection of Legionella species in respiratory specimens using PCR with sequencing confirmation. *J Clin Microbiol.* 2000;38:1709–1712.

42. van Loo IH, Heuvelman KJ, King AJ, et al. Multilocus sequence typing of Bordetella pertussis based on surface protein genes. *J Clin Microbiol.* 2002;40:1994–2001.

43. Rota PA, Oberste MS, Monroe SS, et al. Characterization of a novel coronavirus associated with severe acute respiratory syndrome. *Science.* 2003;300:1394–1399.

Chapter 9

Bacterial Pathogens

Ruth Ann Luna and James Versalovic

Introduction

Bacterial infections represent important diseases worldwide despite decades of antibiotic therapy. Diverse microbial pathogens continue to rapidly evolve and present challenges for medical practice that will require ongoing refinements in laboratory-based diagnostic strategies. Since the 1970s, the steady parade of bacterial pathogen discoveries such as *Legionella pneumophila*, *Helicobacter pylori*, and *Bartonella henselae* have highlighted the ongoing importance of bacterial evolution in human infectious diseases. Established bacterial pathogens such as *Streptococcus pyogenes* and *Mycobacterium tuberculosis* have reemerged during the past two decades. Drug-resistant pathogens including multidrug-resistant organisms spread to different geographic areas, ignoring regional boundaries with the assistance of global immigration and travel. Advances in medicine including oncology and transplantation have resulted in greater numbers of immunocompromised patients with increased risks for invasive bacterial infections.

During the 20th century, clinical microbiology developed into an important part of clinical laboratory services and modern laboratory medicine. Since the advent of the Gram stain in the late 1800s, microbiologists visualized bacterial morphology. Bacteriologic culture on plated or in liquid media usually represented the gold standard for the diagnosis of bacterial infections. Continual development of new media formulations resulted in the improved ability to cultivate diverse bacterial pathogens. Challenges with difficult-to-culture or unculturable pathogens were partly addressed with the development of culture-independent serologic and antigen-detection methods.

Despite the established utility of different methods in clinical microbiology, the advent of molecular microbiology methods has resulted in many improvements in the ability to diagnose and monitor bacterial infections. During the past two decades, molecular methods and applications have gained acceptance by the clinical microbiology community. The successful integration of molecular methods with other laboratory approaches in clinical microbiology requires careful evaluation of existing techniques and clinical relevance.

Bacterial Identification and Culture Confirmation

Conventional clinical microbiology depends on microbial culture and subsequent biochemical testing for accurate identification of bacterial pathogens. DNA probe–based solution hybridization with chemiluminescent signal detection represents a widely accepted strategy for bacterial identification using molecular methods. DNA:RNA hybridization assays, especially those using synthetic oligonucleotide probes targeting ribosomal RNA (rRNA), have been used widely for the identification of a number of medically important microorganisms either following culture, as confirmation, or directly in specimens, as detection. The AccuProbe technology (Gen-Probe Inc, San Diego, CA) is the most widely used method and is based on acridinium ester-labeled DNA probes that are complementary to species-specific 16S rRNA sequences.[1] The AccuProbe method includes DNA:RNA hybridization by the hybridization protection assay (HPA) in a liquid format and chemiluminescence for rapid signal detection. These assays are limited by the availability of commercial DNA probes, and each assay enables identification of a single pathogen or closely related pathogens.

Nucleic acid genotyping and sequencing methods have provided alternative strategies for bacterial identification (Figure 9-1). Sequence and chromosomal DNA profile approaches facilitate identification that is database driven and not limited to particular pathogens for individual assays. Novel pathogens also may be detected by these methods, as sequences or DNA profiles may not match entries in databases and represent unique patterns.

The characterization and comparisons of small and large subunit rRNA sequences (5S, 16S, and 23S) for bacterial identification and phylogenetic studies[2] have facil-

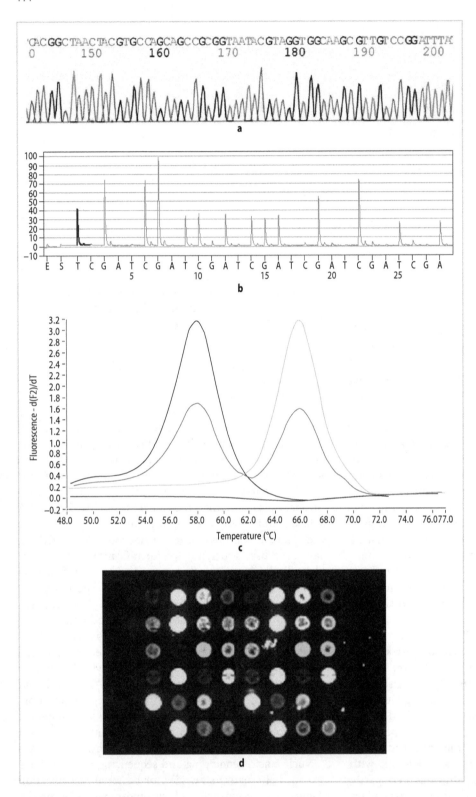

Figure 9-1. Genotyping strategies. (a) Chromatogram generated by DNA sequencing and fluorescent signal detection. (b) Pyrogram generated by pyrosequencing and bioluminescence detection. (c) Melting-curve analyses for characterization of amplicon sequences generated by real-time PCR. (d) Microarray data generated by gene expression profiling of two cell populations.

itated research and development of diagnostic applications. Bacterial rRNA sequences have been compiled into separate sequence databases (e.g., Ribosomal Database Project II) and combined with software tools for bacterial identification and phylogenetic studies (e.g., http://rdp.cme.msu.edu).[3,4] DNA sequencing of all or part of the 16S and 23S rRNA genes has been useful for identification of diverse bacterial pathogens[5] and has resulted in the

development of commercial sequencing platforms (e.g., MicroSeq, Applied Biosystems, Foster City, CA) for microbial identification. Genotypic comparisons based on sequencing of the first 527 base pairs (bp) of the 16S rRNA gene resulted in successful genus- and species-level identification (100% and 93.1%, respectively) of unusual aerobic pathogenic gram-negative bacilli.[6] The juxtaposition of highly conserved and variable sequences within the 16S or 23S rRNA genes[7,8] has culminated in subsequence-based strategies for cost-effective and streamlined identification. Pyrosequencing of selected variable regions, specifically the variable 1 and 3 (V1 and V3) regions, within the 16S rRNA gene provides successful identification of staphylococcal and streptococcal species with 50 bp or less of sequence information.[9] The combination of broad-range polymerase chain reaction (PCR) with cloning and pyrosequencing of V1 and V3 target sequences in the 16S rRNA gene enabled the detection of multiple bacterial contaminants in molecular biology reagents.[10] Targeted genotyping approaches offer the possibility of practical molecular strategies for sequence-based bacterial identification. Finally, future molecular identification strategies may include microarray and microfluidics chromosomal DNA profiling methods that will scan multiple genes and intergenic sequences in parallel.

BLOODSTREAM AND INVASIVE INFECTIONS

The incidence of sepsis and the number of sepsis-related deaths have consistently increased from 1979 to 2000,[11] making sepsis one of the top ten causes of death in the United States. The annualized incidence of sepsis increased 8.7 percent, from 83 cases per 100,000 population in 1979 to 240 cases per 100,000 population in 2000.[11] The diagnosis of bacteremia in cases of sepsis requires the growth of pathogenic bacteria in liquid media, optimally with continuous monitoring by automated detection systems. Blood samples from infected individuals typically contain low levels of organisms (1–10 organisms/ml in adults) so that incubations with continuous monitoring usually require a minimum of 8 to 12 hours prior to detection.

Broad-range PCR has been used for the evaluation of positive blood culture specimens in the clinical microbiology laboratory. Peripheral blood specimens are typically added to bacteriologic liquid media in a glass bottle format, and the blood:media mixtures are monitored continuously in automated blood culture systems. Upon signal (e.g., fluorescence) detection, Gram stain visualization of positive blood cultures and subculturing on plated media are performed for identification. Alternatively, molecular methods may be used for the direct identification of bacterial pathogens in positive blood cultures prior to subculturing specimens on plated media (Table 9-1).

PCR amplification of 16s rRNA gene sequences combined with amplicon sequencing effectively identifies bacteria in blood culture specimens and correlates completely with Gram stain or BACTEC 9240 instrument (Becton Dickinson, Franklin Lakes, NJ) true-positive and true-negative results. Interestingly, the blood culture instruments yielded a 1.3% false-positive signal rate in this study, and all instrument false positives (negative Gram stain and cultures) lacked evidence of bacterial DNA.[12] Several isolates of gram-negative bacilli, including *Acinetobacter* and *Bordetella* organisms, that were difficult to analyze by conventional methods were identified only by DNA sequencing of the 16S rRNA gene using MicroSeq[6] (Applied Biosystems).

Alternative strategies support the potential utility of short subsequences of the 16S rRNA gene for rapid bacterial identification by pyrosequencing.[13] Successful identification of 28 *S. aureus* and 18 streptococcal isolates was achieved by interrogation of 10 nucleotides in the V1 region of 16S rDNA.[9] Pyrosequencing data from the V1 and V3 regions were combined (approximately 30 bp of sequence data) to generate species identification of related enterobacteria. Alternatively, bacterial pathogens may be specifically identified in positive blood cultures by fluorescence in situ hybridization (FISH).[14]

Staphylococcus aureus and coagulase-negative staphylococci (CoNS) represent the most common bacterial isolates from human blood cultures in the United States. In

Table 9-1. Principal Bacterial Pathogens and Molecular Targets

Pathogen	Specimen(s)	Gene (detection)	Gene (drug resistance)
B. henselae	Lymph node aspirates and biopsies	*ribC*	
B. parapertussis	Nasopharyngeal secretions, nasal swabs, sputa, throat swabs	IS*1001*	
B. pertussis	Nasopharyngeal secretions, nasal swabs, sputa, throat swabs	IS*481*	
Brucella species	Blood cultures, tissues, abscess material, bone marrows	IS*711*	
C. pneumoniae	Bronchoscopic washes, nasopharyngeal secretions, sputa, throat swabs	*pmp4*, Pst-1 fragment	
CoNS	Blood cultures, nasal swabs, wound swabs	16S rRNA	*mecA*
EHEC	Stool cultures	*stx*	
ETEC	Stool cultures	LT, ST genes	
H. pylori	Gastric biopsies	*ureC*	*rdxA*, 23S rRNA
L. pneumophila	Bronchoscopic washes, lung biopsies, sputa	*mip*	
M. pneumoniae	Bronchoscopic washes, CSF, lung biopsies, nasopharyngeal secretions, sputa, throat swabs	P1 gene, ATPase Operon gene	
N. meningitidis	Blood cultures, CSF, throat swabs	*ctrA, porA*	
S. aureus	Blood cultures, nasal swabs, wound swabs	*Sa442*	*mecA*
S. pneumoniae	Blood cultures, CSF, nasal swabs	*ply, lytA*	
S. pyogenes	Throat swabs	*ptsI*	
T. whippelii	CSF, intestinal biopsies, lymph node biopsies, synovial fluids	16S rRNA	

CSF, cerebrospinal fluid; CoNS, coagulase-negative staphylococci; EHEC, enterohemorrhagic *E. coli*; ETEC, enterotoxigenic *E. coli*.

addition to species identification, the detection of methicillin-resistant *S. aureus* (MRSA) is important for patient management (Table 9-1). The presence of the *mecA* gene effectively confers methicillin resistance in staphylococci and is a convenient molecular target for PCR-based drug resist ance detection. Real-time PCR can rapidly identify MRSA within 4 hours (DNA preparation, amplification, and detection) by the concurrent application of species-specific and *mecA*-specific DNA probes in parallel or multiplex testing strategies. Real-time PCR strategies have successfully identified MRSA among a panel of bacterial isolates from clinical specimens,[15,16] using both species-specific and *mecA*-specific primer-probe combinations. Investigators have demonstrated that real-time PCR enables rapid MRSA detection directly from smear-positive blood culture bottles, including the BACTEC[17] (Becton Dickinson) and BacT/ALERT[18] (bioMérieux, Hazelwood, MO) systems. The *mecA* gene was detected in 108 of 109 known MRSA isolates, which highlights the potential utility of combining real-time species identification with *mecA* gene detection.[15] Based on the methods already published, appropriate therapies could be instituted 24 to 36 hours earlier if smear-positive blood culture bottles were directly assessed for MRSA. The presence of MRSA dictates the antibiotic treatment strategies, as glycopeptides (e.g., vancomycin) are commonly used in this setting. Differences of 24 to 36 hours may significantly improve patient management by reducing the use of inappropriate antibiotics and diminishing the spread of resistant organisms.

CoNS represent a diverse group of more than 30 different species. The identification of particular species may have clinical implications such as the determination of the presence of *Staphylococcus epidermidis* from a sterile site. Identification of CoNS represents a challenge for development of multiplex real-time PCR methods and melting-curve analyses. A creative primer-biprobe combination resulted in the identification of 15 different CoNS species with only three different real-time PCR reactions.[19]

Streptococcus agalactiae (group B streptococci) remains the leading cause of neonatal sepsis and meningitis and is frequently transmitted as a perinatal infection. Rapid and accurate diagnosis using molecular methods (Table 9-1) facilitates timely management with antimicrobial therapy to prevent perinatal transmission.[20] Although *S. agalactiae* can be successfully cultured from maternal anal or vaginal specimens using enrichment broth culture techniques, the 24- to 48-hour delay in culture detection reduces the utility of group B streptococcal cultures at the time of delivery. For this reason, empiric ampicillin therapy has gained acceptance in obstetrics practice. Real-time PCR assays for rapid detection of *S. agalactiae* directly in vaginal specimens have been developed, targeting species-specific sequences in the *cfb*, or CAMP factor, gene.[21] As bacterial concentrations have not been correlated with different risks of transmission, qualitative real-time PCR detection is sufficient. The Food and Drug Administration (FDA) approved a real-time PCR assay (i.e., IDI-Strep B assay, Becton, Dickinson, and Company, Franklin Lakes, NJ) for detection of *S. agalactiae* directly in anal or vaginal specimens. PCR assays also will be useful for direct detection of invasive group B streptococci in peripheral blood in cases of neonatal sepsis.

CENTRAL NERVOUS SYSTEM INFECTIONS

Rapid diagnosis of central nervous system (CNS) infections may have a dramatic impact on patient outcomes. The most important causes of acute bacterial meningitis are *Neisseria meningitidis* and *Streptococcus pneumoniae*. Childhood vaccination strategies have diminished the risk of meningitis due to *Haemophilus influenzae* serotype b in North America. If acute bacterial meningitis is suspected, cerebrospinal fluid (CSF) specimens are submitted for Gram stain and culture. Immediate Gram stain evaluation is useful, but has limited sensitivity because 10^5 organisms/ml for are required visualization. Laboratory evaluation requires waiting 24 to 48 hours for culture results and a definitive diagnosis.

Although meningococci can be visualized by microscopy and may be cultured in the clinical microbiology laboratory, these organisms present diagnostic challenges with serious implications for patients. PCR testing for detection of *N. meningitidis* infection has been proposed as a strategy for the rapid diagnosis of meningococcal meningitis[22] (Table 9-1) and has been embraced in the United Kingdom and Australia as an important element of laboratory testing. Real-time PCR has been used for direct detection of meningococcal DNA and genogrouping of meningococci for epidemiological purposes in Sweden.[23] *N. meningitidis* DNA was amplified directly from CSF or peripheral blood specimens using the 16S rRNA gene for species detection and the *porA* gene for genogrouping.

Broad-spectrum molecular approaches have been advocated for molecular screening of CSF specimens independent of Gram stain and culture methods (Table 9-1). The conserved 16S rRNA gene contains species-specific target sequences for *N. meningitidis* and has been used in molecular screening strategies. Broad-range PCR based on the 16S rRNA gene has been used successfully to evaluate CSF specimens directly for the presence of bacterial DNA, with a sensitivity and specificity of 100% and 98.2%, respectively.[24] An alternative approach for molecular screening is the multiplex strategy, whereby different genes are used for detection of each species. Corless et al.[25] demonstrated the simultaneous detection of *Neisseria meningitidis*, *Haemophilus influenzae*, and *Streptococcus pneumoniae* by real-time PCR with different genetic targets. A 5′ nuclease (TaqMan) multiplex approach was used to directly amplify bacterial DNA from CSF and peripheral blood specimens. The respective sensitivities of real-time PCR for detection of *N. meningitidis*, *H. influenzae*, and *S. pneumoniae* were 88.4%, 100%, and 91.8%, respectively. More than 4000 CSF specimens were screened in this study,[25] and the improvement in the meningococcal detection rate was 2.9%. That is, 87 additional cases of meningococcal meningitis were identified by PCR alone. Refinements in primer selection targeting less variable sequences in the capsular transport (*ctrA*) gene of *N. meningitidis* accounted for improvements in the sensitivity of the real-time PCR assay.[25] Endpoint PCR detection of *N. meningitidis* increased the laboratory confirmation of clinically suspected cases by 36% when compared to culture and antigen detection.[22]

Molecular methods may yield benefits for the diagnosis of other CNS bacterial infections. *Mycoplasma pneumoniae* is an important cause of atypical pneumonia and is difficult to culture, in contrast to the genital mycoplasmas. In addition to its role in respiratory infections, *M. pneumoniae* may cause meningoencephalitis or transverse myelitis in pediatric patients. PCR tests for the detection of *M. pneumoniae* have been useful for the provision of timely and accurate diagnoses of *M. pneumoniae* CNS infections in children.[26]

GASTROINTESTINAL INFECTIONS

Enteric bacterial pathogens cause well-recognized gastric and intestinal infections. Pathogens such as *Campylobacter*, *Salmonella*, and *Shigella* represent important causes of gastroenteritis and bacillary dysentery and may be cultured from freshly collected stool specimens in infected patients. Successful culture and biochemical identification of enteric pathogens from fecal specimens provide cost-effective diagnoses. However, specific diagnostic challenges that require subspecies or toxigenic strain identification highlight the limitations of current approaches (Table 9-1).

Intestinal *E. coli* is recognized as a commensal organism and pathogen of the human intestine, so the ability to distinguish nonpathogenic and pathogenic isolates is important. Specific pathogenic *E. coli* strains or clones have been associated with human enteric infections. Enterohemorrhagic *E. coli* (EHEC) causes hemorrhagic colitis and hemolytic uremic syndrome. Candidate EHEC isolates can be serotyped as O157:H7 by latex agglutination or tested for Shiga-like toxin production by antigen detection. The limitation of serotyping is highlighted by the fact that more than 20% of EHEC isolates lack the O157:H7 serotype. The Shiga-like toxin genes may be directly detected by DNA amplification and may reduce the turnaround time for diagnosis of this potentially fatal infection.[27] Enterotoxigenic *E. coli* (ETEC) is the most important cause of traveler's diarrhea and, with *Campylobacter jejuni*, remains one of the two most common causes of nonviral gastroenteritis. Culture methods cannot distinguish toxigenic from nontoxigenic strains except by antigen detection. Molecular methods that enable the specific detection of either the heat-labile (LT) or heat-stable (ST) toxin genes provide options for direct ETEC detection in stool isolates.[28]

Tropheryma whippelii is the etiologic agent of Whipple's disease, a rare multisystemic disease primarily involving the small intestine and characterized by inclusion-rich macrophages in the lamina propria. Patients with Whipple's disease may present with diarrhea, weight loss, arthralgias, abdominal pain, and dementia. As up to 15% of cases may not involve the intestinal tract, sampling of extraintestinal sites (e.g., CSF, synovial fluid) may be important for molecular diagnosis of this disorder. Intestinal biopsy specimens, lymph node biopsy specimens, and synovial fluid may be tested directly by PCR amplification of *Tropheryma*-specific DNA.[29,30] As this organism is generally nonculturable, bacterial DNA detection is very useful for the establishment of a specific diagnosis. Importantly, this organism often persists in asymptomatic individuals and its DNA may be detected in healthy individuals using fecal or oral specimens.[30] Colonization of the intestinal tract may be difficult to distinguish from infection, and thus the molecular data should be interpreted in the context of the intestinal histology.

In addition to intestinal infections, *Helicobacter pylori* and other gastric *Helicobacters* may cause chronic gastritis and peptic ulcer disease.[31] Long-term infections with *H. pylori* have been associated with gastric adenocarcinomas and mucosa-associated lymphoid tissue (MALT) lymphomas. Serologic tests are useful for IgG screening, and fecal antigen testing is effective for direct detection. The bacteria reside adjacent to the gastric mucosa and require biopsy sampling by endoscopy for successful culture. In addition to histology and rapid urease testing, endpoint PCR provided strategies for successful detection of *H. pylori* and macrolide resistance mutations in gastric biopsies[32,33] (Table 9-1). Endpoint PCR studies using the 16S rRNA gene for genus-specific PCR detection yielded novel findings such as the detection of *Helicobacter cinaedi* in gastric biopsy specimens obtained from patients with gastritis.[34] More recently, real-time PCR assays have been used for detection and molecular resistance testing of *H. pylori* in gastric biopsies.[35] He et al.[36] described real-time quantitative PCR of *H. pylori* with the *ureC* gene as the target in an assay spanning 6 logs of DNA concentrations. Interestingly, 24 of 27 specimens that were negative by culture were positive by real-time PCR, although contamination could not be excluded.[36]

RESPIRATORY INFECTIONS

Bacterial pathogens represent important causes of respiratory tract infections. Pneumonias caused by various pathogens have overlapping features and are not clinically distinguishable with respect to etiologic agent. Diagnosis of upper or lower respiratory tract infections may require sampling and culture of different sites. Respiratory specimens include throat or nasopharyngeal swabs, sputa, tracheal aspirates, and bronchoscope-assisted collections of fluid or tissue of the lower respiratory tract. In addition to effective differentiation among pathogenic and commensal organisms, colonization must be distinguished from infection. Among bacterial pathogens that cause respiratory infections, several organisms continue to be impractical to culture, and indirect serologic tests may be used.

The diagnosis of *Mycoplasma pneumoniae* as a cause of atypical pneumonia requires IgM serologic testing or molecular methods for direct detection. The utility of PCR has been demonstrated for the detection of *M. pneumoniae* DNA in throat swabs, sputa, and lower respiratory specimens[37,38] (Table 9-1). The risk for pneumonia is especially prominent among children 5 to 15 years of age, in whom 30% of infections progress to pneumonia if untreated.[39] Molecular methods have altered our view of *M. pneumoniae* as a cause of both atypical and acute bacterial pneumonia. PCR methods for detection have been recommended alone and in combination with IgM serologic tests for the diagnosis of respiratory infections caused by *M. pneumoniae*.[38,40] Sensitivities and specificities of PCR tests have ranged from 78% to 92% and 92% to 100%, respectively.[40] In one study, the positive predictive value of endpoint PCR was 100% and contrasted sharply with the relatively low positive predictive value (50%) of IgM detection by the indirect immunofluorescence assay (IFA).[41] Real-time detection of *M. pneumoniae* DNA enhanced molecular diagnostic strategies by improving speed and test handling.[42] Multiplex quantitative real-time PCR has been employed for the simultaneous assessment of atypical pneumonia caused by *Chlamydia pneumoniae*, *Legionella pneumophila*, or *M. pneumoniae*.[43] A comparison of results obtained by real-time PCR with 73 specimens yielded an overall 98.3% agreement with conventional PCR.[43]

Pertussis or whooping cough caused by *Bordetella pertussis* or *Bordetella parapertussis* is an important disease in children and adults. As *B. pertussis* is a fastidious pathogen and requires specialized media for culture, PCR amplification has been adopted as a strategy for diagnosis (Table 9-1). Direct fluorescence assay (DFA) and microbiologic culture have reduced sensitivities when compared to PCR assays in multiple studies. Endpoint and real-time PCR methods are commonly used for the detection of *B. pertussis* or *B. parapertussis* DNA in nasopharyngeal swabs[44-47] from patients. Documented sensitivities for endpoint PCR (95.0%) and real-time PCR (100%) compared favorably with microbiologic culture (11.6% and 36.0%) and DFA tests (11.4%).[44,45] Insertion sequences IS481 and IS1001 have been useful for the detection of *B. pertussis* and *B. parapertussis*, respectively. In addition to IS481, the pertussis toxin promoter contains species-specific target sequences for PCR detection. A systematic comparison of real-time PCR, endpoint PCR, culture, and DFA studies indicated that real-time PCR based on insertion sequence detection had the highest sensitivity and best overall performance.[47] Careful PCR assay selection and quality assessment procedures must be emphasized, as a published investigation presented evidence for substantial over- and misdiagnosis of pertussis cases in two disease outbreaks in New York.[48]

The detection of *Streptococcus pyogenes* (group A streptococci) in throat swabs represents an important strategy for the diagnosis of streptococcal pharyngitis. The typical strategy includes rapid antigen testing with culture confirmation of all specimens negative by antigen testing. This strategy is currently recommended by the American Academy of Pediatrics.[49] DNA probe hybridization methods for the detection of *S. pyogenes* DNA have been proposed as a stand-alone approach instead of the established two-tiered testing procedure.[50] Uhl et al.[51] recommended real-time PCR methods for detection of *S. pyogenes* DNA in throat swabs as a stand-alone test. Real-time PCR matched culture, outperformed rapid antigen testing, and could be performed more rapidly than culture for confirmatory testing. The high prevalence of this disease and potential impact for patient management supports the consideration of molecular testing for the diagnosis of streptococcal pharyngitis (Table 9-1).

Molecular Resistance Testing

Molecular resistance testing refers to the direct detection of genes or mutations conferring antimicrobial resistance. The detection of the *mecA* gene was previously discussed as a strategy for identifying MRSA isolates (see "Bloodstream and Invasive Infections"). Gene detection is relatively straightforward and akin to qualitative bacterial pathogen detection. In contrast, mutation detection requires different methods designed to identify the presence of nucleotide substitutions, deletions, or insertions (Figure 9-1). Parallel identification and detection of drug resistance mutations in bacteria may be complicated by the presence of many different mutations in single or several genes. The ability to detect multiple mutations in parallel may require microarray or high-throughput sequencing strategies in the future.

Detection of the *vanA* and *vanB* glycopeptide resistance genes in enterococci represents a useful molecular strategy for surveillance testing of vancomycin-resistant enterococci (VRE). Like *mecA* detection in MRSA, the presence of *vanA* or *vanB* is sufficient for the reporting of VRE isolates in patients. Endpoint multiplex PCR has been used to detect VRE directly in surveillance specimens and compared favorably with culture and biochemical testing.[52] The sensitivity and specificity of multiplex PCR were 98.4% and 96.1%, respectively.[52] Use of multiplex PCR methods resulted in a turnaround time reduction of approximately 48 hours and resulted in cost savings of approximately 40%.[52] Reductions in turnaround times and labor costs may be further reduced by the implementation of real-time PCR detection of *vanA* or *vanB* target sequences.[53] Cost savings in laboratory testing for *vanA* and *vanB* detection were calculated over time and, when combined with training costs, generated a payback period of 3 years for laboratory costs alone. Further cost benefits for the healthcare system caused by more timely adjustments in patient management and reductions in spread of resistant organisms due to changes in isolation practices were not computed.

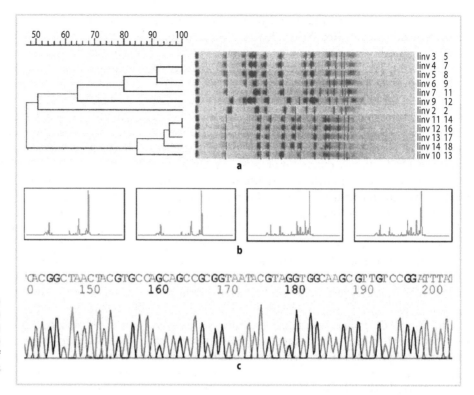

Figure 9-2. DNA typing of bacterial pathogens. (a) Gel image of pulsed field gel electrophoresis (PFGE) data. (b) Peak profiles of DNA fragments generated by repetitive extragenic palindramic PCR (rep-PCR) and microfluidics fragment resolution. (c) One of multiple chromatograms generated by multilocus sequence typing (MLST).

Detection of particular nucleotide substitutions associated with drug resistance may be practical if small sets of mutations are responsible for the vast majority of resistance in particular organisms. Since two point mutations in the 23S rRNA gene account for greater than 90% of macrolide resistance in *Helicobacter pylori*,[54,55] convenient polymerase chain reaction–restriction fragment length polymorphism (PCR-RFLP) methods[33,54] and reverse hybridization[32] assays have been developed for direct mutation detection (Table 9-1). Gastric biopsy specimens may be obtained directly from rapid urease tests and used for molecular resistance testing several weeks following tissue collection.[33]

Molecular Epidemiology

Nosocomial, or hospital-acquired, infections represent the most common complication affecting hospitalized patients and comprise an important category of adverse events in hospitals.[56] Nosocomial infection surveillance activities and epidemiologic studies in hospitals are essential aspects of infection control efforts. Classical epidemiology, usually performed by infection control personnel, includes traditional case-based outbreak investigations that correlate microbiologic identification and antimicrobial susceptibility testing patterns with reviews of case clusters. Molecular epidemiology requires the correlation of classical epidemiology with molecular data for delineation of outbreak-related clones. Molecular epidemiology refers to clonal investigations of bacterial pathogens by genotypic

methods and includes methods such as DNA fingerprinting, DNA profiling, and DNA typing (Figure 9-2 and Table 9-2). Molecular methods yield patterns of different-sized DNA fragments or aggregate sequence information that may be useful for epidemiologic or clonal investigations. Studies have demonstrated the importance of real-time molecular typing strategies for the control of nosocomial infections. Hacek et al. demonstrated hospital savings of

Table 9-2. DNA Typing Strategies

Method	Instrument(s)	Time
AFLP	Thermal cycler, electrophoresis equipment	1–2 days
MLST	DNA sequencer	1–2 days
PFGE	PFGE apparatus	2–3 days
RAPD (AP-PCR)	Thermal cycler, electrophoresis equipment	1 day
rep-PCR	Thermal cycler, electrophoresis equipment, microfluidics device	4 hours–1 day
Ribotyping	Electrophoresis/blotting system	1 day
Spoligotyping	Thermal cycler, miniblotter apparatus	2 days

AFLP, amplified fragment length polymorphism; MLST, multilocus sequence typing; PFGE, pulsed field gel electrophoresis; RAPD, random amplification polymorphic DNA; AP-PCR, arbitrarily primed PCR; rep-PCR, repetitive extragenic palindromic PCR.

greater than $4.3 million during a 2-year period following implementation of routine molecular epidemiologic investigations.[57]

The established gold standard of molecular epidemiology is pulsed field gel electrophoresis (PFGE; Table 9-2), a method that depends on the electrophoretic separation of large DNA fragments created by digestion of bacterial DNA with rare-cutting restriction enzymes.[58,59] Cultivation of bacteria is required prior to initiation of typing studies, and the PFGE studies require approximately 2 days for completion. Several multicenter studies have been published that document the relative abilities of laboratories to perform PFGE and participate in interlaboratory comparisons.[60–62] In one study,[60] four of 12 laboratories failed to generate interpretable PFGE data with *S. aureus*, which highlights the formidable technical challenges of this test. Centralized computer studies of data obtained from four selected laboratories generated similarities of 85% with a group of identical *S. aureus* isolates.[60] Improved harmonization of PFGE protocols recently was achieved by focusing on several critical parameters, but only seven of ten laboratories provided data of sufficient quality for interlaboratory comparisons.[62] Although PFGE has evolved as the historical standard for molecular typing of bacterial pathogens, data comparability and reproducibility represent ongoing challenges due to lack of standardization.

Chromosomal or plasmid RFLP studies, based on conventional electrophoretic separation of DNA fragments, have been less useful for typing bacterial pathogens. Plasmids represent nonessential extrachromosomal DNA molecules that often are absent in bacterial pathogens and limit unique identification with this method. Chromosomal RFLP approaches produce highly complex patterns that are difficult to interpret and limit interlaboratory comparisons.

Ribotyping is a variant of chromosomal RFLP methods and is performed by digestion of chromosomal DNA and hybridization with rRNA operon probes.[63] Generally, ribotyping is less discriminatory compared with other methods due to the limited complexity of ribotyping patterns. A commercial ribotyping method, the Riboprinter Microbial Characterization System (DuPont Qualicon, Wilmington, DE), is available, but the reduced discrimination with this assay continues to be a disadvantage relative to other typing methods such as PFGE and DNA fingerprinting by PCR.[64,65]

DNA typing methods using PCR include amplified fragment length polymorphism (AFLP),[66,67] arbitrarily primed PCR (AP-PCR) or random amplification polymorphic DNA (RAPD) studies,[68,69] multilocus sequence typing (MLST),[70] repetitive extragenic palindromic-PCR (rep-PCR),[71,72] and spoligotyping.[73,74] PCR methods facilitate DNA typing by providing nucleic acid amplification for specimens with limited amounts of target DNA. AFLP yields complex DNA profiles with relatively high discriminatory capabilities when testing various bacterial pathogens.[67] AP-PCR and RAPD methods are similar to AFLP but utilize short random

oligonucleotide primers and fortuitously anneal to multi-copy chromosomal DNA sequences. Multiple amplicons generated by PCR amplification can be separated by conventional agarose gel electrophoresis. Rep-PCR yields different-sized DNA fragments that are separated by various distances between interspersed repetitive DNA elements.[72] Amplicons generated by rep-PCR may be separated by agarose gel electrophoresis or in microfluidic channels with laser-based fragment detection (DiversiLab, Bacterial Barcodes, Houston, TX).[75] Rep-PCR studies suggest that particular MRSA clones are more frequently associated with disease outbreaks.[76] Development of rep-PCR DNA profile databases can be combined with digitized microfluidic channel data to facilitate Internet pattern matching with sophisticated clustering algorithms. MLST has been proposed as a next-generation molecular typing strategy[70] and, in selected studies, MLST matches PFGE for relative discriminatory abilities.[77] High-throughput sequencing capabilities are required for MLST to be practically useful in a diagnostic laboratory setting. As diagnostic laboratories migrate toward more strain- or subspecies-level identification, molecular typing methods may have a prominent role in the diagnosis of bacterial infections.

Summary and Future Trends

Molecular methods have matured and gained acceptance as an important component of laboratory testing for the diagnosis of infectious diseases caused by bacterial pathogens. The initial hype has been supplanted by practical and selective data-driven molecular strategies for diagnosis and patient monitoring. Rapid advances in microbial genomics and bioinformatics have created many opportunities for the development of molecular assays with improved specificity over earlier assays. As the entire genomes of many important bacterial pathogens have been sequenced, it is possible to use multistrain genomic sequencing and comparative genomics for identification of individual pathogens. The greatly increased quantities of genomic data will be translated into the selection of optimal genetic targets for species-specific and strain-specific detection by DNA amplification methods. The development of comprehensive gene and mutation databases will drive the development of new tests for specific virulence genes, toxin genes, and drug resistance genotypes. The next generation of molecular technologies will include developments in high-throughput sequencing, custom microarray applications, and microfluidics or chromatography chromosomal scanning approaches. The rapid change in testing methods will challenge laboratories to maintain leading-edge technical proficiencies and provide clinically relevant information in clinically useful reporting formats. Demands for quality control and quality assessment will require new approaches to keep pace with the rapid evolution of molecular diagnostics and its applications in medicine.

References

1. Arnold LJ Jr, Hammond PW, Wiese WA, et al. Assay formats involving acridinium-ester-labeled DNA probes. *Clin Chem.* 1989;35:1588–1594.

2. Olsen GJ, Woese CR. Ribosomal RNA: a key to phylogeny. *FASEB J.* 1993;7:113–123.

3. Cole JR, Chai B, Marsh TL, et al. The Ribosomal Database Project (RDP-II): previewing a new autoaligner that allows regular updates and the new prokaryotic taxonomy. *Nucleic Acids Res.* 2003;31:442–443.

4. Devulder G, Perriere G, Baty F, et al. BIBI, a Bioinformatics Bacterial Identification Tool. *J Clin Microbiol.* 2003;41:1785–1787.

5. Kolbert CP, Persing DH. Ribosomal DNA sequencing as a tool for identification of bacterial pathogens. *Curr Opin Microbiol.* 1999;2:299–305.

6. Tang YW, Ellis NM, Hopkins MK, et al. Comparison of phenotypic and genotypic techniques for identification of unusual aerobic pathogenic gram-negative bacilli. *J Clin Microbiol.* 1998;36:3674–3679.

7. Gray MW, Sankoff D, Cedergren RJ. On the evolutionary descent of organisms and organelles: a global phylogeny based on a highly conserved structural core in small subunit ribosomal RNA. *Nucleic Acids Res.* 1984;12:5837–5852.

8. Van de PY, Chapelle S, De Wachter R. A quantitative map of nucleotide substitution rates in bacterial rRNA. *Nucleic Acids Res.* 1996;24:3381–3391.

9. Jonasson J, Olofsson M, Monstein HJ. Classification, identification and subtyping of bacteria based on pyrosequencing and signature matching of 16S rDNA fragments. *APMIS.* 2002;110:263–272.

10. Grahn N, Olofsson M, Ellnebo-Svedlund K, et al. Identification of mixed bacterial DNA contamination in broad-range PCR amplification of 16S rDNA V1 and V3 variable regions by pyrosequencing of cloned amplicons. *FEMS Microbiol Lett.* 2003;219:87–91.

11. Martin GS, Mannino DM, Eaton S, et al. The epidemiology of sepsis in the United States from 1979 through 2000. *N Engl J Med.* 2003;348:1546–1554.

12. Qian Q, Tang YW, Kolbert CP, et al. Direct identification of bacteria from positive blood cultures by amplification and sequencing of the 16S rRNA gene: evaluation of BACTEC 9240 instrument true-positive and false-positive results. *J Clin Microbiol.* 2001;39:3578–3582.

13. Ronaghi M, Karamohamed S, Pettersson B, et al. Real-time DNA sequencing using detection of pyrophosphate release. *Anal Biochem.* 1996;242:84–89.

14. Oliveira K, Procop GW, Wilson D, et al. Rapid identification of *Staphylococcus aureus* directly from blood cultures by fluorescence *in situ* hybridization with peptide nucleic acid probes. *J Clin Microbiol.* 2002;40:247–251.

15. Grisold AJ, Leitner E, Muhlbauer G, et al. Detection of methicillin-resistant *Staphylococcus aureus* and simultaneous confirmation by automated nucleic acid extraction and real-time PCR. *J Clin Microbiol.* 2002;40:2392–2397.

16. Elsayed S, Chow BL, Hamilton NL, et al. Development and validation of a molecular beacon probe-based real-time polymerase chain reaction assay for rapid detection of methicillin resistance in *Staphylococcus aureus. Arch Pathol Lab Med.* 2003;127:845–849.

17. Tan TY, Corden S, Barnes R, et al. Rapid identification of methicillin-resistant *Staphylococcus aureus* from positive blood cultures by real-time fluorescence PCR. *J Clin Microbiol.* 2001;39:4529–4531.

18. Shrestha NK, Tuohy MJ, Hall GS, et al. Rapid identification of *Staphylococcus aureus* and the *mecA* gene from BacT/ALERT blood culture bottles by using the LightCycler system. *J Clin Microbiol.* 2002;40:2659–2661.

19. Edwards KJ, Kaufmann ME, Saunders NA. Rapid and accurate identification of coagulase-negative staphylococci by real-time PCR. *J Clin Microbiol.* 2001;39:3047–3051.

20. Noya FJ, Baker CJ. Prevention of group B streptococcal infection. *Infect Dis Clin North Am.* 1992;6:41–55.

21. Ke D, Menard C, Picard FJ, et al. Development of conventional and real-time PCR assays for the rapid detection of group B streptococci. *Clin Chem.* 2000;46:324–331.

22. Pollard AJ, Probe G, Trombley C, et al. Evaluation of a diagnostic polymerase chain reaction assay for *Neisseria meningitidis* in North America and field experience during an outbreak. *Arch Pathol Lab Med.* 2002;126:1209–1215.

23. Molling P, Jacobsson S, Backman A, et al. Direct and rapid identification and genogrouping of meningococci and *porA* amplification by LightCycler PCR. *J Clin Microbiol.* 2002;40:4531–4535.

24. Saravolatz LD, Manzor O, VanderVelde N, et al. Broad-range bacterial polymerase chain reaction for early detection of bacterial meningitis. *Clin Infect Dis.* 2003;40:40–45.

25. Corless CE, Guiver M, Borrow R, et al. Simultaneous detection of *Neisseria meningitidis*, *Haemophilus influenzae*, and *Streptococcus pneumoniae* in suspected cases of meningitis and septicemia using real-time PCR. *J Clin Microbiol.* 2001;39:1553–1558.

26. Bitnun A, Ford-Jones EL, Petric M, et al. Acute childhood encephalitis and *Mycoplasma pneumoniae. Clin Infect Dis.* 2001;32:1674–1684.

27. Wang G, Clark CG, Rodgers FG. Detection in *Escherichia coli* of the genes encoding the major virulence factors, the genes defining the O157:H7 serotype, and components of the type 2 Shiga toxin family by multiplex PCR. *J Clin Microbiol.* 2002;40:3613–3619.

28. Tsen HY, Jian LZ. Development and use of a multiplex PCR system for the rapid screening of heat labile toxin I, heat stable toxin II and Shiga-like toxin I and II genes of *Escherichia coli* in water. *J Appl Microbiol.* 1998;84:585–592.

29. Fenollar F, Fournier PE, Raoult D, et al. Quantitative detection of *Tropheryma whippelii* DNA by real-time PCR. *J Clin Microbiol.* 2002;40:1119–1120.

30. Dutly F, Altwegg M. Whipple's disease and "*Tropheryma whippelii.*" *Clin Microbiol Rev.* 2001;14:561–583.

31. Versalovic J, Fox JG. *Helicobacter.* In: Murray P, Baron EJ, Jorgensen JH, et al., eds. *Manual of Clinical Microbiology.* Washington, DC: ASM Press; 2003:915–928.

32. van Doorn LJ, Henskens Y, Nouhan N, et al. The efficacy of laboratory diagnosis of *Helicobacter pylori* infections in gastric biopsy specimens is related to bacterial density and *vacA*, *cagA*, and *iceA* genotypes. *J Clin Microbiol.* 2000;38:13–17.

33. Pena JA, Fox JG, Ferraro MJ, et al. Molecular resistance testing of *Helicobacter pylori* in gastric biopsies. *Arch Pathol Lab Med.* 2001;125:493–497.

34. Pena JA, McNeil K, Fox JG, et al. Molecular evidence of *Helicobacter cinaedi* organisms in human gastric biopsy specimens. *J Clin Microbiol.* 2002;40:1511–1513.

35. Chisholm SA, Owen RJ, Teare EL, et al. PCR-based diagnosis of *Helicobacter pylori* infection and real-time determination of clarithromycin resistance directly from human gastric biopsy samples. *J Clin Microbiol.* 2001;39:1217–1220.

36. He Q, Wang JP, Osato M, et al. Real-time quantitative PCR for detection of *Helicobacter pylori. J Clin Microbiol.* 2002;40:3720–3728.

37. Buck GE, Eid NS. Diagnosis of *Mycoplasma pneumoniae* pneumonia in pediatric patients by polymerase chain reaction (PCR). *Pediatr Pulmonol.* 1995;20:297–300.

38. Daxboeck F, Krause R, Wenisch C. Laboratory diagnosis of *Mycoplasma pneumoniae* infection. *Clin Microbiol Infect.* 2003;9:263–273.

39. Taylor-Robinson D. Infections due to species of *Mycoplasma* and *Ureaplasma*: an update. *Clin Infect Dis.* 1996;23:671–682.

40. Ferwerda A, Moll HA, de Groot R. Respiratory tract infections by *Mycoplasma pneumoniae* in children: a review of diagnostic and therapeutic measures. *Eur J Pediatr.* 2001;160:483–491.

41. Dorigo-Zetsma JW, Zaat SA, Wertheim-van Dillen PM, et al. Comparison of PCR, culture, and serological tests for diagnosis of *Mycoplasma pneumoniae* respiratory tract infection in children. *J Clin Microbiol.* 1999;37:14–17.

42. Hardegger D, Nadal D, Bossart W, et al. Rapid detection of *Mycoplasma pneumoniae* in clinical samples by real-time PCR. *J Microbiol Methods.* 2000;41:45–51.

43. Welti M, Jaton K, Altwegg M, et al. Development of a multiplex real-time quantitative PCR assay to detect *Chlamydia pneumoniae*, *Legionella pneumophila* and *Mycoplasma pneumoniae* in respiratory tract secretions. *Diagn Microbiol Infect Dis*. 2003;45:85–95.

44. Tilley PA, Kanchana MV, Knight I, et al. Detection of *Bordetella pertussis* in a clinical laboratory by culture, polymerase chain reaction, and direct fluorescent antibody staining; accuracy, and cost. *Diagn Microbiol Infect Dis*. 2000;37:17–23.

45. Chan EL, Antonishyn N, McDonald R, et al. The use of TaqMan PCR assay for detection of *Bordetella pertussis* infection from clinical specimens. *Arch Pathol Lab Med*. 2002;126:173–176.

46. Qin X, Turgeon DK, Ingersoll BP, et al. *Bordetella pertussis* PCR: simultaneous targeting of signature sequences. *Diagn Microbiol Infect Dis*. 2002;43:269–275.

47. Sloan LM, Hopkins MK, Mitchell PS, et al. Multiplex LightCycler PCR assay for detection and differentiation of *Bordetella pertussis* and *Bordetella parapertussis* in nasopharyngeal specimens. *J Clin Microbiol*. 2002;40:96–100.

48. Lievano FA, Reynolds MA, Waring AL, et al. Issues associated with and recommendations for using PCR to detect outbreaks of pertussis. *J Clin Microbiol*. 2002;40:2801–2805.

49. Committee on Infectious Diseases AAP. Group A streptococcal infections. In: Pickering LK, Peter G, Baker C, et al., eds. *Red Book 2000: Report of the Committee on Infectious Diseases*. Elk Grove Village, IL: American Academy of Pediatrics; 2000:526–536.

50. Chapin KC, Blake P, Wilson CD. Performance characteristics and utilization of rapid antigen test, DNA probe, and culture for detection of group A streptococci in an acute care clinic. *J Clin Microbiol*. 2002;40:4207–4210.

51. Uhl JR, Adamson SC, Vetter EA, et al. Comparison of LightCycler PCR, rapid antigen immunoassay, and culture for detection of group A streptococci from throat swabs. *J Clin Microbiol*. 2003;41(1):242–249.

52. Petrich A, Luinstra K, Page B, et al. Effect of routine use of a multiplex PCR for detection of *vanA*- and *vanB*- mediated enterococcal resistance on accuracy, costs and earlier reporting. *Diagn Microbiol Infect Dis*. 2001;41:215–220.

53. Palladino S, Kay ID, Costa AM, et al. Real-time PCR for the rapid detection of *vanA* and *vanB* genes. *Diagn Microbiol Infect Dis*. 2003;45:81–84.

54. Versalovic J, Shortridge D, Kibler K, et al. Mutations in 23S rRNA are associated with clarithromycin resistance in *Helicobacter pylori*. *Antimicrob Agents Chemother*. 1996;40:477–480.

55. Versalovic J, Fox JG. *Helicobacter*. In: Murray P, Baron EJ, Jorgensen JH, et al., eds. *Manual of Clinical Microbiology*. Washington, DC: ASM Press; 2003:915–928.

56. Burke JP. Patient safety: infection control—a problem for patient safety. *N Engl J Med*. 2003;348:651–656.

57. Hacek DM, Suriano T, Noskin GA, et al. Medical and economic benefit of a comprehensive infection control program that includes routine determination of microbial clonality. *Am J Clin Pathol*. 1999;111:647–654.

58. Goering RV. Molecular epidemiology of nosocomial infection: analysis of chromosomal restriction fragment patterns by pulsed-field gel electrophoresis. *Infect Control Hosp Epidemiol*. 1993;14:595–600.

59. Tenover FC, Arbeit RD, Goering RV, et al. Interpreting chromosomal DNA restriction patterns produced by pulsed-field gel electrophoresis: criteria for bacterial strain typing. *J Clin Microbiol*. 1995;33:2233–2239.

60. van Belkum A, van Leeuwen W, Kaufmann ME, et al. Assessment of resolution and intercenter reproducibility of results of genotyping *Staphylococcus aureus* by pulsed-field gel electrophoresis of *Sma*I macrorestriction fragments: a multicenter study. *J Clin Microbiol*. 1998;36:1653–1659.

61. Deplano A, Schuermans A, Van Eldere J, et al. Multicenter evaluation of epidemiological typing of methicillin-resistant *Staphylococcus aureus* strains by repetitive-element PCR analysis. The European Study Group on Epidemiological Markers of the ESCMID. *J Clin Microbiol*. 2000;38:3527–3533.

62. Murchan S, Kaufmann ME, Deplano A, et al. Harmonization of pulsed-field gel electrophoresis protocols for epidemiological typing of strains of methicillin-resistant *Staphylococcus aureus*: a single approach developed by consensus in 10 European laboratories and its application for tracing the spread of related strains. *J Clin Microbiol*. 2003;41:1574–1585.

63. Grimont F, Grimont PA. Ribosomal ribonucleic acid gene restriction patterns as potential taxonomic tools. *Ann Inst Pasteur Microbiol*. 1986;137B:165–175.

64. Price CS, Huynh H, Paule S, et al. Comparison of an automated ribotyping system to restriction endonuclease analysis and pulsed-field gel electrophoresis for differentiating vancomycin-resistant *Enterococcus faecium* isolates. *J Clin Microbiol*. 2002;40:1858–1861.

65. Aarnisalo K, Autio T, Sjoberg AM, et al. Typing of *Listeria monocytogenes* isolates originating from the food processing industry with automated ribotyping and pulsed-field gel electrophoresis. *J Food Prot*. 2003;66:249–255.

66. D'Agata EM, Gerrits MM, Tang YW, et al. Comparison of pulsed-field gel electrophoresis and amplified fragment-length polymorphism for epidemiological investigations of common nosocomial pathogens. *Infect Control Hosp Epidemiol*. 2001;22:550–554.

67. Fry NK, Bangsborg JM, Bergmans A, et al. Designation of the European Working Group on Legionella Infection (EWGLI) amplified fragment length polymorphism types of *Legionella pneumophila* serogroup 1 and results of intercentre proficiency testing using a standard protocol. *Eur J Clin Microbiol Infect Dis*. 2002;21:722–728.

68. Williams JG, Kubelik AR, Livak KJ, et al. DNA polymorphisms amplified by arbitrary primers are useful as genetic markers. *Nucleic Acids Res*. 1990;18:6531–6535.

69. Welsh J, McClelland M. Fingerprinting genomes using PCR with arbitrary primers. *Nucleic Acids Res*. 1990;18:7213–7218.

70. Clarke SC. Nucleotide sequence-based typing of bacteria and the impact of automation. *Bioessays*. 2002;24:858–862.

71. Versalovic J, Koeuth T, Lupski JR. Distribution of repetitive DNA sequences in eubacteria and application to fingerprinting of bacterial genomes. *Nucleic Acids Res*. 1991;19:6823–6831.

72. Versalovic J, Schneider M, de Bruijn FJ, Lupski JR. Genomic fingerprinting of bacteria using repetitive sequence-based polymerase chain reaction. *Methods Mol Cell Biol*. 1994;5:25–40.

73. Warren RM, Streicher EM, Sampson SL, et al. Microevolution of the direct repeat region of *Mycobacterium tuberculosis*: implications for interpretation of spoligotyping data. *J Clin Microbiol*. 2002;40:4457–4465.

74. van der Zanden AG, Kremer K, Schouls LM, et al. Improvement of differentiation and interpretability of spoligotyping for *Mycobacterium tuberculosis* complex isolates by introduction of new spacer oligonucleotides. *J Clin Microbiol*. 2002;40:4628–4639.

75. Healy M, Huong J, Bittner T, et al. Microbial DNA typing by automated rep-PCR. *J Clin Microbiol*. 2005;43:199–207.

76. van der ZA, Verbakel H, van Zon JC, et al. Molecular genotyping of *Staphylococcus aureus* strains: comparison of repetitive element sequence-based PCR with various typing methods and isolation of a novel epidemicity marker. *J Clin Microbiol*. 1999;37:342–349.

77. Peacock SJ, de Silva GD, Justice A, et al. Comparison of multilocus sequence typing and pulsed-field gel electrophoresis as tools for typing *Staphylococcus aureus* isolates in a microepidemiological setting. *J Clin Microbiol*. 2002;40:3764–3770.

Chapter 10

Mycobacterial Infections

Betty A. Forbes

Clinical Utility

Microbiology laboratories have developed and introduced clinical molecular assays for mycobacteria during the last several years because of the need for a reliable and rapid means of diagnosing tuberculosis (TB) for public health and therapeutic reasons. Molecular tests are used for identification of mycobacteria directly in clinical specimens, for mycobacterial identification, and for determination of drug susceptibilities.

Direct Detection

The limitations of routine acid-fast bacilli (AFB) smear and culture are well known. Although rapid, a sputum AFB smear has a reported sensitivity range of 22% to 78%. In recent years, the specificity of AFB smears has been a problem if specimens are obtained from individuals with a high incidence of disease due to nontuberculous mycobacteria (NTM), such as HIV-infected individuals. Similarly, culture of sputum is positive in the majority of patients with pulmonary TB if multiple specimens are obtained;[1] however, almost 30% of patients reported to have TB, including 22% of patients with pulmonary TB, are not culture confirmed.[2] Moreover, due to the slow growth rate of mycobacteria, cultures usually take at least a week, and in some instances as long as 6 to 8 weeks, to become positive.

Initially, amplification techniques were expected to dramatically reduce turnaround time and to have better sensitivity and specificity compared to conventional AFB smear and culture methods. However, despite numerous and significant advances, molecular methods have not replaced AFB smears and cultures for the diagnosis of mycobacterial infections from respiratory or extrapulmonary sites. Conventional tests remain a primary means of establishing a diagnosis as well as for drug susceptibility testing for optimal therapy.

Respiratory Specimens

The appropriate clinical use of nucleic acid amplification (NAA) assays has been difficult to delineate. (Only commercially available NAA assays are discussed here; however, similar issues also are pertinent to laboratory-developed amplification assays.)

Commercially available NAA assays were initially evaluated as screening tests (i.e., all specimens were tested regardless of the suspected risks for TB). When testing smear-positive specimens, these assays performed well (sensitivity 95% to 96%, specificity, 99% to 100%), but with smear-negative specimens, the sensitivity was much lower (48% to 53%).[3] Based on the results of these early trials, the Food and Drug Administration (FDA) limited the use of two commercially available NAA kits, the Amplified Mycobacterium Tuberculosis Direct (AMTD) test (Gen-Probe, Inc, San Diego, CA) and the Amplicor Mycobacterium tuberculosis test (Roche Diagnostic Systems, Inc, Indianapolis, IN) to AFB smear-positive respiratory specimens only from patients who had not received antituberculosis drugs for 7 or more days or had not been treated for TB within the last 12 months.

The utility of NAA assays for the detection of the 20% to 30% of culture-negative cases was difficult to determine from these early studies because culture growth was used as the gold-standard method.[4] In 1998, a clinical trial was performed to evaluate a reformulated AMTD test (AMTD 2, Gen-Probe, Inc, San Diego, CA) compared to a physician estimation of the probability that a patient had TB, with review by a physician panel of experts for cases that were not proven TB.[5] The enhanced AMTD2 test was performed on respiratory specimens from 339 patients, and results were compared with culture and clinical diagnosis results. The AMTD2 test had an overall sensitivity of 85.9%, a specificity of 97.8%, a positive predictive value (PPV) of 91.0%, and a negative predictive value (NPV) of 96.6%. The FDA approved the new version AMTD2 test in 1999 for testing respiratory specimens regardless of the AFB smear results.

Table 10-1. Evaluation of the Enhanced AMTD2 Test Based on Comprehensive Clinical Diagnosis

Clinical Suspicion of TB	AFB Smear: PPV and NPV (%)	AMTD Test: Sensitivity, Specificity, PPV, NPV (%)
Low (<10%)	36, 96	83, 97, 59, 99
Intermediate (10–80%)	30, 71	75, 100, 100, 91
High (>80%)	94, 37	87, 100, 100, 91

Source: Data from Reference 6.
AMTD2, Amplified Mycobacterium Tuberculosis Direct test (Gen-Probe, Inc, San Diego, CA); AFB, acid-fast bacilli; NPV, negative predictive value; PPV, positive predictive value; TB, tuberculosis.

Subsequent clinical trials of the enhanced AMTD2 test demonstrate the importance of using not only mycobacterial culture results but also multiple other parameters including clinical signs and symptoms, response to therapy, and other laboratory results to interpret the results of NAA tests.[6–9] Data from these studies support the use of the enhanced AMTD2 test as a rapid method for the diagnosis of pulmonary TB in patients for whom there is a moderate to high suspicion of TB, regardless of the AFB smear result.

In another study,[6] enrolling physicians were asked to quantify their degree of clinical suspicion for TB using a scale from 0% to 100%; subjects were broken down into three major groups. In addition, a conservative consensus standard for the diagnosis of pulmonary TB was established and an independent expert panel reviewed all cases with a clinical suspicion of less than 80% and only one culture or no cultures positive for *M. tuberculosis* (Table 10-1). NAA tests were most useful for cases with a higher clinical suspicion.

As more of these studies are published, optimal use of NAA tests in conjunction with clinical information and other test methods will become manifest, allowing NAA tests to be utilized in a cost-effective manner with positive impact on patient management. Clearly, based on recent studies, decisions about when and how to use NAA tests for TB diagnosis should be individualized according to the clinical setting and NAA results interpreted within the context of the clinical suspicion for TB and on the basis of laboratory performance. To help laboratories and clinicians in this regard, guidelines (Table 10-2) for the use of NAA tests in the diagnosis of TB were set forth by the Centers for Disease Control and Prevention (CDC).[10,11]

Nonrespiratory Specimens

Both laboratory-developed and commercially available NAA assays have been used to test nonrespiratory specimens, although no commercially available test kit is approved by the Food and Drug Administration (FDA) for this purpose. Because clinical diagnosis often is uncertain, and AFB smear and culture lack sensitivity, the use of NAA tests is particularly attractive for suspected cases of extrapulmonary TB.

In particular, NAA assays have been evaluated in patients suspected of having tuberculous meningitis.[12–14] Signs and symptoms of this disease are nonspecific. AFB smears in patients with TB meningitis are positive in only 10% of cases. Isolation of *M. tuberculosis* is positive in only approximately 50% of adults[15] and is insufficiently timely to aid clinical judgment with respect to treatment. Although promising, results of these NAA studies have varied with respect to sensitivity, while specificity was greater than 98% in most instances.

Similar results with other extrapulmonary specimens have been obtained. In many studies, the performance of NAA tests with extrapulmonary specimens has been similar to their performance with respiratory specimens,[7,16,17] while in other studies, the sensitivity was quite low. Based on studies published to date, it is clear that more studies must be performed to establish optimal

Table 10-2. Guidelines for the Use of NAA Tests on Respiratory Specimens for TB

AFB Smear	Specimen No.	NAA Result	Action
Positive	1	Positive	Presumed to have TB*
Positive	1	Negative	Test for inhibitors. If inhibitors are detected, NAA is no diagnostic help. If no inhibitors are detected, repeat NAA on no more than 2 additional specimens
	2, 3 (repeats)	Negative	Presumed to have NTM
		Positive	Clinician must rely on clinical judgment
Negative	1	Positive	Repeat NAA
	2, 3 (repeats)	Positive	Presumed to have TB
		Negative	Clinician must rely on clinical judgment
Negative	1	Negative	Repeat NAA
	2, 3 (repeats)	Negative	Presumed not to be infectious†
		Positive	Clinician must rely on clinical judgment

Source: Data from Reference 7.
* Unless there is concern about NTM, the NAA test adds little to the diagnostic workup.
† Clinician must rely on clinical judgment regarding the need for antituberculous therapy and further diagnostic workup.
NAA, nucleic acid amplification; TB, tuberculosis; NTM, nontuberculous mycobacteria.

Table 10-3. Commercially Available, Molecular-Based Amplification Assays for the Diagnosis and Treatment of Mycobacterial Infections

Test (Manufacturer)	Method	Applications/Comments
Amplified *Mycobacterium tuberculosis* Direct test (Gen-Probe, Inc, San Diego, CA)	TMA	FDA approved for testing respiratory specimens Target: rRNA Direct detection of *M. tuberculosis* in broth cultures
Amplicor *Mycobacterium tuberculosis* test (Roche Diagnostics, Indianapolis, IN)	PCR	FDA approved for testing AFB smear-positive respiratory specimens only Automated version: COBAS Amplicor MTB Target: 16S rDNA Direct detection of *M. tuberculosis* in broth cultures
BDProbe Tec (Becton Dickinson Diagnostic Instrument Systems, Sparks, MD)	SDA	Fully automated Targets: IS6110 and 16S rDNA
LCx *M. tuberculosis* test (Abbott Laboratories, Abbott Park, IL)	LCR	Semiautomated
INNO-LiPA Mycobacteria v2 (Innogenetics, Gent, Belgium)	PCR with reverse hybridization	Identifies genus *Mycobacteria* and 16 mycobacterial species Target: 16S-23S ribosomal spacer gene region
INNO-LiPA Rif. TB (Innogenetics, Gent, Belgium)	PCR with reverse hybridization	Detects *M. tuberculosis* complex plus rifampin resistance Target: region of the *rpoB* gene
GenoType Mycobacteria (Hain, Diagnostica, Nehren, Germany)	PCR with reverse hybridization	Identifies 13 mycobacterial species and a supplemental kit with 16 additional species Target: 23S rRNA gene

FDA, Food and Drug Administration; LCR, ligase chain reaction; PCR, polymerase chain reaction; rRNA, ribosomal RNA; SDA, strand displacement amplification; TMA, transcription-mediated amplification.

sample volume, nucleic acid extraction and amplification procedures, and uniform criteria for interpretation of results for each specimen type, including formalin-fixed, paraffin-embedded tissues. However, based on current data, a negative NAA result does not rule out extrapulmonary TB, particularly if the AFB smear for the specimen is negative.

NAA tests appear to be useful for early identification of *M. tuberculosis* complex for all specimen types grown in liquid cultures, except blood.[18,19] Sensitivity and specificity of NAA assays using this approach are both greater than 98%. In addition, the INNO-LiPA Mycobacteria assay (Innogenetics NV, Ghent, Belgium) (Table 10-3) successfully identifies mycobacteria directly from aliquots of culture medium from the MB/BacT ALERT 3D System (MB/BacT) (Organon Teknika, Boxtel, the Netherlands).[20]

NAA tests also have been evaluated for their usefulness in monitoring therapeutic efficacy. Although beneficial for initial diagnosis, most NAA assays appear to be unsuitable for monitoring treatment of TB patients since nucleic acid targets persist long after AFB smears and cultures become negative.[21,22] However, detection of *M. tuberculosis* messenger RNA (mRNA) may prove to be a potentially useful method for monitoring therapeutic efficacy,[23] although more studies are required to determine its clinical utility.

Identification

Mycobacterial isolates have traditionally been identified to the species level based on phenotypic and biochemical

tests. These methods are slow and cumbersome and may fail to obtain an identification, with results varying among different isolates of the same species. Therefore, laboratories are increasingly using molecular methods for identification. Rapid identification of *M. tuberculosis* is of paramount importance for therapeutic and public health reasons. Rapid detection and identification of NTM, for which there are currently at least 100 species, is becoming more important since NTM lung disease is caused by many NTM species with a range of clinical presentations.[24] Toward this goal, a variety of molecular approaches have been published for identification of not only *M. tuberculosis* complex organisms, but NTM as well (e.g., References 25 and 26). Finally, two commercially available systems using amplification of a region of the 16S-23S ribosomal RNA (rRNA) gene spacer region, or the 23S rRNA gene with subsequent hybridization to a membrane strip containing probes to the most commonly isolated mycobacterial species, have been used to identify mycobacteria.[27]

Susceptibility Testing

To successfully control the spread of TB, cases must be detected and treated in a timely manner. At best, conventional susceptibility testing methods for *M. tuberculosis* are available within 7 to 14 days, after a culture result is positive. Thus, molecular methods that can rapidly detect drug resistance are attractive. Mutations have been delineated that are responsible for resistance to the primary drugs used to treat TB, including rifampin (RIF), isoniazid (INH), ethambutol (EMB), streptomycin (STR), and

Table 10-4. Examples of Laboratory-Developed Methods for Mycobacterial Infections

Application	Methods	Comments
Direct detection	PCR: single or multiplex Real-time PCR Peptide nucleic acids	Targets include *IS6110*, *MPB64* and protein antigen B
Identification	PCR-RFLP with agarose gel or CE SSCP High-density DNA probe arrays	Targets include *hsp65*, 16S rDNA, *recA*, *rpoB*, *dnaJ*, and 32-kDa protein Numerous techniques and targets for identification of *M. tuberculosis* complex
Drug susceptibility	PCR-RFLP Heteroduplex analysis RT-PCR Real-time PCR Sequencing SSCP High-density DNA probe arrays Oligonucleotide arrays	To date, DNA sequencing is a more successful method for detecting RIF resistance

Epidemiology	*IS6110* RFLP
	Secondary markers
	   Polymorphic guanine-cytosine-rich repetitive
	   RFLP typing
	   Spoligotyping (PCR-based)
	
	Mixed-linker PCR
	Variable number tandem repeat analysis
	Mycobacterial interspersed repetitive units analysis
		IS6110 RFLP has high discriminatory power
		
		Spoligotyping is useful when discriminating isolates of *M. tuberculosis* with few *IS6110* bands, and is economical, easy to perform, and rapid

CE, capillary electrophoresis; PCR, polymerase chain reaction; PCR-RFLP, PCR–restriction fragment length polymorphism; RIF, rifampin; SSCP, single-strand conformation polymorphism.

pyazinamide (PZA). Because RIF resistance is an excellent marker for multidrug-resistant TB and 95% of all RIF-resistant strains have mutations localized in an 81 base pair (bp) region of the bacterial RNA polymerase gene, *rpoB*, which encodes the active site of the enzyme,[28] numerous molecular strategies have been developed to successfully detect RIF resistance. In contrast, research has shown that more than a single gene mutation is frequently responsible for resistance to INH, EMB, and STR. Although numerous molecular formats have been used to detect RIF drug resistance, the complexity of the drug resistance mechanisms for other agents combined with the complexity of the technology has hampered their broader acceptance in the clinical laboratory setting. Nevertheless, relevant mutations for resistance to most of the primary antituberculosis drugs have been described; most commonly, conventional or real-time polymerase chain reaction (PCR) in conjunction with identification of specific mutations within the amplicon using a variety of methods are employed to detect drug resistance mutations.

Epidemiology

Molecular epidemiological methods have made significant contributions to our understanding of the pathogenesis and transmission of TB within populations. For example, molecular fingerprinting techniques have provided epidemiological evidence of exogenous reinfection as well as

quantification of the level of infectiousness among AFB smear-negative patients.[29] Of great significance has been the use of DNA fingerprinting of *M. tuberculosis* isolates to determine the occurrence of laboratory cross-contamination of cultures. Laboratory cross-contamination represents a significant problem that can result in unnecessary treatment and drug toxicity for a patient. Molecular typing also has provided insight into the pathogenesis of cavitary and noncavitary disease caused by NTM.[24]

Available Tests

There are hundreds of publications in which molecular methods, using a variety of formats, have been used to directly detect mycobacteria in clinical specimens, identify mycobacteria, and detect drug resistance mutations in *M. tuberculosis*. Examples of NAA methods used for mycobacteria are provided in Tables 10-3 and 10-4.

Interpretation of Results

As with any laboratory test, prior to the interpretation of results of molecular tests on patient specimens or AFB clinical isolates, results of controls included with each run must be interpreted first. Selection and use of appropriate controls is an essential feature of any NAA test. Regardless of the format, positive and negative controls must be run in parallel with patient samples. If the test is a laboratory-developed assay to directly detect *M. tuberculosis*, the concentration of the positive control should be near the lower limit of detection of the assay. If the run is large, multiple negative controls should be included to monitor for cross-contamination. As with any other laboratory test, if these controls do not perform as expected, the run must be repeated. Optimally, an internal inhibition control with upstream and downstream primer recognition sequences should be added to each patient sample reaction to monitor for inhibition. If an internal inhibition control is not included (some commercially available assays do not include an inhibition control, e.g., the AMTD test), a second reaction should be performed with addition and amplification of a known target nucleic acid. If inhibition is detected, a test result cannot be reported. For assays using gel or capillary electrophoresis (CE), molecular-weight markers are used.

Inherent problems and limitations associated with NAA tests are false-positive results due to cross-contamination, as well as false-negative results due to inhibition or inadequate sample collection, transport, and processing. In addition, sampling error due to low numbers of mycobacteria (paucibacillary) or inadequate sample volumes also can lead to false-negative test results. Results should be interpreted in the context of the patient's history, physical examination, and clinical course. Thus, it is imperative that clinicians as well as clinical microbiologists have a thorough understanding of the advantages and limitations of the particular NAA assay used for patient testing as well as the specific microbiology and pathogenesis of the identified mycobacterium.

Sequenced-based or PCR-RFLP methods for identification of NTM provide a rapid tool for identification of this vast group of organisms. However, paradoxically, the identification of mycobacteria has become even more complex with the introduction of these techniques, since these methods have uncovered greater complexity of mycobacterial species. In a study of 72 mycobacterial isolates that did not belong to any officially recognized species, only three cases had agreement of species identification by conventional tests, high-performance liquid chromatography, and genetic sequencing.[30] Further complicating the interpretation of molecular identification results were findings that specific species identification was not the rule using analysis of the 16S rRNA gene of patient strains.[31] Based on these results, identification of mycobacteria will mandate attention to quality control of available databases used for mycobacterial identification, coupled with the realization that the taxonomy of the genus *Mycobacterium* is far from elucidated. Thus, interpretation of identification results using molecular-based methods will require constant changes and updates to available databases.[30,32]

In conclusion, molecular-based diagnostic tests should be interpreted within the context of clinical information and test performance characteristics. Of great importance

is strict adherence to guidelines for method validation that include the determination of clinical utility for accurate interpretation of results.

Laboratory Issues

There are numerous laboratory issues that pertain to the development, introduction, and performance of any clinical molecular test. Unfortunately, only guidelines, not universal standards, currently exist for the validation and subsequent quality control and assurance of laboratory-developed tests.[33,34] For example, all NAA methods require adequate and appropriately designed space, as well as other measures, is to minimize cross-contamination of samples.[35,36] This section addresses those laboratory issues that are specific to the diagnosis of mycobacterial infections by molecular assays.

False-positive amplification results can occur from carryover of amplicon while setting up and performing the molecular assay, as well as from cross-contamination of clinical specimens during processing for AFB smear and culture.[37] A review of 14 studies revealed a median false-positive rate of AFB culture of 3.1%.[38] Of 236 patients reported with false-positive cultures, 67% of patients were subsequently treated, and some had toxicity from therapy as well as unnecessary hospitalizations, tests, and contact investigations. Thus, performance of NAA tests to directly detect and identify *M. tuberculosis*, with their inherent potential for false-positive results, underscores the critical need for adherence to strict laboratory technique, inclusion of appropriate negative controls, and careful interpretation of results within the context of the clinical presentation.

As is the case with molecular testing for other infectious agents, the lack of a perfect gold standard complicates the interpretation of a positive amplification result with a negative culture. Likewise, false-negative amplification results can occur because of inhibition, sampling error, and inadequate sample preparation. The theoretical detection of one AFB has not generally been achieved in reality, which is a particular issue for the diagnosis of *M. tuberculosis* infection where there are often few organisms present in the clinical sample. This coupled with the tendency of mycobacteria to clump and thereby cause an uneven distribution of organisms in a sample can result in duplicate tests with discrepant results that are difficult to interpret.

Owing to the nature of NAA methods, quality control is essential for these procedures. A quality control program should consist of an internal quality control program, as well as participation in an external quality control program such as that offered by the CDC. The critical need for strict adherence to quality control measures was underscored when 20 unknowns were sent to 30 laboratories performing NAA tests; only five laboratories correctly identified the presence or absence of *M. tuberculosis* DNA in all samples.[39]

Specific to molecular-based identification methods, laboratories performing these techniques must be aware of the multiple problems with present sequence repositories such as base errors, ambiguous base designation, and incomplete sequences.[31] It is becoming apparent that visual inspection is becoming more cumbersome and challenging due to the growing number of hsp65 alleles described in the literature.[32] Another issue slowly arising from PCR-RFLP analysis for identification is the lack of standardization for electrophoresis conditions, which makes comparison of data from different laboratories challenging. For example, difficulties in PCR-RFLP interpretation stemming from similarities in a number of band sizes needed to discriminate species via agarose gel electrophoresis could be alleviated using 10% polyacrylamide gel electrophoresis.[40]

As previously mentioned, the complexity of drug resistance in M. tuberculosis has hindered the utility of molecular tests. However, this limitation may be ultimately overcome by development of other molecular approaches (see "Future Applications"). Another caveat to testing is that the presence of a resistance gene does not always imply expression of that gene and phenotypic resistance.

Cost-effectiveness is another laboratory issue associated with the performance of NAA tests for the diagnosis of TB and identification of mycobacteria. Since NAA tests cannot currently replace conventional methods for the diagnosis and management of TB, a NAA test is an additional test with associated costs. Although cost savings may be realized because of possibly preventing more invasive and costly diagnostic procedures (e.g., bronchoalveolar lavage), limiting unnecessary or potentially toxic empiric antituberculous therapy, shortening hospital stays in costly isolation rooms, and limiting transmission, this type of outcomes research has yet to be systematically done. Our understanding of the natural history of infection caused by M. tuberculosis will continue to evolve as different applications are explored and evaluated in the clinical setting. Many questions must be answered to fully exploit and utilize the potential of molecular tests for the diagnosis of mycobacterial infections. Toward this end, continued objective evaluation of the analytic and clinical performance of molecular tests, and the impact on patient outcomes, is imperative.

Future Applications

Continued advances in nucleic acid-based technologies will serve only to enhance capabilities for the diagnosis of mycobacterial infections. Efforts employing a variety of strategies are already well under way.

Miscellaneous Methods

Different strategies and formats to allow for easier and more rapid means by which to detect and identify mycobacteria are continually being published. To illustrate, DNA extracted directly from slides of AFB smear-negative specimens was tested for M. tuberculosis by PCR and sequence analysis for RIF resistance; this technique was 100% sensitive and specific for the detection of M. tuberculosis and RIF resistance.[41]

Another recent approach is the use of fluorescently labeled peptide nucleic acids (PNAs) to directly detect M. tuberculosis microscopically.[42] PNAs are DNA-like molecules in which the sugar-phosphate backbone is replaced with a peptidelike structure that can hybridize to specific DNA sequences with specific base pairing. PNAs can be labeled with a fluorescent dye to allow for visualization of PNA binding to specific DNA sequences present on a slide. Of significance, the PNA can easily pass through an intact cell wall and bind specifically to intracellular nucleic acid sequences. This strategy for the direct microscopic identification of M. tuberculosis and NTM appears to hold some promise. Finally, new rapid phenotypic methods, such as the luciferase phage assay or the PhaB assays[43] (Biotec Laboratories, Ipswich, UK), avoid some pitfalls associated with genotypic methods for detecting drug resistance in M. tuberculosis. New strategies will continue to be developed and evaluated in direct detection and identification of mycobacteria as well as drug susceptibility testing.

Automation and Miniaturization

The development of real-time PCR assays and other amplification formats in which single or multiple nucleic acid targets can be amplified and analyzed in a single closed tube in minutes rather than hours is particularly suited for subsequent automation. Instruments that automate the extraction of either RNA or DNA also have been introduced, allowing for the performance of a greater number of molecular-based assays while also providing a more consistent quality of nucleic acid for analysis.

In addition to automation of NAA assays for the diagnosis of mycobacterial infections, there will be miniaturization of analytical devices by micromachining technology that will perform PCR in microreactors consisting of either silicon or silicon and glass microchips.[44] Advances in this area will have a major impact on the ability to diagnose TB in the field and might prove to be particularly attractive for use in underdeveloped countries where the prevalence of TB is high.

Microarrays

High-density oligonucleotide arrays can rapidly examine large numbers of DNA sequences with a single hybridization step. DNA microarrays can be employed in two modes: (1) DNA-based comparison of the genomic content of different strains and (2) RNA-based monitoring of gene expression. Preliminary work has begun in the simultaneous detection, species identification, drug resistance profiling, and strain genotyping of mycobacteria involved in human disease.[45,46] Utilizing a high-density array, simultaneous species identification of 121 isolates was achieved, as well as detection of RIF resistance in 41 isolates of *M. tuberculosis*.[46] Similarly, high-density probe arrays for species identification and RIF resistance using sequences from the 16S rDNA gene and the *rpoB* gene, respectively, were used to evaluate 51 *M. tuberculosis* RIF resistance-causing rpoB mutations; arrays also included 2.2 kilobases (kb) of the *M. tuberculosis* wild-type *katG* gene, previously shown to confer INH resistance.[47] The total process from culture, including sample preparation and amplification, took less than 4 hours manually. As *M. tuberculosis* drug resistance determinants are gradually delineated, this type of platform could be expanded, even with the addition of epidemiological markers.

Clinical Knowledge

In addition to further technological innovation, epidemiologic and operational research is needed to develop algorithms for optimal use of molecular-based assays for patient management, particularly in light of test expense. In developed countries, TB remains a low-prevalence disease, and the most rapid way to improve test performance is to select patients for testing in whom results will have the greatest predictive value. Toward this end, there is a need for well-designed, patient-based clinical trials with NAA tests. Numerous questions need to be answered regarding the use of these tests in previously treated individuals, children, and other subpopulations, in paucibacillary forms of TB, as well as regarding how to assess the infectiousness of individual patients, when to isolate a patient, and when to begin contact investigations.[3] Additional questions remain as to whether NAAs can ultimately be used to distinguish latent from active *M. tuberculosis* infections and monitor response to chemotherapy. As the natural history of mycobacterial infections becomes better understood in conjunction with the advancement of molecular test methods, significant potential for rapid, sensitive, specific, and cost-effective diagnosis of mycobacterial infections will become a reality.

References

1. Bradley SP, Reed SL, Cantanzaro A. Clinical efficacy of the amplified *Mycobacterium tuberculosis* direct test for the diagnosis of pulmonary tuberculosis. *Am J Resp Crit Care Med.* 1996;153:1606–1610.

2. Nardell E, Bautolte S, Shampra P, et al. Tuberculosis without culture confirmation (abstract). *Am Rev Respir Dis.* 1995;151:A336.

3. American Thoracic Society Workshop: rapid diagnostic tests for tuberculosis. What is the appropriate use? *Am J Resp Crit Care Med.* 1997;155:1804–1814.

4. Barnes PF. Rapid diagnostic tests for tuberculosis. *Am J Respir Crit Care Med.* 1997;155:1497–1498.

5. Jonas V, Acedo M, Clarridge JE, et al. A multi-center evaluation of MTD and culture compared to clinical diagnosis [abstract]. In: *Abstracts of the 98th General Meeting of the American Society for Microbiology*; May 17–21, 1998; Atlanta, GA. Abstract L-31.

6. Cantanzaro A, Perry S, Clarridge JE, et al. The role of clinical suspicion in evaluating a new diagnostic test for active tuberculosis. *JAMA.* 2000;283:639–645.

7. O'Sullivan CE, Miller DR, Schneider PS, et al. Evaluation of Gen-Probe Amplified *Mycobacterium tuberculosis* Direct Test by using respiratory and nonrespiratory specimens in a tertiary care center laboratory. *J Clin Microbiol.* 2002;40:1723–1727.

8. Bergmann JS, Yuoh G, Fish G, et al. Clinical evaluation of the enhanced Gen-Probe Amplified *Mycobacterium tuberculosis* Direct Test for rapid diagnosis of tuberculosis in prison inmates. *J Clin Microbiol.* 1999;37:1419–1425.

9. Peirsimoni C, Callegaro A, Scarparo C, et al. Comparative evaluation of the new Gen-Probe *Mycobacterium tuberculosis* Direct Test and the semiautomated Abbott LCx *Mycobacterium tuberculosis* assay for the direct detection of *Mycobacterium tuberculosis* complex in respiratory and extrapulmonary specimens. *J Clin Microbiol.* 1998;36:3601–3604.

10. Centers for Disease Control and Prevention. Nucleic acid amplification tests for the diagnosis of tuberculosis. *MMWR Morb Mortal Wkly Rep.* 1996;45:950–952.

11. Centers for Disease Control and Prevention. Update: nucleic acid amplification tests for tuberculosis. *MMWR Morb Mortal Wkly Rep.* 2000;49:593–594.

12. Baker CA, Cartwright CP, Williams DN, et al. Early detection of central nervous system tuberculosis with the Gen-Probe nucleic acid amplification assay: utility in an inner city hospital. *Clin Infect Dis.* 2002;35:339–342.

13. Bonington A, Strang JIG, Klapper PE, et al. Use of Roche AMPLICOR *Mycobacterium tuberculosis* PCR in early diagnosis of tuberculous meningitis. *J Clin Microbiol.* 1998;36:1251–1254.

14. Lang AM, Feris-Iglesias J, Pena C, et al. Clinical evaluation of the Gen-Probe Amplified Direct Test for detection of *Mycobacterium tuberculosis* complex organisms in cerebrospinal fluid. *J Clin Microbiol.* 1998;36:2191–2194.

15. Roos KL. *Mycobacterium tuberculosis* meningitis and other etiologies of the aseptic meningitis syndrome. *Semin Neurol.* 2000;20:329–335.

16. Peirsimoni C, Scarparo C, Piccoli P, et al. Performance assessment of two commercial amplification assays for direct detection of *Mycobacterium tuberculosis* complex from respiratory and extrapulmonary specimens. *J Clin Microbiol.* 2002;40:4138–4142.

17. Scarparo C, Piccoli P, Rigon A, et al. Comparison of enhanced *Mycobacterium tuberculosis* Amplified Direct Test with COBAS AMPLICOR *Mycobacterium tuberculosis* assay for direct detection of *Mycobacterium tuberculosis* complex in respiratory and extrapulmonary specimens. *J Clin Microbiol.* 2000;38:1559–1562.

18. Forbes BA, Hicks KE. Ability of PCR assay to identify *Mycobacterium tuberculosis* in BACTEC 12B vials. *J Clin Microbiol.* 1994;32:1725–1728.

19. Katila ML, Katila P, Erkinjuntti-Pekkanen R. Accelerated detection of mycobacteria with MGIT 960 and COBAS AMPLICOR systems. *J Clin Microbiol.* 2000;38:960–964.

20. Scarparo C, Piccoli P, Rigon A, et al. Direct identification of mycobacteria from MB/BacT Alert 3D bottles: comparative evaluation of two commercial probe assays. *J Clin Microbiol.* 2001;39:3222–3227.

21. Bennedsen J, Thosen V, Pfyffer GE, et al. Utility of PCR in diagnosing pulmonary tuberculosis. *J Clin Microbiol.* 1996;34:1407–1411.

22. Desjardin LE, Chen Y, Perkins MD, et al. Comparison of the ABI 7700 System (TaqMan) and competitive PCR for quantitation of IS6110 DNA in sputum during treatment of tuberculosis. *J Clin Microbiol.* 1998;36:1964–1968.

23. Hellyer TJ, Desjardin LE, Hehman GL, et al. Quantitative analysis of mRNA as a marker for viability of *Mycobacterium tuberculosis*. *J Clin Microbiol*. 1999;37:290–295.

24. Griffith DE, Brown-Elliott BA, Wallace RJ. Diagnosing nontuberculous mycobacterial lung disease. *Infect Dis Clin N Am*. 2002;16: 235–249.

25. Kirschner P, Springer B, Vogel U, et al. Genotypic identification of mycobacteria by nucleic acid sequence determination: report of a two year experience in a clinical laboratory. *J Clin Microbiol*. 1993;31:2882–2889.

26. Brunello F, Ligozzi M, Cristelli E, et al. Identification of 54 mycobacterial species by PCR-restriction fragment length polymorphism analysis of the hsp65 gene. *J Clin Microbiol*. 2001;39:2799–2806.

27. Padilla E, Gonzalez V, Manterola JM, et al. Comparative evaluation of the new version of the INNO-LiPA mycobacteria and GenoType *Mycobacterium* assays for identification of *Mycobacterium* species from MB/BacT liquid cultures artificially inoculated with Mycobacterial strains. *J Clin Microbiol*. 2004;42:3083–3088.

28. Ramaswamy S, Musser JM. Molecular genetic basis of antimicrobial agent resistance in *Mycobacterium tuberculosis*: 1998 update. *Tuber Lung Dis*. 1998;79:3–29.

29. Burgos MV. Molecular epidemiology of tuberculosis. *Eur Respir J*. 2002;20(suppl 36):54s–65s.

30. Tortolli E, Bartoloni A, Böttger EC, et al. Burden of unidentifiable mycobacteria in a reference laboratory. *J Clin Microbiol*. 2001;39: 4058–4065.

31. Turenne CY, Tschetter L, Wolfe J, et al. Necessity of quality-controlled 16S rRNA gene sequence databases: identifying nontuberculous *Mycobacterium* species. *J Clin Microbiol*. 2001;39:3637–3648.

32. da Silva Rocha A, Barreto AM, Campos CED, et al. Novel allelic variants of mycobacteria isolated in Brazil as determined by PCR-restriction enzyme analysis of hsp65. *J Clin Microbiol*. 2002;40: 4191–4196.

33. National Committee for Clinical Laboratory Standards. *Molecular Diagnostic Methods for Infectious Diseases: Approved Guidelines [MM3-A]*. Wayne, PA: National Committee for Clinical Laboratory Standards; 1993.

34. National Committee for Clinical Laboratory Standards. *Quantitative Molecular Methods for Infectious Disease: Proposed Guidelines*. Wayne, PA: National Committee for Clinical Laboratory Standards; 2001. NCCLS Document MM6-P.

35. Lisby G. Application of nucleic acid amplification in clinical microbiology. *Mol Biotechnol*. 1999;12:75–99.

36. Wolk D, Mitchell S, Patel R. Principles of molecular biology testing methods. *Infect Dis Clin N Am*. 2001;15:1157–1204.

37. Chang CL, Kim HH, Son HC, et al. False-positive growth of *Mycobacterium tuberculosis* attributable to laboratory contamination confirmed by restriction fragment length polymorphism analysis. *Int J Tuberc Lung Dis*. 2001;5:861–867.

38. Burman WJ, Reves RR. Review of false-positive cultures for *Mycobacterium tuberculosis* and recommendations for avoiding unnecessary treatment. *Clin Infect Dis*. 2000;31:1390–1395.

39. Noordhoek GT, vanEmbden JDA, Kolk AH. Reliability of nucleic acid amplification for detection of Mycobacterium tuberculosis: an international collaborative quality control study among 30 laboratories. *J Clin Microbiol*. 1996;34:2522–2525.

40. Brunello F, Ligozzi M, Cristelli E, et al. Identification of 54 mycobacterial species by PCR-restriction fragment length polymorphism analysis of the hsp65 gene. *J Clin Microbiol*. 2001;39:2799–2806.

41. Patnaik M, Liegmann K, Peter JB. Rapid detection of smear-negative *Mycobacterium tuberculosis* by PCR and sequencing for rifampin resistance with DNA extracted directly from slides. *J Clin Microbiol*. 2001;39:51–52.

42. Stender H, Lund K, Petersen KH, et al. Fluorescence in situ hybridization assay using peptide nucleic acid probes for differentiation between tuberculous and nontuberculous *Mycobacterium* species in smears of *Mycobacterium* cultures. *J Clin Microbiol*. 1999;37:2760–2765.

43. Riska PF, Su Y, Bardarov S, et al. Rapid film-based determination of antibiotic susceptibilities of *Mycobacterium tuberculosis* strains by using a luciferase reporter phage and the Bronx box. *J Clin Microbiol*. 1999;37:1144–1149.

44. Park DJ, Drobniewski FA, Meyer A, et al. Use of a phage-based assay for phenotypic detection of mycobacteria directly from sputum. *J Clin Microbiol*. 2003;41:680–688.

45. Schneegass I, Köhler JM. Flow-through polymerase chain reactions in chip thermocyclers. *J Biotech*. 2001;82:101–121.

46. Gingeras TR, Ghandour G, Wang E, et al. Simultaneous genotyping and species identification using hybridisation pattern recognition analysis of generic *Mycobacterium* arrays. *Genome Res*. 1998;8:435–448.

47. Troesch A, Nguyen H, Miyada CG, et al. *Mycobacterium* species identification and rifampin resistance testing with high-density DNA probe arrays. *J Clin Microbiol*. 1999;37:49–55.

Chapter 11

Molecular Pathology Laboratory Management

Hanna Rennert and Debra G.B. Leonard

Introduction

Currently more than 800 laboratories perform nucleic acid–based tests of human samples for the identification of genetic diseases, malignancies, infectious organisms, patient or sample identification, and human leukocyte antigen (HLA) typing.[1] The operation of a clinical molecular pathology laboratory requires integration of expertise in medical, scientific, and clinical molecular pathology, resources including facilities, equipment, and personnel, and skills in organization, administration, management, and communication. Quality service is achieved by adherence to clinical laboratory regulations, from specimen collection and processing to reporting of patient results. This chapter reviews fundamental knowledge important for the management and operation of a clinical molecular pathology laboratory.

The Role of the Molecular Pathology Laboratory

Molecular pathology laboratories perform tests for different clinical purposes, including genetics, cancer, and infectious diseases. Although all applications share the use of nucleic acids as the main analyte, the different types of testing require different management considerations (Table 11-1). Considerations relevant for each type of test performed in molecular pathology are reviewed.

Genetic Disorders

All diseases have a genetic contribution, whether it is a specific genetic disease or an increased likelihood for developing a medical condition. Genetic disorders are primarily caused by mutations present in every cell of an individual. Molecular testing for neoplasia or an infectious disease requires a sample of the tumor or the infected tissue, respectively, while molecular testing for a genetic disease can be performed on most accessible tissue types. In addition, because genetic testing examines germline mutations, it has important implications not only for the individual but also for family members that may have inherited the same mutation. Genetic testing also raises ethical concerns, including informed consent, potential for employment or insurance discrimination based on test results, and beginning-of-life issues with prenatal testing. Genetic test results often are not definitive, requiring complex risk-assessment calculations for interpretation. The American College of Medical Genetics (ACMG) and the American Society of Human Genetics (ASHG) have published guidelines and recommendations for many of the more common single-gene disorders (Table 11-2).

Genetic Testing

Molecular genetic testing is currently used for the following major clinical purposes: diagnostic, carrier, prenatal, and presymptomatic DNA testing.[2]

Diagnostic testing is performed on affected individuals for establishing or confirming a clinical diagnosis. Because these DNA tests are gene specific, the patient should have symptoms consistent with the disorder to justify performing the test. Genetic tests may be useful for diagnosis with an early atypical clinical presentation, or when other diagnostic procedures are more expensive or complex. For example, molecular testing for the absence of the survival motor neuron 1 (*SMN1)* gene for spinal muscular atrophy (SMA) in hypotonic newborns is a simple procedure performed on peripheral blood lymphocytes (PBL), replacing the need for a more painful and complex muscle biopsy.

Carrier testing is used to detect recessive mutations in healthy individuals to identify the risk of having an affected child. This application can be used for individuals with a family history of a genetic disorder, or for population screening. Testing of an affected family member can identify the specific mutation present in a family, thus

Table 11-1. Special Considerations in Molecular Pathology Testing Stratified by Clinical Application

Application	Considerations
Genetics	Ethical issues (presymptomatic and prenatal testing)
	Consequences for family members
	Informed consent requirements
	Requirements for family-related information (ethnicity, pedigree, specimens)
	Time sensitivity (prenatal diagnosis)
	Complex risk-assessment calculations
Oncology	Many types of samples
	Extensive use of paraffin-embedded tissue samples (familiarity with limitations)
	Need for diagnostic samples for optimal interpretation of minimal residual disease test results
Infectious diseases	High-volume testing
	Use of automated platforms
	High cost of commercial in vitro diagnostic test kits
	Increased need for quantitative testing with a wide dynamic range and low detection limit
Identity testing	Chain-of-custody documentation for specimens
	Special patient-identification requirements
	Complex calculations
	Special accreditation for paternity and forensic testing
	Special qualifications required for the laboratory director
HLA testing	Time sensitivity (≤24 hour-turnaround-time)
	Complex analyses
	Special accreditation by the American Society for Histocompatibility and Immunogenetics (ASHI)

allowing directed testing for other family members and improving the accuracy of the risk assessment for individuals with a negative test result. In contrast, population screening focuses on the most prevalent mutations, often with different sensitivity of mutation detection for different ethnic populations.

Prenatal testing refers to the detection of disease mutations in a fetus, using fetal cells obtained by amniocentesis or chorionic villus sampling (CVS). To overcome some of the problems associated with pregnancy termination of an affected fetus, some laboratories offer preimplantation genetic testing in the setting of in vitro fertilization for couples with a family history of a specific genetic disease. Preimplantation genetic testing is performed on a single blastomere from an early embryo, allowing selection of only unaffected embryos for implantation.

Presymptomatic testing is used primarily for the identification of adult-onset dominant disorders prior to the onset of clinical symptoms, in which the offspring of an affected parent has a 50% chance of inheriting the disease. This category includes neurological diseases such as Huntington disease and some types of cancer. Presymptomatic testing is the most problematic and challenging in terms of its psychological effect on the individual and hence requires extensive protocols for pre- and post–genetic test counseling.

Genetic testing requires special attention to informed consent issues, the appropriateness of the testing, and the urgency of testing. Many laboratories choose to require documentation of informed consent for the specific genetic test being requested prior to performing the genetic test. Informed consent can be documented by obtaining the completed consent form or a copy of the completed consent form, or by confirmation by the physician on the requisition form that informed consent is on record in his or her medical office. Until informed consent is documented, the laboratory can extract and store the appropriate nucleic acid, but only after confirmation of informed consent can the laboratory perform testing. The diagnostic laboratory also should review the requisition form to determine whether the test is appropriate for the specific patient. For example, carrier testing of a minor should be deferred until the minor is an adult, so should prompt a call to the referring clinician. Similarly, a request for testing of an asymptomatic individual for a dominant disease requires confirmation of adequate presymptomatic genetic counseling. For prenatal test requests, gestational age should be assessed to assure that the test result is available to allow for termination of the pregnancy if this is the family's choice. Finally, the laboratory should understand and communicate to healthcare providers the sensitivities and limitations of the tests performed.

Ethical Considerations, Genetic Counseling, and Informed Consent

Despite the tremendous advances in understanding of the human genome, the benefit of genetic testing for the patient is not always clear. Testing may be warranted, even if the results are inconclusive or preventive strategies or treatments are not available.[3] The availability of individual genetic information raises critical ethical, legal, and social issues because genetic testing examines the patient's own genetic makeup, rather than acquired (somatic) genetic abnormalities or infectious agents, with implications for other family members. Recently, after intensive lobbying by various advocacy organizations including health professionals and industry leaders, the Senate passed the Genetic Information Nondiscrimination Act of 2005 (S 306),[4] although the House of Representatives version of the nondiscrimination bill (HR 1227) has yet to be passed. This federal legislation would prevent health insurers and employers from using information to determine eligibility, set premiums, or hire and fire employees, and would ensure that genetic information is used for the benefit of the patient. The bills also encourage individuals to take advantage of genetic screening, counseling, testing, and new therapies that will result from the scientific advances in the field of genetics.

Table 11-2. Professional Organizations and Standards for Molecular Pathology Laboratories

Organization	Standards and Guidelines
Centers for Medicare and Medicaid Services (CMS; http://www.hcfa.gov) (formerly Health Care Finance Association, HCFA)	Mandatory federal guidelines for regulating laboratory testing via the Clinical Laboratory Improvement Amendments of 1988 (CLIA'88)
American College of Medical Genetics (ACMG; http://www.acmg.net)	Standards and guidelines for clinical genetic laboratories Gene patents and accessibility of genetic testing Policy regarding genetic testing of minors Storage and use of genetic materials Recommended standards for interpretation of sequence variations Recommendations and guidelines regarding genetic testing for fragile X syndrome, apolipoprotein testing for Alzheimer disease, Prader Willi-Angelman syndrome, Canavan disease, cystic fibrosis, Huntington disease, venous thromboembolism (factor V Leiden and prothrombin), congenital hearing loss, colon cancer, and breast and ovarian cancer
American Society of Human Genetics (ASHG; http://www.ashg.org)	Educational resources in human genetics Legislation for genetic information nondiscrimination
American Society for Histocompatibility and Immunogenetics (ASHI; http://www.ashi-hla.org)	Standards for molecular histocompatibility and immunogenetic testing
Clinical and Laboratory Standards Institute (http://www.clsi.org) (formerly National Committee for Clinical laboratory Standards, NCCLS)	Molecular diagnostic methods for genetic diseases (MM1-A2) Immunoglobulin and T-cell receptor gene rearrangement assays (MM2-A) Molecular diagnostic methods for infectious diseases (MM3-A2) Nucleic acid–amplification assays for hematopathology (MM5-A) Quantitative molecular diagnostics for infectious diseases (MM6-A)
The College of American Pathologists (CAP; http://www.cap.org)	Recommendations for in-house development and performance of molecular tests Molecular pathology checklist for laboratory accreditation
Food and Drug Administration (FDA; http://www.fda.gov)	Guidelines for industry registration and listing of analyte-specific reagents (ASRs) Guidelines for laboratory development and reporting of tests using ASR Premarket review templates for in-house-developed genetic tests Guidelines for industry for manufacturing and validating molecular tests for the detection of HIV-1 and hepatitis C virus (HCV)
National Institutes of Health (NIH; http://www.nih.gov)	Promoting safe and effective genetic testing in the Unites States: final report of the task force in genetic testing
Secretary's Advisory Committee on Genetics, Health and Society (SACGHS; http://www.4.od.nih.gov/oba/sacghs.htm) (formerly Secretary's Advisory Committee on Genetic Testing, SACGT)	Recommendations to the secretary through the assistant secretary for health on all aspects of the development and use of genetic tests
Clinical Laboratory Improvement Advisory Committee (CLIAC; http://www.phppo.cdc.gov/cliac/default.asp)	Setting new CLIA regulations for genetic testing
Centers for Disease Control and Prevention (CDC; http://www.cdc.gov)	Guidelines and recommendations for laboratory testing of HCV and HIV Data collection of genetic testing and results

Molecular genetic testing often requires interpretation using complex risk-assessment calculations.[5] Healthcare professionals must correctly interpret laboratory test results and be able to accurately convey the test results and interpretation to the patient, and the patient's family, as appropriate. Accurate communication of results to patients and families, however, can be complex and time-consuming and therefore may be performed by genetic counselors or clinicians trained in medical genetics, rather than physicians without genetics expertise. The benefits of this approach are illustrated by a study in which one third of physicians misinterpreted a negative genetic test result for familial adenomatous polyposis (FAP) and inappropriately suggested that the patients dis-

continue recommended aggressive surveillance.[6] For these reasons, most genetic tests should be ordered through healthcare professionals trained in genetics to ensure that the benefits and risks of testing have been explained to the patient during the informed consent process.[7] This also ensures that genetic testing is voluntary. Although obtaining consent is primarily the responsibility of the referring clinician, the diagnostic laboratory should consider requiring documentation of informed consent.[2] There are now proposed changes to the Clinical Laboratory Improvement Amendments of 1988 (CLIA) regulations specific for genetic testing that include a requirement for laboratories to document informed consent prior to performing a genetic test.[8]

Confidentiality

In view of the risks of discrimination in health insurance and employment associated with genetic testing, confidential handling of genetic test results is important. Discussion and communication of results must be limited to authorized healthcare providers. Genetic test results should be communicated verbally or faxed only to the referring physician or genetic counselor. Faxing of results is, in general, considered to be less confidential.[2] Release of any patient information, especially to nonhealthcare entities, must be authorized by the patient and documented. To ensure the confidentiality of genetic test results, some patients choose to personally pay for genetic testing rather than use health insurance, which should be accepted by the laboratory. The US Department of Health Human Services has issued guidelines for ensuring the privacy of patients' health information as part of the Health Insurance Portability and Accountability Act of 1996 (HIPAA).[9] Breech of patients' confidentiality for any type of healthcare information, not just for genetic information can result in litigation against the individual or the institution.

Cancer

Hematopoietic Neoplasms

Molecular hematopathology refers to molecular testing for leukemias and lymphomas to identify somatic DNA alterations.[10] These DNA changes are present only in the affected population of hematolymphoid cells and are not a part of the genetic makeup of the individual. The recent development in polymerase chain reaction (PCR)-based techniques has provided greater diagnostic sensitivity and specificity for diagnostic testing, as well as for monitoring of disease during and after therapy. Likewise, the ability to test very small amounts of nucleic acid has enabled the use of a wide range of sample types, including paraffin-embedded tissues (PETs). For molecular testing, however, formalin fixation is optimal. In contrast to genetic tests, which need be performed only once for an individual, molecular oncology tests often are performed repeatedly for initial diagnosis and during and after treatment. If testing is not performed at the time of diagnosis, later testing of the diagnostic specimen may be useful to confirm a molecular marker for minimal residual disease (MRD) testing. Molecular hematopathology results, whenever possible, are interpreted in the context of histopathology, flow cytometry, and clinical findings.

Solid Tumors

As the molecular rearrangements and mutations that cause specific solid tumor types are identified, the detection of these mutations is used for diagnosis and MRD assessment.[11] Many of these molecular rearrangements were identified through molecular characterization of specific chromosomal translocations identified by cytogenetic analysis of solid tumors, including bone and soft tissue sarcomas, such as alveolar rhabdomyosarcoma, Ewing sarcoma, and synovial sarcoma. The expression of the fusion transcripts for the more common translocations can be detected by reverse transcription–polymerase chain reaction (RT-PCR) testing. The preferred specimen for sarcoma testing is frozen tissue because the optimal analyte is RNA.

Specific somatic changes in solid tumors are used to predict response to treatment. For example, genetic analysis for loss of heterozygosity on chromosomes 1p and 19q is used to predict response to treatment for oligodendroglioma tumors, the presence of which correlates with a better outcome.[12]

Laboratory issues specific to solid tumor testing include the use fresh or frozen tissue for RNA-based testing, the use of microdissection to reduce the nonmalignant cell population in the specimen, and working with small tissue specimens such as needle biopsies.

Infectious Diseases

As molecular techniques have become routine, more and more microorganisms are detected or characterized by molecular testing.[13] Molecular tests are especially suitable for infectious agents which are difficult to culture and for drug-resistance testing. Molecular methods also are useful for viral quantitation as a part of monitoring response to therapy, such as human immunodeficiency virus (HIV) and hepatitis C virus (HCV) infections. Because some infectious disease tests are high volume, and automated instrumentation is being developed, commercial test kits for many pathogen types are available. However, these commercial infectious disease test kits are expensive. Although improved patient outcome due to early diagnosis and treatment may outweigh laboratory expenses, such savings have not been fully demonstrated. Finally, the need for confidentiality protections for patients having HIV testing has prompted specific federal and state legislation to ensure the protection of patients and their families.

Identity Testing and HLA Typing

Identity tests use polymorphic DNA markers to establish the identity of an individual or to determine an inheritance pattern.[14] Identity testing is used for several clinical applications including analysis of bone marrow engraftment following bone marrow transplantation, maternal cell contamination (MCC) studies for prenatal genetic testing, paternity testing, and forensic identity testing. Paternity and forensic identity testing, in particular, require additional considerations, including special accreditation (reviewed in Table 11-2), director qualifications, chain-of-custody documentation, verification of identity, familiarity with complex probability calculations, reporting of results, and legal proceedings.

HLA typing is time-sensitive, requires 24-hour laboratory staffing, and involves complex anlysis of the test results. Laboratories performing HLA typing require special accreditation (see Table 11-2).

Regulatory Agencies

Laboratories performing clinical testing must comply with numerous regulations. With the advent of the Clinical Laboratory Improvement Amendments of 1988 (CLIA),[15] all laboratories are required to implement minimum quality standards. Proof of meeting these standards (accreditation), which may be done through voluntary accreditation programs offered by professional organizations, is critical to providing high-quality laboratory services. Molecular diagnostic laboratories are faced with special challenges due to the complex technical issues and ethical considerations involved in DNA-based testing. Several regulatory agencies are currently developing guidelines and standards for molecular pathology tests (Table 11-2). Some of these regulatory agencies and regulations are discussed.

CLIA and CLIA '03

All clinical laboratory testing is regulated by CLIA. The Congress passed CLIA to establish quality standards for all clinical laboratory testing to ensure the accuracy, reliability, and timeliness of patient test results.[16] CLIA is "test-site neutral," meaning that the same regulations apply to any location performing testing. Every laboratory examining "material derived from the human body for the purpose of providing information for the diagnosis, prevention, or treatment of any disease" is subject to CLIA. Final regulations to meet the law were published in 1992 in the *Federal Register*.[17] In 2003, new, extensively revised CLIA regulations were published and nicknamed CLIA '03. The changes include major reorganization and consolidation of the regulations by basing requirements on the flow of a patient sample through the laboratory, and updating the requirements to accommodate new technologies.[18]

The Centers for Medicare and Medicaid Services (CMS), formerly known as the Health Care Financing Administration (HCFA), in conjunction with the Centers for Disease Control and Prevention (CDC), were originally charged with developing and enforcing the CLIA regulations. CMS continues to oversee much of these regulatory activities, including laboratory registration, on-site inspection, training, and accreditation.

CLIA certificates are based on the complexity of the test method and are divided into three main categories: waived, moderate complexity, and high complexity. The level of complexity is determined by assigning a numerical score for each test or methodology based on numerous criteria

including the knowledge, training, and experience required to perform the test, complexity of reagent and material preparation, characteristics of the operational steps, availability of calibrators, controls and proficiency testing, equipment and test system troubleshooting, and interpretation of results. Under the new CLIA '03 regulations, however, all quality control and quality assessment requirements now apply equally to high- and moderate-complexity laboratories, although some of the personnel qualifications remain more stringent for high-complexity laboratories.[18] These criteria are considered to be key elements in performing clinical testing and can be found on the Food and Drug Administration (FDA) Web site (http://www.fda.gov/).

Molecular pathology tests are considered high-complexity tests and as such must comply with CLIA requirements. Some of the requirements for high-complexity tests include qualifications of personnel performing and overseeing the testing, procedure manual specifications, method verification of performance specifications, proficiency testing, quality assurance, patient test management, and inspection. CLIA, however, does not provide specific guidelines for molecular testing, and, therefore, each molecular pathology laboratory is responsible for the development of a test management program according to CLIA criteria.

Voluntary Accreditation Organizations

CLIA regulations allow CMS to approve nonprofit, professional organizations that have laboratory testing and inspection standards equivalent to or more stringent than CLIA to inspect clinical testing laboratories in place of CLIA inspection. The two major organizations providing CLIA inspections are the Joint Commission on Accreditation of Healthcare Organizations (JCAHO), which accredits more than 80% of the US healthcare organizations, and the Laboratory Accreditation Program of the College of American Pathologists (LAP-CAP). The majority of molecular pathology laboratories are inspected and accredited by LAP-CAP. When a test site meets the accrediting agency's requirements, as assessed by inspection, the laboratory, in essence, is meeting CLIA requirements and receives a CLIA license.

The College of American Pathologists

LAP-CAP accredits only laboratory test sites and not entire healthcare organizations. LAP-CAP does not base its requirements for accreditation on the different CLIA complexity levels of testing; instead it requires that all testing laboratories adhere to the same guidelines. LAP-CAP lists its requirements and guidelines in checklists, each consisting of a series of laboratory guideline questions. All laboratories must follow the Laboratory General checklist and the specific laboratory checklist, which corresponds to each specific laboratory section. In addition to general requirements concerning personnel qualifications, quality control, test performance verification, and operation-related guidelines similar to CLIA, the Molecular Pathology checklist also includes test- and application-specific guidelines. LAP-CAP also requires laboratories to have a procedure manual for each test or process, which complies with the Clinical and Laboratory Standards Institute (CLSI; formerly National Committee for Clinical Laboratory Standards, NCCLS) GP2-3A.[19] LAP-CAP-accredited laboratories must also participate in a proficiency testing program when available, or perform internal proficiency checks when an external proficiency testing program is not available, for each test performed.

The Food and Drug Administration

In the United States, the FDA oversees regulation of medical devices under the 1938 Federal Food, Drug, and Cosmetics Act and subsequent amendments. Unless specifically exempted, medical devices must "be properly labeled and packaged, be cleared for marketing by the FDA, meet their labeling claims, and be manufactured under Good Manufacturing Practices (GMP), which is a mandated quality assurance system." These rules concerning the design, manufacturing, marketing, and surveillance of medical devices can be found in the Code for Federal Regulations (CFR). The FDA also oversees some of the functions related to laboratory operation, including classification of tests as required by CLIA and review of clinical laboratory test kits or systems.

The FDA and Genetic Testing

The recent growth of genetic testing, mostly developed and performed by individual laboratories without FDA review, has raised public concerns about the quality and clinical usefulness of these tests. The Secretary's Advisory Committee on Genetic Testing (SACGT) was established in 1998 to advise the secretary of the Department of Health and Human Services (DHHS) on medical, scientific, ethical, legal, and social issues raised by the development and use of genetic testing. The SACGT, in conjunction with the Clinical Laboratory Improvement Advisory Committee (CLIAC), recommended that the FDA provide regulatory oversight of laboratory-developed genetic testing. The vast majority of genetic testing is performed using laboratory-developed assays rather than by commercial FDA-approved test kits, raising concerns about the quality and clinical usefulness of these tests. As the first step in developing a review process for laboratory-developed tests, the FDA developed a "test review template" for gathering data on the use, performance, interpretation, and reporting of laboratory-developed tests.[20] Although this template was well received by SACGT, the FDA determined that laboratory-developed tests were part of medical practice, which is not regulated by the FDA, and did not develop a review

mechanism for laboratory-developed tests. A new committee has been formed, called the Secretary's Advisory Committee on Genetics, Health, and Society (SACGHS), and the committee has determined to monitor the activities of CLIA and FDA for regulatory oversight of laboratory-developed genetic tests.

Analyte-Specific Reagents

Although the majority of the FDA regulations for clinical assays target commercially developed in vitro diagnostic test kits intended for clinical use, the FDA issued regulations for commercial reagents used in laboratory-developed tests in 1997. The phrase "home-brew" assay[21,22] has been used to describe a laboratory-developed test used by clinicians for patient management. Although these regulations are not specific for molecular tests, almost all tests in the molecular pathology laboratory are developed, validated, and performed without the use of FDA-approved test kits. These tests are distinct from research assays that have unproven clinical utility and cannot be used for patient care. In 1997, the FDA developed regulations for manufacturers of reagents used in laboratory-developed tests. These reagents, termed "analyte-specific reagents" (ASRs), serve as the key component for laboratory-developed tests including molecular pathology tests, and include primers or probes that hybridize to specific DNA sequences. The manufacturers of ASRs are prohibited from making statements about the analytic or clinical performance of the reagents, and validation of tests using ASRs is the responsibility of the laboratory. The laboratory must include a disclaimer in the patient report stating, "This test was developed and its performance characteristics determined by (laboratory name). It has not been cleared or approved by the U.S. Food and Drug Administration." The result of the ASR regulations has been an increase in the availability of commercial reagents for molecular pathology tests.

Elements of Laboratory Design

Successful laboratory operation requires optimal utilization of space, appropriate equipment, qualified personnel, adequate information system services, and financial management.

Facilities

The power of molecular testing is achieved by the use of PCR as the main diagnostic procedure. A serious problem in the clinical use of PCR is false-positive amplification or PCR contamination. Because the product of PCR amplification serves as the substrate for the generation of additional products, PCR amplification produces a very large number of amplicons that can potentially contaminate subsequent amplifications of the same target sequence. This kind of contamination has been termed "carryover" to differentiate it from contamination by genomic DNA. This potential for PCR product contamination requires special precautions. Therefore, the single most important step in designing laboratory space for molecular pathology testing is meticulous attention to the physical separation of the pre-PCR and post-PCR work areas to minimize PCR contamination.[23]

The pre-PCR area, also referred to as a "clean room" or "preamplification area," is used for the pre-PCR steps of sample receiving and processing, including extraction of nucleic acids and setting up amplification reactions. The post-PCR area, also considered a "dirty room" or "post-amplification area," is used for PCR amplification and analysis of PCR products. The pre-PCR laboratory ideally contains separate work areas for nucleic acid extractions and PCR setup to minimize cross-contamination of patient nucleic acid samples. Additionally, a containment unit, such as a biosafety cabinet, may be used for setting up PCR reactions. These cabinets usually are equipped with ultraviolet light for reducing DNA contamination of the work area at the end of reaction setup.

If possible, the air system for the pre-PCR and post-PCR laboratories should be independent. Otherwise, air filters can be installed in the inflow to the pre-PCR room air system, which can be cleaned routinely. An additional measure to limit PCR contamination is to maintain the pre-PCR and post-PCR rooms at different air pressures. The pre-PCR area is maintained at positive pressure, reducing the entrance of airborne contaminants and PCR products, while the post-PCR room is maintained at negative pressure, reducing contaminants from exiting the room. If installation of a pressure system is not possible, then the two work areas can be located at a relative distance from each other.

To comply with universal blood-borne pathogen precautions, nucleic acid extraction from patient specimens can be performed in a closed safety cabinet. Specimens known to contain infectious agents such as HIV and HCV can be preferentially processed in a separate biological safety hood. If organic solvents such as phenol, chloroform, or xylenes are used, a chemical fume hood should be available in the work area. Within the pre-PCR laboratory, RNA extractions should be physically separated from DNA extraction if DNA extraction uses RNase, which can degrade RNA. All work areas should be cleaned daily with 10% bleach solution. In addition to pre-PCR and post-PCR areas, the molecular pathology laboratory also may have a neutral reagent preparation area (unless reagents are separately prepared in both rooms) and a data management room for the processing, review, and reporting of test results, which also may be performed in the post-PCR area.

To maximize use of space, equipment, technical expertise, and trained technologists, all types of molecular pathology testing (genetics, infectious disease, cancer, and identity testing) can be consolidated into a single laboratory. Implementing a core molecular pathology laboratory can reduce labor costs by approximately 30%[24] as well as reduce equipment costs and space requirements due to duplication of these resources in several laboratories.

PCR Contamination Control

In addition to physical separation of the pre-PCR and post-PCR areas, specific procedures are recommended for use of PCR in the clinical laboratory. To ensure that PCR products are not transferred from the post-PCR to the pre-PCR laboratory, each should contain separate supplies and equipment. Pipettes, instruments, and supplies should not be transferred from the post-PCR to the pre-PCR area. This separation of supplies and equipment also dictates the workflow in the laboratory. PCR samples are first set up in the pre-PCR room and then transferred to the post-PCR room for PCR amplification and post-PCR analysis. Worksheets, once moved to the post-PCR area for post-PCR analysis, can no longer be taken back into the pre-PCR area and must be processed and filed in the post-PCR area or a neutral area.

Reagents and solutions for sample preparation and PCR work should be prepared with type I water only in the designated work areas. All reagents, except primers, deoxynucleotide triphosphates (dNTPs), and enzymes, should be purchased as sterile reagents or sterilized to prevent bacterial growth. Reagents, including autoclaved type I water and 10 mM Tris-1 mM EDTA buffer (TE) used to dissolve DNA, should be stored as small aliquots to minimize the number of samplings from the same aliquot. Similarly, oligonucleotides used for PCR amplification should be synthesized and purified in a clean environment. To minimize the number of sample transfers and the chance of sporadic contamination and errors, PCR reagents, including primers, dNTPs and buffers, can be combined into a "premixture master mix" (MM), divided into aliquots that are appropriately labeled, and stored frozen at −20°C.[23] Before using for clinical testing, the MM aliquot must be tested to ensure that it specifically amplifies the target sequence without producing PCR products in the negative "minus DNA" controls. A "minus DNA" negative control tested last in each run ensures the lack of DNA contamination in PCR reagents.

Although carryover of amplified sequences contributes to the majority of false positives, cross-contamination between samples can also be a factor. Consequently, precautions must be taken not only during the setup of PCR amplification reactions but also in all aspects of sample handling, from sample collection to sample extraction. For good laboratory practice, gloves should be changed frequently, at least when entering or reentering the pre-PCR area and whenever the technologist notes the gloves to have been contaminated. Technologists should wear protective clothes to prevent operator-borne spread of contaminating DNA products, with separate protective clothes (i.e., laboratory coats) for the pre-PCR and post-PCR areas.

To minimize aerosolization of PCR products, PCR tubes should be pulse-centrifuged before opening. Microcentrifage tube caps should be opened using both hands, and not flicked open with the thumb of the same hand, to prevent aerosilization. Because cross-contamination of pipettors can lead to false-positive results and to minimize aerosolization, aerosol barrier tips are used for all pre-PCR steps. MM and other nonsample components should be added to the reaction tubes before the DNA samples are added; DNA should be added last and each tube capped before the technologist proceeds to the addition of the next sample. Positive and negative control DNA or RNA should be the last reaction tubes to be set up, after the patient sample reactions are set up and closed.

Another approach to minimize carryover of PCR products is to synthesize all PCR products with deoxyuridine triphosphate (dUTP) in place of deoxythymidine triphosphate (dTTP). Prior to amplification, the PCR reactions are treated with uracil-N-glycosylase (UNG), which will degrade uracil-containing amplicons, allowing amplification only from thymidine-containing target DNA.[25] Some commercially available test kits incorporate this process into the kits.

Equipment

The equipment required for molecular pathology testing is rarely manufactured for clinical use. Most equipment is designed for research and adapted for clinical use.[23] Nucleic acid extractions may be performed manually, although for higher-volume testing, automated extraction instruments are available and have demonstrated variable success for the clinical laboratory. PCR can be set up manually in biosafety cabinets; for higher-volume testing, robotic systems are available. Robotic systems, however, have reagent dead volumes that increase reagent wastage. Thermal cyclers are standard equipment in the molecular pathology laboratory, and the number required depends on the work volume. Post-PCR analysis is highly variable, although electrophoresis apparatus is commonly used.

New specialized equipment for post-PCR analysis includes automated sequencers or capillary electrophoresis instruments, chemiluminescent or colorimetric plate readers, real-time PCR instruments, and denaturing high-performance liquid chromatography (DHPLC) instruments for mutation screening. Most of the available viral load tests are performed using commercial kits, which require the use of specific instruments supplied by the test kit manufacturer. Because of the high level of testing complexity and the concern of PCR contamination, researchers or personnel not trained in molecular pathology should not use the clinical molecular pathology equipment.

Because these instruments are used for clinical testing, they require rigorous surveillance and prompt technical support by manufacturers who are not always aware of the critical clinical testing issues. In addition, these instruments require ongoing maintenance. Most maintenance procedures are defined by the manufacturer and include temperature checks of the PCR wells for thermal cyclers and calibration of pipetters. In the absence of manufacturer's guidelines, the laboratory should set up its own maintenance program in consultation with the manufacturer.

Personnel

Personnel Qualifications

Effective laboratory operation requires well-trained staff and a good management team. CLIA regulations specify that for high-complexity testing, individuals for the positions of director, technical supervisor, and testing staff must have specific qualifications.

The director, as listed on the CLIA certificate, in addition to having 2 years' experience supervising a high-complexity laboratory, must be a licensed doctor of medicine, osteopathy, or podiatry or have a doctoral degree in one of the biological, chemical, physical, or medical sciences. The laboratory director is responsible for the overall operation and administration of the laboratory, including the development and implementation of new tests, current procedure manuals, quality control and training programs for staff, and teaching residents.

The technical supervisor establishes the quality standards of the laboratory by selecting and monitoring methods and instrumentation and documenting the competency of laboratory personnel, while the general supervisor provides day-to-day supervision of testing, personnel, and reporting of results. The qualifications for these positions range from a licensed doctor to an individual holding a bachelor's degree in science plus specific training or experience or both. The laboratory also may have clinical consultants, who must hold a medical or doctoral degree in a relevant discipline with appropriate experience in molecular testing. The Genetic Workgroup (GW) of CLIAC, created in 1998, reviewed personnel qualifications and recommended including specific genetic experience and board certification for supervisors who oversee genetic testing.[20]

Testing personnel who perform high-complexity testing must have an associate's degree in laboratory science or medical laboratory technology, or education and training equivalent to an associate's degree. The laboratory technologists are responsible for all tasks associated with the daily operation of the laboratory, including specimen receiving and processing, testing, identifying problems and troubleshooting, maintaining equipment, and documenting quality control procedures. In addition, they are required to work according to established procedures in adherence with the quality control standards implemented in the laboratory to comply with CLIA, CAP or other regulations. Because there are very few commercially available molecular test kits, molecular pathology technologists perform much of the development of new tests, as well as validation of commercial molecular kits used for clinical testing.

Because of the high level of desired expertise, technologists also need to be encouraged to attend educational courses to obtain the appropriate background in molecular pathology and the skills required for performing these tests. For the same reason, it is also crucial for the senior management of the laboratory to acknowledge the staff, encourage personal growth, and create new mechanisms for promotion. Although some of these recommendations represent the authors' personal views and may present a burden in the stringent financial environment of many healthcare institutions, the cost of training new technologists is higher than that of creating an environment that promotes job satisfaction and employee retention.

Genetic Counselors

The role of the genetic counselor is to assess the need for genetic testing through family history, inform the patient about the specific risks and benefits of specific genetic tests, order the tests, and communicate the results to the patient. Although the genetic counselor is traditionally a part of the clinical medical genetics service, an increasing number of test sites use genetic counselors as a link between the patient and healthcare providers and the laboratory.

Resident and Fellow Training in Molecular Pathology

Pathology residency programs are required to provide molecular pathology training to residents. Because the molecular biology knowledge and practical experience of pathology residents is highly variable, the Association for Molecular Pathology (AMP) Training and Education Committee generated general goals for molecular pathology resident training programs. AMP molecular pathology training recommendations for residents include basic knowledge in human genetics and molecular biology, which are relevant to all aspects of molecular testing, specific technology information, as well as knowledge of specific molecular pathology tests.[26] Because molecular pathology training time can be brief (1 to 3 months), training may need to be accomplished through didactic lectures that encompass the tests performed in the laboratory as well as basic concepts in molecular pathology and technology, rather than more extensive practical experience.

Education of fellows requires broader training, resources, and time. The increasing importance of this field for clinical practice and the desire to undergo formal molecular pathology training led to the development of fellowship training programs and professional certification by several professional boards, specifically the American Board of Medical Genetics (ABMG) and the American Board of Pathology (ABP). Official training programs in clinical molecular genetics by the ABMG and in molecular genetic pathology (jointly by the ABMG and the ABP) are accredited by the Accreditation Committee on Graduate Medical Education (ACGME). Official accreditation of either of these training programs requires filing of a program application with review and on-site formal inspection by an ACGME representative.[27] The goal of these programs is to provide structured educational training for qualified individuals seeking to integrate molecular genetic pathology into their clinical practice experience in all current aspects of the field, including basic science, diagnostic laboratory procedures, laboratory management, and consultation. To be eligible for the examination, fellows should have a strong background in molecular biology and molecular genetics as well as practical experience, and should be able to use this information for diagnosis and management of genetic disorders, infectious diseases, malignancies, identity testing, and HLA typing.

Residents and fellows can contribute significantly to the daily operation of the laboratory, including acquisition of clinical information and communication of test results. In addition, they can assist with the development and implementation of new tests, according to the skill level of the trainee and as time permits. In return, they gain new expertise that may be an advantage when seeking employment.

Staff Training and Accreditation Programs

Appropriate technical staff training is vital to the successful operation of a molecular pathology laboratory.[27] Accreditation programs in medical genetics and molecular pathology ensure that members of the laboratory staff are well trained for performing their assigned roles. Individuals who want to practice clinical molecular pathology have several options, depending on their initial education.

Individuals who hold a medical or doctoral degree and are interested in directing a molecular pathology laboratory can be certified by the ABMG. ABMG is a member of the American Board of Medical Specialists (ABMS) that provides certification in all medical specialties. Certification in clinical molecular genetics requires passing of a general examination in medical genetics as well as a subspecialty examination in clinical molecular genetics. Individuals must have a doctoral degree (MD or PhD) and must have completed 2 years in an accredited genetics program to be eligible to take the ABMG examination for certification. In addition, candidates must provide a record (logbook) documenting their involvement in 150 clinical molecular genetic cases, which is approved by the fellowship program director. The examination is offered every 3 years.

In 1999, the ABMS approved a new subspecialty in molecular genetic pathology (MGP) offered jointly by the ABMG and the ABP. Candidates for this certification must hold a medical degree, have board certification in their specific field of medical genetics or pathology, have a valid license to practice medicine in the United States, and have completed a year of training in an accredited MGP fellowship training program. The first MGP examination was given in 2001; the test is given biannually. MGP training programs are accredited based on standards developed jointly by the ABP and the ABMG.

The American Board of Clinical Chemistry (ABCC) has a certification program in molecular diagnosis, which was offered for the first time in 2000. This certification is offered biannually to individuals who hold doctoral degrees and practice in any one of several clinical laboratory specialties.

Certification in molecular diagnosis is offered to medical and molecular biology technologists by the National Credentialing Agency for Laboratory Personnel, Inc (NCA). The examination is given biannually and is useful for clinical molecular laboratory staff, particularly the senior technical staff who become certified laboratory specialists in molecular biology. The American Society of Clinical Pathology certifies technical staff as a technologist in molecular pathology, based on qualification for the examination by several routes.

Financial Management

Molecular pathology testing is a market with growing gross revenue, which requires an understanding of the influence of finances on the technical aspects of the laboratory. Because many clinical molecular pathology laboratories are part of healthcare systems, they are constantly subjected to limiting managed care contracts and reduced reimbursements, and as such, they are often viewed as cost centers. Molecular pathology laboratory management should develop cost-effective business plans that present molecular pathology testing in the context of the clinical programs this testing supports, if the testing is not independently cost-effective, such that hospital administration views the laboratory as a revenue center.

Cost Analysis

In the current restrictive medical economic environment, the decision to perform a specific test must include business (financial) as well as medical considerations. The evaluation process for deciding to implement a new test or deciding to discontinue a current test should include a cost analysis. The charges for a test are determined mostly by the costs of performing the test and the value of the test in the market (demand). A cost analysis should account for all expenses associated with performing a given test. In a

structured approach, a standard template can be developed and used to price any new test based on the cost for each step of the testing process.

Cost analysis involves two main types of expenses: direct expenses and indirect expenses.[28] The direct expenses enumerate all costs directly related to the testing, including equipment, reagents, consumables, salary, and benefits. The calculation of reagent costs is based on the known volume of reagent used and the cost per volume, including reagents for controls and dead volumes. For manual, low-volume testing, the largest component of direct cost is labor, which can comprise up to 90% of the total direct test cost. Laboratory labor cost calculations are generally done using the hands-on technologist time needed to perform the test multiplied by an average hourly salary rate plus the appropriate benefit rate. For example, the cost for a PCR-RFLP test should take into consideration the time required for specimen accessioning and storage, DNA extraction, PCR setup, post-PCR analysis, interpretation, and reporting of results, usually an average of 6 to 8 hours of technologist time, which is divided by the number of samples tested at the same time to reach the labor cost per test.

Indirect costs include overhead, such as licensing fees, royalties, supervisory and administrative salaries, equipment maintenance fees, building services (such as electricity, phones, heating, etc.), marketing, and information system requirements. These costs are more difficult to determine and are not usually a part of the routine cost analysis for academic laboratories. Accurate determination of laboratory costs is important for assessing profitability.

Billing

Billing for molecular pathology tests follows the same guidelines as billing for other pathology laboratory services, requiring a Current Procedural Terminology (CPT) code and an International Classification of Diseases (ICD-9-CM) diagnostic code. The ICD-9 code, which is required for payment, should be provided by the requesting physician when a test is ordered, while the pathologist is responsible for using the appropriate CPT codes for billing of test services. CPT coding of molecular pathology tests, other than most molecular infectious disease tests which have single test-specific CPT codes, is based on a combination of several CPT codes for the various procedural steps that are performed as part of a molecular test. For example, nucleic acid extraction, amplification, and electrophoresis all have separate CPT codes. A single test using all of these procedures is billed using a combination of all the appropriate CPT codes, used multiple times as needed, with the addition of a modifier code following a hyphen at the end of the primary CPT code. Most molecular CPT codes describe a molecular procedure rather than a specific method. For example, a nucleic acid extraction can be performed for RNA or DNA, using different procedures, each bearing a different cost. Therefore, the same CPT code can be associated with different billing fees, although the Medicare reimbursement rate remains fixed. Additionally, each procedure (or CPT code) can be billed more than once within a single test, depending on the number of times the procedure was performed. For example, a PCR-RFLP test for the detection of two mutations associated with hereditary hemochromatosis would be coded using one DNA extraction code, two PCR amplification codes, two restriction enzyme digestion codes, one gel electrophoresis code, and one interpretation and report code. A complete list of the CPT codes can be found in the *Physician's Current Procedural Manual*, published by the American Medical Association.[29]

Pathogen-specific codes are available for molecular infectious disease tests, such as HIV-1, HCV, and hepatitis B virus viral loads, for which all steps of the procedure (extraction, amplification, detection, and reagents) are covered by a single CPT code. When specific CPT codes are available for a pathogen type, three coding options are available based on the testing method used, specifically for probe hybridization, amplification, or quantification. Infectious disease tests without pathogen-specific CPT codes are coded using a combination of method-based CPT codes.

For molecular pathology tests requiring professional interpretation, the professional component is coded using the interpretation and report CPT code (83912) with a modifier, "-26," to differentiate the billing from the technical component, reported with a "TC."

Reimbursement for molecular pathology tests is dictated, to a large extent, by the reimbursement policies of CMS, which are generally followed by third-party payers such as insurance companies. FDA approval is not necessary for billing of molecular pathology tests; however, some third-party payers may not reimburse for tests that are not FDA approved. In addition, billing Medicare for tests using a non-FDA-approved commercial test kit is fraudulent; while billing for tests performed using ASRs is not. Due to the low reimbursement rates for molecular tests, some molecular pathology laboratories will not perform tests for patients from other institutions without billing the sending institution or pre-payment by the patient, which usually guarantees full payment.

Patent

Another consideration prior to the implementation of a new test is the patent status of the test. Patents can cover a specific method of testing for an analyte, any method of testing for an analyte, or a mutation-gene-disease association in general. The most common royalty payments for molecular pathology laboratories are payments for the use of the PCR method and Taq polymerase, licensed by Roche Diagnostics, Inc. Many diagnostic tests use PCR. Royalty payments for use of Taq polymerase range from 9% to 15% of the amount billed or reimbursed for a test, and generally are higher for commercial laboratories than for academic laboratories.

Of special concern are patenting and licensing of patents for mutations in specific genes associated with disease. Examples of such patents include apolipoprotein E genotyping for Alzheimer disease, Canavan disease, and Charcot-Marie-Tooth disease type 1A. Patenting imposes a significant risk to the molecular pathology laboratory because the number of diagnostic patents, particularly in the area of medical genetics, has greatly increased in recent years. Many clinically relevant DNA sequences are patented, and the terms of use offered by the holders vary considerably; in some instances, a laboratory will be unable to perform a test because the patent is exclusively licensed to another laboratory. Thus, a laboratory considering implementation of a new molecular test first may conduct searches of existing patents and patent applications to see whether the new test infringes on existing or pending patents. Typically, patent attorneys employed by the medical center conduct patent searches. Internet resources provided by the US Patent and Trademark Office (http://www.uspto.gov) allow laboratories to perform searches directly. If a patent exists that covers any part of the molecular test to be implemented, the laboratory or medical center must negotiate an agreement for clinical testing with the patent holder or licensee, if the patent holder will grant a license. Licensing agreements may include royalty payments that increase the cost of the test, and limitations on the use of the test or the volume of testing the laboratory can perform. For this reason, many molecular pathology leaders argue that patented genetic tests should be broadly licensed at affordable costs to allow any qualified clinical laboratory to perform the tests.

Laboratory Information Systems

Most molecular pathology laboratories require a computer information system to handle the large volume of data that is both received and reported. Selecting and installing a laboratory information system (LIS) is a lengthy and labor-intensive process, usually performed by the department or institution rather than by the laboratory. The application software allows users to perform tasks that are specific to the laboratory operations. These tasks include registering patients and accessioning specimens, ordering laboratory tests, reporting test results, and tracking quality control data (Figure 11-1). In addition, the LIS facilitates use of appropriate templates for billing and reporting of results. The primary function of the LIS application is management of the database of patients and laboratory test results. The most-used system is a relational database management system, which links all the data in tables related to one another by common elements. This kind of structure allows the technologist, for example, to quickly produce a list of only those patient specimens that are going be tested for a particular test. When two or more tables contain the same primary field (patient identifier), information can be retrieved from multiple tables. For example, to monitor

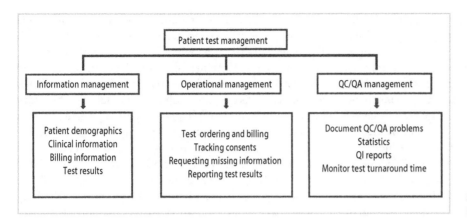

Figure 11-1. Organizational chart for LIS-based molecular pathology testing management.

engraftment after allogeneic bone marrow transplant, the entire list of test results and dates of testing can be obtained for any particular patient. Because departmental LIS systems are not designed to meet the specific information requirements of the molecular pathology laboratory, many molecular pathology laboratories also use networked personal computers (PCs) for data management. These PCs are mostly used as tools for running standard applications, such as word processing, spreadsheets, and other specialized applications, for example, sequencing and genetic risk-assessment applications. Since, however, molecular pathology laboratories have unique data management requirements, a separate patient database may be maintained on the laboratory PCs. To reduce transcription errors and eliminate the labor-intensive work of retyping patient information and test results, laboratory PCs should be interfaced with the LIS system to allow direct transfer of test results for each patient. Furthermore, some molecular pathology instruments, such as the COBAS system (Roche Diagnostics) for HIV-1 and HCV testing, can be interfaced directly to the LIS. The results, collated with specimen identification, are automatically transferred to the LIS, followed by verification by laboratory personnel and report release for clinical use.

To improve laboratory operations, many quality control activities can be performed using the LIS, including monitoring of turnaround time, control results, and statistics. Procedures and other documentation can be maintained and managed by the laboratory computer as well. Security and access control are crucial components of the LIS. Access control (passwords) and patient confidentiality (limiting access to only those who need specific information) are some of the tools required to maintain patient confidentiality.

Test Management

Choice of Test Menu

The menu of tests for molecular pathology laboratories varies significantly and is determined by three principal factors: clinical requirement and usefulness, laboratory competency, and test costs. Other factors that affect the decision about adding a new test include the prevalence of the disease, the mutation(s) causing the disease, the number of different mutations associated with the disease, availability of ASR or FDA-approved test kits, complexity of testing, equipment requirements, and existence of patents that apply to the test. Each of these items requires serious consideration and support on behalf of the institution.

The clinical requirement and usefulness of a test are defined by the significance of the test result for disease diagnosis and clinical management. For example, HIV viral load testing is widely used because it provides immediate information regarding the patient response to treatment and prognosis. Likewise, population-based genetic screening for cystic fibrosis (CF), now offered to all individuals and couples of childbearing age, provides immediate information about a couple's risk for an affected child.[30]

"Competency" refers to the availability of skilled laboratory personnel who can perform, supervise, troubleshoot, and correctly interpret molecular tests. For example, RT-PCR-based tests require knowledge not only of PCR but also of RNA processing in the clinical laboratory.

Test costs are another important factor for selection of tests to offer. Generally, when the cost of a test is low and the volume is high, a test will have a profit margin. A common issue is deciding whether to perform the test or to use a reference laboratory for a specific test. This usually requires a break-even analysis to determine the point (threshold) at which there is no profit or loss for performing the test, taking into consideration the cost of the test, the expected revenue, and the expected volume of testing. Rare or urgent tests may be more expensive since tests are run individually rather than batched analyses, as can be done in a reference laboratory, with combined testing from many sites. In contrast, high-volume tests are likely to be profitable when performed by an individual laboratory.

The prevalence of the disease or mutation in the population affects the testing volume and therefore the number of laboratories that perform a specific test. The laboratory, however, may choose to test for less-common diseases or mutations if it receives a sufficient specimen volume to make the testing cost-effective. For example, some laboratories offer comprehensive testing for neurological diseases when there is specific clinical expertise at their medical center, or with inclusion of clinical samples referred to the laboratory from other sites in the United States or internationally.

The number of different mutations in one or more genes accounting for a disease is a consideration for testing. In general, the greater the number of mutations in a single gene or the number of different genes that can cause a disease, the more complex and labor-intensive testing becomes. Therefore, for common disorders, such as CF, commercial kits are available that detect 25 of the more common mutations in the *CFTR* gene, requiring substantially less time for test development than laboratory-developed methods or complete *CFTR* gene analysis.

Ease of testing and equipment are two important considerations. Tests requiring lengthy procedures, such as Southern blot analysis, or complex analyses (SMA carrier testing, for example) are less likely to be performed by many laboratories, especially if the test volume is low or commercial test kits are not available. The use of ASRs or FDA-approved tests is preferred by many laboratories because they simplify the laboratory workflow and facilitate quality assurance, even though these tests are often more expensive relative to laboratory-developed tests.

Finally, patents that cover the disease mutations, genes, or testing methods for a test can be a consideration when deciding to implement and perform a test. Patent or license exclusivity may be enforced, licensing or sublicensing fees may be too costly, or other conditions of licensing may not be reasonable for the laboratory, such that the laboratory cannot or chooses not to implement and perform a test covered by one or more patents. This may be even more significant for complex genetic disease tests that require testing of multiple genes, each of which may be covered by patents.

Choice of Test Method

Several factors influence the selection of the testing method, including the mutation type, the degree of mutation heterogeneity, the anticipated test volume, the available resources, such as equipment and expertise, and patent issues. The majority of clinical tests target specific mutations or sequences. The greater the number of sequence variations that need to be detected by a test, the more difficult and labor-intensive the test becomes. The most-frequently used method in molecular pathology laboratories is amplification, usually by PCR. Some of the more common factors affecting the choice of methods from nucleic acid extraction through PCR and post-PCR analysis are discussed.

Nucleic acid extraction is a principal part of most molecular tests. Numerous extraction methods are currently available. Some of the issues to consider in choosing an extraction method for DNA or RNA are yield, quality of the nucleic acid required for the subsequent testing steps, storage, processing speed, and costs. Laboratories may use more than one method for DNA or RNA purification. Some of the more common methods currently utilized are desalting methods and silica-gel membrane columns. Columns are particularly convenient for processing of small volumes of blood for a large number of samples and are available for either DNA or RNA. Organic-based methods can be used but are labor-intensive and have significant safety risks for the clinical laboratory, so are less commonly used now than in the past. Quick lysis methods (alkaline or boiling) generate crude DNA, which may be suitable for some test applications.

The most common method in the molecular pathology laboratory is PCR, which has enabled the implementation of hundreds of clinical molecular tests. The method is particularly suitable for detection of point mutations and other small sequence variations, for detection of chromosomal rearrangements, for detection or quantification of pathogens by amplification, or for sequence analysis. Variations of PCR include RT-PCR for amplification of RNA sequences, multiplex PCR for the simultaneous amplification of two or more sequences, and real-time PCR for quantification of specific sequences (see chapter 2).

While PCR amplification is relatively standard, many methods are used to analyze the resulting PCR products. The simplest method for analysis of PCR products is gel electrophoresis to determine the size of the PCR products that have been synthesized with comparison to a sizing standard that has been run on the same gel. A second common method for analysis of PCR products is digestion with a restriction enzyme followed by analysis of the DNA fragments by gel electrophoresis. PCR products can be hybridized to allele-specific oligonucleotide (ASO) probes complementary for either the normal or mutant allele. A variation on this approach is the reverse dot-blot, in which numerous allelic probes are fixed to specific locations on a solid membrane and hybridized with multiplex PCR products. Methods using hybridization steps are more labor-intensive and expensive than enzymatic digestions and are used less frequently than other post-PCR analysis methods.

Small length changes and genetic rearrangements present in PCR products can be detected by size variations using agarose or acrylamide gel electrophoresis with ethidium-bromide staining, or by a fluorescent-dependent detection method using either a plate- or capillary-based automated sequencer. Automated sequencers are especially useful for the simultaneous analysis of numerous PCR products labeled either with a single or multiple fluorophores, or when quantitation of a PCR product is required.

A significant portion of PCR testing is being transitioned to real-time PCR, which monitors the generation of the PCR product throughout the amplification process. This approach can be used for either point mutation detection or quantitation, eliminating the need for time-consuming post-PCR analysis and decreasing opportunities for PCR contamination.

Table 11-3. Specimen Types and Handling for Molecular Pathology Testing

Specimen Type	Test Type	Requirements	Shipment	Storage
Blood	Genetics, cancer, identity, HLA typing	EDTA (0.5–10 ml)*	RT	4°C
Bone marrow	Cancer, identity testing	EDTA (0.5–1 ml)	RT	4°C
Plasma	Infectious diseases	EDTA (10 ml)	Dry ice	–80°C
Cerebrospinal fluid	Cancer, infectious diseases	None (0.5–2 ml)	Dry ice	–80°C
Sputum	Cancer, infectious diseases	None (0.5–2 ml)	RT	4°C
Amniotic fluid (<15 weeks gestation)	Genetics	None (10–15 ml)	RT	4°C
Chorionic villus sampling (CVS)	Genetics	5–15 mg	RT	4°C
Cultured amniocytes or CVS	Genetics	2 T25 flasks	RT	4°C
Buccal cells	Genetics, cancer, identity	2 swabs	RT	4°C
Fresh tissue	Cancer, identity	50–100 mg	Dry ice	–80°C
Paraffin-embedded tissue	Cancer, identity	2–5 μm sections	RT	RT
DNA	Genetics, cancer, identity, HLA typing	<1–100 μg	RT	4°C
RNA	Genetics, cancer	<1–20 μg	Dry ice	–80°C

*Sample volume is based on application and age of patient.
RT, room temperature.

When the disease gene is known but the mutations are unknown, mutation-scanning methods are used. The most common scanning methods are single-strand conformation polymorphism (SSCP) and DHPLC, both of which detect single base pair variations with high sensitivity.

Automated platforms for molecular tests are becoming available and are more significant for the clinical laboratory as test volume increases. Currently available automated systems include extraction systems, and instruments that combine PCR amplification and detection. Some automated systems are routinely used in many molecular pathology laboratories for viral load testing, such as for HIV-1. Automated instrumentation can reduce turnaround time and human error.

Clinical Information Requirements

Preanalytic clinical information is essential for determining the appropriateness of the test and is critical for interpretation of results. Clinical information usually is obtained from the requisition form or an electronic test order system. A complete requisition contains patient demographic information to allow for identification of the patient, the ordering healthcare provider's name and contact information, the type of sample, the name of the ordered test(s), relevant clinical information, and any other information essential for appropriate interpretation of test ordered results. For some genetic disorders, such as CF, ethnic background is particularly important because disease prevalence can vary significantly with ethnic background, while a pedigree is required for linkage analysis studies and risk assessment. Laboratories should document informed consent for genetic tests (as discussed in the Genetic Testing section), which may be required by state regulation. For cancer or infectious disease testing, indication of the purpose for testing (diagnosis or minimal residual disease assessment) is needed for appropriate interpretation of the test result.

Specimen Requirements

Molecular pathology testing can be performed using a variety of patient sample types. A list of the more common specimen types, applications, handling and storage requirements is presented in Table 11-3. The most common sample for genetic testing is peripheral blood (PB); buccal cells may be acceptable for some tests. Prenatal testing is performed on cultured or direct amniotic cells and chorionic villus sampling (CVS). A maternal sample may be required for prenatal testing to rule out maternal cell contamination (MCC) of the fetal specimen, to ensure that the test result reflects the fetal genotype rather than the maternal genotype, usually by identity testing of the fetal and maternal samples. Samples for molecular oncology and infectious disease testing may include PB, bone marrow, tissues, and other body fluid (cerebral spinal fluid, sputum, etc). Paraffin-embedded tissues (PET) are used predominantly for DNA-based testing such as gene rearrangement studies for lymphomas, while fresh or frozen tissue generally is used for RNA-based testing, such as the detection of specific fusion transcripts in cancers.

Sample requirements and collection and shipment information for molecular tests should be provided by the laboratory to ensure that samples are collected, handled, shipped, and stored appropriately before shipment, during transit, and during storage in the laboratory before sample processing.

Laboratory Operations

Workflow includes the steps of testing from specimen collection to reporting of results. This process can be divided into preanalytic, analytic and postanalytic phases. The preanalytic phase consists of collecting, transporting, accessioning, and storage of the sample(s) prior to testing. The analytic phase is the process of performing the test. The postanalytic phase consists of all steps after the test is performed, including analysis of the test result, generation of the test report, and communication of the results. Although the preanalytic phase is difficult to control since the steps are performed by individuals outside the laboratory, most errors occur in the analytic phase because of the multistep, predominantly manual nature of molecular testing.

Preanalytic Phase

Samples are usually transported to a central receiving area of the laboratory or directly to the molecular pathology laboratory, either by a local hospital transport system or by overnight carrier if the samples are sent from remote sites. Upon arrival, samples are accessioned into the LIS and assigned a unique identifier or accession number, allowing the sample to be tracked in the laboratory and hospital database. Information entered during accessioning includes patient demographics, test(s) requested, specimen type, and time and date a specimen is collected and received by the laboratory. If available, bar-coded labels can be attached to the requisition form and specimen container.

The clinical information and specimen type are reviewed for appropriateness of the test requested. Missing clinical information can be obtained by contacting the healthcare provider. Genetic test requests are reviewed for ethical considerations.

Some sample types require additional processing prior to nucleic acid extraction. For example, PET blocks are sectioned to allow efficient extraction, and CVS tissue is examined by a qualified cytogeneticist to remove contaminating maternal tissue. Similarly, prenatal cultured cells are examined for confluence; low numbers of cells may not produce sufficient DNA for some analyses, such as Southern blot analysis. For HIV and HCV viral load tests, for example, the plasma must be separated from the blood cells within 4 to 6 hours of collection. The specimen is appropriately stored until processing begins (Table 11-3).

Analytic Phase

For laboratory efficiency and cost-effectiveness, testing is performed on batches of specimens, and the frequency of testing depends on test volume and clinical urgency. The first step in molecular-based testing is nucleic acid isolation. DNA or RNA can be extracted from the patient specimens using a variety of laboratory-developed methods or commercial kits, and the nucleic acid stored appropriately (see Table 11-3). Most tests use PCR, which is set up in the pre-PCR area of the laboratory. To verify sample identity throughout all the steps of testing and prevent possible mix-up and cross-contamination, a worksheet can be used to indicate sample identifiers and numerical locations in the run, as well as reagent information such as lot numbers

and expiration dates. The same worksheet can be used later for documentation of test results for patient samples and controls. The patient samples should be set up first, followed by the controls, as discussed in the PCR Contamination Control section. Regardless of the procedure used, certain principles are essential. Specimen and reagent identifications should be checked with every manipulation performed. Expiration dates and identification of reagents should be checked before each use. Test results should be documented, either by photographing the gel or by printing out the data from the instrument. It is very important at this point to label and correctly identify the samples on pictures or data sheets to prevent interpretation errors.

Postanalytic Phase

After the test is performed, the results are analyzed, the test results and interpretation are entered into the laboratory computer manually or by electronic transfer from an instrument, and the results are communicated verbally to the healthcare provider, if appropriate. To reduce errors, results should be interpreted by two independent reviewers, which may include a technologist previously certified to interpret the specific test through the laboratory's training program, a resident or fellow, or the laboratory director or appropriate designee. Results must comply with the established criteria for result analysis and interpretation as defined in the test procedure manual. Control results are reviewed for accuracy before analysis of patient test results. For PCR-based tests analyzed by electrophoresis, the water/no template control should not have bands other than primer dimers, and control samples must demonstrate expected results. For quantitative assays, control results must fall within the established assay ranges. Patient test results are interpreted as positive or negative, or a quantitative result is obtained by comparison with the assay controls and by comparison to size markers, as appropriate for the specific test method. Unexpected results are assessed for errors in the analytic process. The identified problems are corrected and testing of all or selected specimens is repeated. Results should be recorded manually or electronically transferred to the assay worksheet by the technologist who performed the assay, signed, dated, and entered in the computer using a report template, if available. Entered reports should then be reviewed and released by a second interpreter. For efficient workflow, use of report templates for the most common test results and interpretations, with revisions for specific specimens, facilitates test reporting.

The information required for test reports is defined in the CAP Molecular Pathology checklist and includes patient demographics, methods, mutation(s) tested, and a clinical interpretation in an easy-to-interpret format. Although the CAP, in compliance with CLIA, does not require supervisory review of all test results, it is recommended that all manual assays be reviewed and approved by the laboratory director or qualified designee before reporting. A final report is generated only after results are verified and electronically signed by the laboratory director or a qualified designee. When laboratory director review is not deemed necessary, such as for tests performed using automated equipment, two separate technologists trained to perform the assay, or the same technologist in duplicate, should review the results after entry into the LIS to ensure accurate entry into the LIS prior to release of the reports. Results most often are communicated by printed report or an electronic information system, but direct discussion of urgent or complex test results may be useful for the clinician. Verbal communication or faxing of test results should be performed in compliance with HIPAA regulations to protect patient confidentiality.

Quality Control and Quality Assessment Programs

The molecular pathology laboratory must establish and maintain quality control (QC) and quality assessment also known as quality assurance (QA) programs that are adequate and appropriate for the validity of the procedures performed. The next few sections focus on the principal aspects of these programs.

Quality Control Program

The QC program focuses on the analytic validity of the testing process with the purpose of assessing and ensuring the reliability of patient results. According to CLIA, "The laboratory must establish and follow written QC procedures for monitoring and evaluating the quality of the analytic testing process of each method to assure the accuracy and reliability of patient test results and reports."[17] Specific requirements include adherence to the manufacturer's instructions for instrument operation and test performance, having a current procedure manual, performing and documenting QC test results, maintaining records of all QC activities, and verifying performance specifications. Test sites, especially high-complexity laboratories, may choose to impose more, but not less, stringent QC requirements for the testing process. Molecular pathology tests are largely manual, laboratory-developed, multistep assays, requiring a variety of commercial or laboratory-produced reagents. QC procedures should be designed to detect and reduce errors in the entire testing process. Special attention should be given to the most common types of errors that occur during testing, such as use of expired reagents, improper preparation and storage of reagents and controls, and clerical errors. Some of the key components of the QC program are discussed below.

Test Validation (Verification of Test Performance Characteristics)

There are major differences, as defined by CLIA, between the implementation of an FDA-approved test and the implementation of a laboratory-developed test. If the test is performed using an FDA-approved in vitro diagnostic test kit, the laboratory needs only to verify the performance characteristics of the test for the population of patients seen at that specific laboratory site. Implementation of a laboratory-developed test requires collection of more extensive analytic data to establish the performance characteristics of the test. The performance characteristics that need to be evaluated include accuracy, precision, sensitivity, specificity, reportable range, reference range, and any other applicable characteristics. Laboratories can use the manufacturer's criteria as long as the director determines that these are appropriate for the laboratory's population of patients. To assist in this process, CLIA also recommends that performance characteristics of a new test be compared to a known "gold standard." This is not always practical, since molecular methods often are developed because of the inadequacy of the currently available test methods. The test method also should be validated for all types of specimens that will be accepted for testing.

Establishing the test accuracy requires determining that the test yields appropriate positive, negative, or quantitative results, based on samples with known characteristics as determined by an independent test method. Samples used to determine accuracy can be obtained from several sources, including proficiency surveys or other laboratories performing the test by the same or a different test method. For example, validation results for new RT-PCR procedures for the diagnosis of certain translocations in leukemias can be supported by cytogenetic results for the same specimens.

Establishing the precision of an assay requires demonstrating that the assay results are reproducible. Testing the control specimens and a variety of patient specimens multiple times in separate runs and comparing the results can demonstrate the precision of a test. For quantitative tests, precision is tested over the range of reportable values.

Analytic sensitivity refers to the lowest amount of analyte (nucleic acid) detected or quantified by a test. Analytic sensitivity is determined as the proportion of patient samples that contain the target nucleic acid sequence that tests positive using the test. In quantitative tests, this represents the smallest amount of analyte that is reliably detected by the test. Sensitivity should be determined for qualitative assays for pathogen detection or for MRD monitoring to establish the utility and limitations of the test.

Analytic specificity measures the degree to which the test reacts with nucleic acids other than the intended sequence. It is measured as the proportion of patient samples that do not contain the target nucleic acid that test negative by the test. The analytic specificity of a test can be determined by analyzing a series of positive and negative samples and calculating the detection rate of the true-negative samples, as defined by samples that do not contain the target of the test. Distinguishing among closely related pathogens, however, requires a precise design of primers specific for the target microorganism. Nonspecific signals can be produced by nonoptimal amplification conditions or inhibitors, which can be overcome by high-quality DNA extraction procedures and optimization of assay conditions.

The development of a new test usually is driven by new molecular information combined with a clinical need for a better test. Once the laboratory director decides that a new molecular test will be implemented, the methodology for the assay, controls, specimen types, costs, and other factors are determined. The method for the assay is chosen based on the type of test information required, clinical utility, current use of the test platform in the laboratory, ease of use, and clinically required turnaround time. Once the test method is chosen, the specific test parameters are designed. Each step of the assay is optimized, including nucleic acid extraction, amplification, detection, and interpretation of results. For laboratories that develop many assays, standard starting conditions and optimization criteria facilitate test implementation. For example, PCR assays can initially use standard reagent concentrations and amplification conditions, followed by fine optimization of the PCR conditions as needed. Once the optimal assay conditions are established, the analytic validation of the assay is performed on clinical specimens and/or controls using those testing conditions.

Initial optimization and performance of the assay must include establishing the controls to be used for testing. Appropriate controls are often commercially available from organizations such as Coriell (Camden, NJ) and the American Type Culture Collection (ATCC; Manassas, VA) as frozen immortalized cell lines or DNA containing the pathogen genome or mutation of interest. With the exception of HIV and HCV, for which standardized reference panels are now available, standardized controls are not available for most of the molecular diagnostic tests currently performed. In the absence of purchased controls, patient samples tested by a different method or provided by another laboratory may be used.

The last step of the test evaluation requires clinical validation of the new test. Clinical validation determines the probability that a sample from a patient with the disease or disease risk will test positive (clinical sensitivity), and that a sample from a patient without the disease or disease risk will test negative (clinical specificity). A final step of the clinical validation may be to obtain a panel of mixed positive and negative patient samples without the known test results from another laboratory that performs the same test. After the testing, results are compared to the results obtained by the other laboratory and documented. Any discrepancies should be resolved by a different test method or a third laboratory.

Test Procedure Manual

Test procedure manuals are essential for molecular pathology laboratory function and are required by CLIA. The manual should be simple, easy to follow, and functional, but should provide sufficient detail to act as a reference for all aspects of testing for laboratory personnel and for training purposes. The manual, in a written or electronic format, must be current and available to all laboratory personnel. Manuals for high-complexity tests include written policies for sample collection, equipment performance evaluation, QC program, and standard operating procedures (SOP) for tests. An example of the contents of a test procedure manual is shown in Table 11-4. The procedures are usually written by laboratory technologists or a supervisor, and

Table 11-4. Contents of a Standard Test Procedure (an example of a PCR-RFLP test)

Item	Content
Background	Theoretical information concerning the disorder and the test
Principle of the assay	Description of how the restriction enzyme detects the specific mutation
Summary of the assay	Characteristics of the restriction-based assay used
Clinical significance	Use of the test for patient care
Strategy for analysis	Overview of the testing steps (i.e., extraction, PCR amplification, digestion, gel electrophoresis)
Specimen collection or acquisition	Description of acceptable specimen type, storage, shipment, and required clinical information
Criteria for rejected samples	Description of unacceptable samples (i.e., specific specimen types, improper labeling, damage)
Equipment and supplies	List of equipment necessary for testing (i.e., PCR machine, gel electrophoresis)
Reagents	List of reagents used for each test step (e.g., PCR, restriction enzyme digestion, gel electrophoresis equipment)
Assay procedure	Description of the testing steps, including general considerations, sample preparation, pre-PCR preparation and setup, thermal cycling, PCR cleanup, PCR product digestion, gel preparation and electrophoresis, gel documentation
Analysis of results	Description of expected results, control results, criteria for gel analysis and interpretation, documentation of results in the LIS and laboratory data base, if used
Turnaround time and schedule for retaining specimen	Expected turnaround time for the specific test, specimen and DNA storage, and schedule for retaining the specimen and DNA
References	Literature or commercial-based information
Addenda	E.g., the worksheet for the specific test, the manufacturers' product insert

Table 11-5. Complete Molecular Pathology Laboratory Procedure Manual: Examples of Required Information, Guidelines, and Protocols

General Information

Staff and contact information
Test information
Requisition forms (genetics, oncology, infectious diseases, identity testing)
Information for clients (shipping, sample type, billing information, consent form, test-specific fax coversheets)
Licenses and permits (CLIA certification and CAP accreditation form)
Reagent handling for molecular testing guidelines
Probe and primer documentation

General Laboratory Operating Procedures

Quality control, quality assurance, and quality improvement programs
Specimen-receiving procedure
Prevention of PCR contamination
Logging-of-primers procedure
Autoclaving of solutions procedure
Use of PCR biosafety chambers
Programming of PCR thermal cyclers
Sequencing using a capillary electrophoresis instrument
Equipment-maintenance procedures
Centrifuges, balance, pH meter, and spectrophotometer: checks and cleanup
Water check procedure
Timer check procedure
Thermometer validation
Temperature-check procedure
Maintenance and validation of PCR thermal cyclers

Nucleic Acid Extraction Procedures

Large-scale DNA extraction from blood by desalting method
Small-scale DNA extraction from blood by column
Fresh- and frozen-tissue DNA extraction
Paraffin-embedded-tissue DNA extraction
Prenatal (amniocytes and CVS) DNA extraction
RNA extraction from blood by column
Nucleic acid quantitation

Test-Specific Procedure Manuals

Genetics

Factor V Leiden analysis
Myotonic dystrophy PCR and Southern analysis
Cystic fibrosis mutation analysis
Spinal muscular atrophy direct testing
Spinal muscular atrophy carrier testing (dosage analysis)
Spinal muscular atrophy linkage analysis

Oncology

IGH gene PCR for detection of B-cell clonality
T-cell receptor PCR for detection of T-cell clonality
BCL2 gene PCR for detection of M-bcr and m-bcr breakpoints
PML-RARA RT-PCR for detection of t(15;17) in APL
BCR-ABL RT-PCR for detection of t(9;22) in CML and ALL
RT-PCR for detection of translocations in sarcomas

Identity Testing

Bone marrow engraftment analysis by genotyping of STR markers
Parentage and identity testing
Maternal cell contamination analysis

Infectious Diseases

HIV-1 viral load assay
HCV viral load assay
HBV viral load assay
Microbial molecular identification analysis

IGH, immunoglobulin heavy chain; *BCL2*, B-cell lymphoma protein 2; M-bcr, major breakpoint cluster region; m-bcr, minor breakpoint cluster region; *PML-RARA*, promyelocytic leukemia-retinoic acid receptor alpha; APL, acute promyelocytic leukemia; CML, chronic myelogenous leukemia; ALL, acute lymphoblastic leukemia; STR, short tandem repeat; HCV, hepatitis C virus; HBV, hepatitis B virus.

then reviewed, edited, and approved by the laboratory director or designee. Any changes to an established procedure manual are documented in writing or electronically and approved by the director. Any laboratory staff members that perform a specific test must review the procedure manual annually, with documentation of the review.

The necessary elements of a test procedure manual are detailed in the CLIA guidelines, which follow closely the items described in CLIS GP2-A3, Clinical Laboratory Technical Procedure Manuals.[19] An example of a complete laboratory procedure manual is presented in Table 11-5. Manufacturer's product inserts or operation manuals can be used as a component of a test procedure manual, but additional information specific to the testing as performed by the laboratory must be provided.

Controls

Every clinical test requires use of appropriate controls. Controls are used to document reproducibility and to ensure that the test is working properly and results are reliable. Several types of controls are used for molecular tests: positive, negative, sensitivity, inhibition, water, and QC controls. Combinations of these controls are used as appropriate based on the method and purpose of the test. A positive control is defined as a sample that contains the target sequence and produces a positive result when tested. Sources of positive controls include positive patient samples and commercially available cell lines or nucleic acids. A negative control is a sample that does not contain the target sequence and produces a negative result when tested. Sensitivity controls are needed for assays that require a specified level of analytical sensitivity. This control is particularly important for MRD tests for cancer and viral load tests to define the lower limit of detection of the specific test. In general, a sensitivity control is included in each run of the test, since the sensitivity of each test run should be documented and not be assumed to be the same as during validation of the test. A no-template control or water control is a control reaction containing all reagents but no template nucleic acid. This control tests for contamination of the PCR reagents and should not produce any PCR products except for primer dimers. An inhibition control (addition of external target nucleic acid or amplification of another template sequence to check for PCR amplification) is used only when the lack of production of a PCR product is interpreted as a negative result for the test. A QC control is a patient sample that was previously tested and is included for repeat testing on a new run. These samples function to assess the accuracy of the reported results as well as to monitor for interassay variability.

The controls should be processed in the same manner as the patient samples during testing; however, their use and storage should be well defined in the test procedure manual to avoid degradation. Controls should be validated for acceptability and approved by the laboratory director or designee before use in clinical testing. Failure of controls to perform as expected should be investigated, with findings and corrective action documented. Some QC results, for example, in HIV viral load testing, should be charted and analyzed on standard Levi-Jennings plots. Deviations and adverse trends indicate that something is changing in the analytic system, and require investigation and corrective action.

Preventive Equipment Maintenance

All instruments used in the molecular pathology laboratory require written standard procedures for normal operation, performance evaluation, and preventive maintenance. Function checks should be performed on a regular schedule to check critical characteristics and detect malfunctions before test results are affected. In the absence of manufacturer's guidelines, the laboratory should establish a maintenance procedure that appropriately reflects the use of the instrument. Of particular importance are the thermal cyclers, because any change in their performance will have a direct impact on many tests. Thermal cyclers should be routinely monitored for cycle time reproducibility, verification of temperature accuracy, and efficiency of heating and cooling rates. These diagnostic checks are usually incorporated into the instrument's software and are a part of the manufacturer's recommendations for instrument maintenance. Temperature logs for each temperature-dependent piece of equipment, including an acceptable temperature range, are required by CLIA. Temperatures of refrigerators, freezers, and incubators must be documented daily if used for reagent storage. Other

instruments, such as water baths, should be documented each day of use. An equipment maintenance and performance evaluation log should be maintained for every laboratory instrument and should be kept for the duration of the clinical use of the instrument.

Quality Assessment Program

CLIA requires each laboratory to have an active QA program to assess various aspects of the technical and nontechnical performance of the molecular pathology laboratory. CLIA requires establishment of guidelines and procedures designated not only "to evaluate the ongoing and overall quality of the testing process," but also to evaluate "the effectiveness of its policies and procedures," followed by requirements to "identify and correct problems, assure reliable and prompt reporting of test reports and assure the adequacy and competence of the staff."[17] In the CLIA '03 version, "quality assurance" was renamed "quality assessment," recognizing that quality cannot always be assured but it can be evaluated or assessed.[18] The laboratory QA program must monitor and evaluate both the ongoing and the overall quality of the total testing process through error detection, corrective actions and their review, and the integration of improvements in procedures. To meet the CLIA requirements, the molecular pathology laboratory must have a QA program that includes numerous laboratory practices, including personnel training and performance evaluation, proficiency testing, inspections, correlation of molecular results with clinical data, and a QC program. Elements monitored by the QA program, such as turnaround time, rejected specimens, and various indicators of test quality, do not relate directly to the analytic validity of the testing process and thus are not a part of the QC program. A complete list of these indicators can be found in the LAP-CAP Molecular Pathology checklist. Table 11-6 lists some of the more important components for which the LAP-CAP requires ongoing surveillance and documentation.

Although CLIA requires that clinical laboratories continually evaluate and improve their work in all areas, some requirements are particularly important from an institutional perspective. CLIA mandates that test results obtained from different methodologies performed under the same certificate be compared, documented, and reviewed for the detection of errors that can affect patient care. This means that molecular oncology test results, for example, should be compared with the results obtained by other laboratories, such as the flow cytometry and cytogenetics laboratories, for the same patient.

Training

Personnel performing high-complexity molecular pathology testing must meet established qualifications in

Table 11-6. Examples of QC and QA Topics That Require Documentation and Corrective Action

Proficiency Testing

Ongoing evaluation of proficiency test results

QC and QA of Testing

Detection and correction of clerical and analytic errors
Recording of failed nucleic acid isolations
Recording of failed hybridization reactions
Monitoring of test turnaround time
Discrepancies between preliminary and final reported results
Discrepancies between the molecular pathology laboratory and other laboratory findings
Performance of statistics and appropriate comparative studies on all molecular pathology tests
Logging of unusual, difficult, and instructive cases

Laboratory-Developed Assay Validation

Performing validation to confirm analytic test performance characteristics
Documenting validation studies for establishing assay performance characteristics
Documenting analytic characteristics including accuracy, sensitivity, specificity, and precision
Demonstrating and documenting clinical validity

Procedure Manual

Annual review of all policies and procedures by the laboratory director or designee
Review of all new policies, procedures, and changes to existing procedures
Knowledge of testing procedures for the tests performed by each technologist in the laboratory
Information for all DNA probes, PCR primers, and other nucleic acid reagents used for testing

Paternity and Forensic Identity

Chain-of-custody (proof of identity)
Genetic characteristics (heterogeneity, recombination rates, etc.) of the DNA markers used
Release of information

Specimen Handling

Disposition of unacceptable specimens
Sample condition, inadequate volumes, and evidence of tampering

Reagents

Validation of reagents used for tests
Characteristics of the specific reagents used in each assay

Controls

Failed control results or when results exceed defined tolerance limits

Instruments

Ongoing evaluation of results of instrument maintenance and function (temperatures, instrument characteristics, cleanliness)
Function checks for detection of problems and malfunctions
Repairs and services
Temperature checks for temperature-dependent equipment

Personnel

Continuing medical laboratory education

Safety

Radioactive area surveys and wipe tests
Radioactive waste disposal

training, experience, job performance, and competency. Training includes competency in performance of the test methodology, calculations, independent judgment, quality control of the method, and knowledge of the instruments. These training requirements cannot be based simply on academic requirements or experience. The on-site training must be sufficient to ensure that staff members have the skills necessary for performing every step of the analytic process, including assay method, preventive maintenance, and quality control measures.

To this end, a training program ensuring that technologists are properly trained to perform laboratory operations must be used. As the first step, technologists can be trained by observing a technologist who knows how to perform the procedure and by reading the procedure manual. Then the technologist should test two to three blind sets of specimens in addition to known controls, with or without observation depending upon the level of experience of the technologist, to ensure that the technologist understands the test and performs it correctly. Monitoring of the training testing ensures the accuracy of the technologist's performance. Finally, the results of training runs must be documented and approved by the laboratory director or designee.

A part of ongoing training is annual competency evaluation. This allows the laboratory director or designee to review different aspects of the technologist's performance, including technical skills, control of PCR contamination, equipment operation, procedure knowledge, and laboratory safety. The overall performance of each technologist is documented, and corrective or additional training measures are implemented as necessary.

Training also includes continuing education programs, which assist the technologist in attaining some of the technical skills and knowledge required to keep up with changes in procedures, instruments, and new tests, as well as improve their ability to perform new assays, troubleshoot, and handle new problems.

Proficiency Testing

Proficiency testing plays a key role in assessing the internal quality of work in CLIA-regulated high-complexity testing laboratories. CLIA requires the laboratory to successfully participate in a CMS-approved proficiency testing program for all analytes tested. CAP provides approved proficiency testing programs in several relevant fields, including genetics, infectious diseases, oncology and identity testing (Table 11-7). Proficiency testing samples are sent at least once per year. In the absence of an external proficiency testing program for a specific test, the laboratory can set up a sample exchange proficiency testing program with another laboratory performing the same test. Proficiency samples must be tested in the same manner as patient samples, by the same technologists performing the clinical testing, using the same interpretation procedures. Laboratories

Table 11-7. CAP Proficiency Surveys for Molecular Pathology Testing

Category/Name	Survey	Type of Testing
Genetics		
MGL	Molecular genetics	Molecular testing for various genetic diseases or genes
Oncology		
MO	Molecular oncology	Molecular analysis of leukemia and lymphomas
MSI	Microsatellite instability	Molecular analysis of PET colorectal carcinoma by DNA amplification of microsatellites
SARC	Sarcoma translocation	Molecular analysis of various sarcoma translocations by RT-PCR
CYH	Fluorescence in situ hybridization	Analysis of FISH for *HER2/NEU* amplification using chromosome-specific DNA probes
Identity		
ME	Monitoring engraftment	Monitoring for bone marrow and stem cell engraftment
PAR, PARF	Parentage testing	DNA testing by PCR and RFLP
ML, DL, DML	HLA molecular typing	Molecular typing of class I and class II HLA markers
FID, FIDM	Forensic sciences—nuclear and mitochondrial DNA	Nuclear and mitochondrial DNA analysis for numerous polymorphic loci
DNA, DNAF	Forensic sciences—DNA database	Analysis of polymorphic loci for the DNA database program
Infectious Disease		
ID	Nucleic acid amplification identification	Analysis of infectious pathogens analyzed by advanced amplification methods (NASBA, bDNA, LCR, PCR)
HIV, HV2	HIV viral load	Quantitative analysis of HIV by nucleic acid amplification and genotyping, respectively
HCVN, HCV2	Hepatitis C viral load	Quantitative analysis of HCV by nucleic acid amplification and genotyping, respectively
HPV	Human papillomavirus	Qualitative analysis of HPV by nucleic acid testing
HC	*C. trachomatis*, herpes, and *N. gonorrhoeae*	Pathogen analysis by nucleic acid amplification and nucleic acid probe methods
NAT	Nucleic acid testing	Qualitative analysis of infectious pathogens designated for blood donor centers
ISH	In situ hybridization	In situ hybridization testing for various viral nucleic acid targets

PET, paraffin-embedded tissue; RT-PCR, reverse transcription–polymerase chain reaction; FISH, fluorescence in situ hybridization; RFLP, restriction fragment length polymorphism; HLA, human leukocyte antigen; NASBA, nucleic acid sequence–based amplification; bDNA, branched DNA technology; LCR, ligase chain reaction; PCR, polymerase chain reaction; HCV, hepatitis C virus; HPV, human papillomavirus.

failing two of three consecutive testing events for any test must submit a plan to the CAP or other proficiency testing agency for and implementation of corrective action.

Laboratory Inspection

Molecular pathology laboratories must be inspected by an external inspection team every 2 years for compliance with CLIA regulations. LAP-CAP inspections are performed by a team of inspectors from an institution other than that of the laboratories being inspected, and the inspection team assesses the quality indicators for continued quality performance as listed in the LAP-CAP checklist.[31] The checklist addresses laboratory procedures including specimen processing and testing, reagents, controls, instrumentation, personnel, physical facilities, and laboratory safety. Inspection also assesses for PCR contamination control, participation in proficiency testing programs, and documentation of the QC and QA program activities (Table 11-6). Failure to comply is documented as a "Phase I" or "Phase II" deficiency. Most items on the molecular pathology check-

list are Phase II, with a serious potential to affect patient care. Phase II deficiencies require immediate attention and correction, documented in writing to the CAP. Phase I deficiencies are less serious but also require documentation of corrective action. On alternate years, the laboratory is required to perform a self-inspection.

Recently, as a part of ongoing efforts to strengthen the laboratory accreditation process, to promote public confidence in the LAP-CAP, and to help assure regulators that CAP-accredited laboratories meet or exceed CLIA requirements, the CAP has made significant changes in its LAP, including unannounced routine inspections beginning in January 2006. This means that laboratories will not know the exact date of the inspection and the identity of the inspection team members prior to the inspection. Instead, the laboratories will be provided with a 90-day window of the anniversary of their last inspection, 45 days prior to and 45 days after, pending CMS approval, in which the inspection will occur. By implementing this process for routine inspections, CAP expects to help ensure that laboratories are in continuous compliance and that they are providing quality patient testing at all times.

Alternatively, laboratories can be inspected directly by CLIA or by JCAHO as an accrediting organization for clinical laboratories under the CLIA program. The CLIA inspection regulations are found in Subpart Q of the *Code of Federal Regulations*, which addresses both basic and specific inspection requirements.[32] CLIA inspections under JCAHO are conducted by CMS. The CMS policy for laboratory inspections includes announced initial and biennial recertification inspections and unannounced complaint and follow-up inspections. The CMS inspection focuses more on outcomes than on laboratory process. The goals of this outcome-oriented survey are not only to determine the laboratory's regulatory compliance but also to assist laboratories in improving patient care by emphasizing those aspects that have a direct impact on the laboratory's overall test performance.

Accreditation by JCAHO meets the conditions required by federal law and regulations. Consequently, laboratories that are accredited by JCAHO in lieu of direct federal oversight and that meet the CLIA requirements for laboratories are not subject to routine inspection by state survey agencies to determine their compliance with federal requirements.[33] To be eligible, JCAHO must apply standards and criteria that are equal to or more stringent than the requirements established by DHHS. The JCAHO accreditation process is more stringent than federal certification requirements in that JCAHO accredits a healthcare organization (for example, a hospital) as a whole, not just the laboratory. As such, an organization that loses JCAHO accreditation for reasons other than poor laboratory performance also would lose the ability to legally test human specimens under the laboratory's existing certificate of accreditation, if JCAHO accreditation is being used to meet the CLIA requirements. The JCAHO also began conducting unannounced inspections in 2006.

Summary

In this chapter, we have summarized many of the issues and considerations that are important for the successful management of a molecular pathology laboratory. Although these issues are addressed separately, many are interconnected. If even one function is weak, the success of testing is compromised. Molecular pathology is a rapidly growing field of anatomic pathology and laboratory medicine. The most significant challenges facing the management team of a molecular pathology laboratory are continuous acquaintance with newly developed technologies, new approaches for data analysis (bioinformatics), changing regulations, and evolving testing considerations for a variety of clinical applications, as well as understanding basic business concepts in marketing and finance. Keeping pace with these challenges ensures that the molecular pathology laboratory will be an even greater driving force of medical practice in the 21st century and beyond.

References

1. Klein M. Marketing research products to molecular pathologists. *BioTactics in Action.* 1998;1:1–5; Online Newsletter at www.biotactis.com/newsletter/v1i5/molbio.htm.
2. Grody WW, Matteson KJ, Murphy PD, et al. Molecular diagnostic methods for genetic diseases; approved guidelines. CLSI, MM1-A2. Vol 26. No. 27. Wayne PA, 2000.
3. Casey DK. Genes, dreams and reality. The promise and risks of the new genetics. *Judicature.* 1999;83:105–111.
4. Genetic Information Nondiscrimination Act of 2005 (S 306). Available at: http://www.govtrack.us/congress/bill.xpd?bill=s109-306.
5. Grody WW, Noll WW. Molecular diagnosis of genetic diseases. In: Henry JB, ed. *Clinical Diagnosis and Management by Laboratory Methods.* Philadelphia: WB Saunders; 2001:1372–1381.
6. Giardiello FM, Bresinger JD, et al. The use and interpretation of commercial APC gene testing for familial adenomatous polyposis. *N Engl J Med.* 1997;336:823–827.
7. National Human Genome Research Institute. *Promoting Safe and Effective Genetic Testing: Final Report of the Task Force on Genetic Testing.* Bethesda, MD: National Human Genome Research Institute; 1997.
8. US Department of Health and Human Services, Centers for Disease Control and Prevention. Notice of intent: genetic testing under the Clinical Laboratory Improvement Amendments. *Fed Regist.* 2000;65:25928–25934.
9. *Health Insurance Portability and Accountability Act of 1996.* Public Law 104–191. 104th Congress (August 21, 1996). Available at: http://aspe.hhs.gov/admnsimp/pl104191.htm.
10. Gulley ML. Leukemias and lymphomas. In: Leonard DGB, ed. *Diagnostic Molecular Pathology.* Philadelphia: WB Saunders; 2003:113–127.
11. Barr FG, Ladanyi M. Sarcomas. In: Leonard DGB, ed. *Diagnostic Molecular Pathology.* Philadelphia: WB Saunders; 2003:53–76.
12. Fallon KB, Palmer CA, Roth KA, et al. Prognostic value of 1p, 19q, 9p, 10q, and EGFR-FISH analyses in recurrent oligodendrogliomas. *J Neuropathol Exp Neurol.* 2004;63:314–322.
13. Unger ER, Guarner J. Infectious diseases. In: Leonard DGB, ed. *Diagnostic Molecular Pathology.* Philadelphia: WB Saunders; 2003:129–141.
14. Van Deerlin V. Identity testing: applications of DNA typing in anatomic pathology. In: Leonard DGB, ed. *Diagnostic Molecular Pathology.* Philadelphia: WB Saunders; 2003:163–188.
15. *Clinical Laboratory Improvement Amendments (CLIA) of 1988.* Public Law 100–578. 100th Congress (October 31, 1988). Available at: http://www.cms.hhs.gov/clia.
16. Ehrmeyer SS, Laessig HR. Compliance issues—the regulations. In: Harmening DM, ed. *Laboratory Management Principles and Processes.* Upper Saddle River, NJ: Prentice-Hall; 2003:225–243.
17. US Department of Health and Human Services. Medicare and CLIA programs. Regulations implementing the Clinical Laboratory Improvement of 1988 (CLIA). *Fed Regist.* 1992;57:7002–7186.
18. US Department of Health and Human Services. Medicare and CLIA Programs. Regulations implementing the Clinical Laboratory Improvement of 1988 (CLIA). *Fed Regist.* 2003;68:3639–3714.
19. Hoeltge GA, Dynek DA, Delaharty DC, et al. Clinical laboratory technical procedure manuals approved guidelines. Wayne, PA: National Committee for Clinical Laboratory Standards; 1996. Document GP-2A3-P.
20. Kaul KL, Leonard DG, Gonzales A, Garrett CT. Oversitght of genetic testing: an update. *J Mol Diag.* 2001;3:85–91.
21. Food and Drug Administration. Medical devices: classification/reclassification: restricted devices: analyte specific reagents. *Fed Regist.* 1997;62:62243–62260.

22. Takes PA, Murray G. The analyte specific reagent rule: a new set of regulations for labs, manufacturers. *Clin Lab News*. 1998;24:10.

23. Ferreira-Gonzales A. Establishing a molecular diagnostics laboratory. In: Henry JB, ed. Clinical Diagnosis and Management by Laboratory Methods. Philadelphia: WB Saunders. 2001:1333–1339.

24. Dadoun R. Impact on human resources: Core laboratory versus laboratory information system versus modular robotics. *Clin Lab Manage Rev*. 1998;12:248–255.

25. Udaykumar E, Epstein JS, Hewlett IK. A novel method employing UNG to avoid carry-over contamination in RNA-PCR. *Nucleic Acids Res*. 1993;21:3917–3918.

26. Dumler S, Fink LM, Frank TS, et al. Goals and objectives for molecular pathology education in residency programs. *J Mol Diag*. 1999;1:5–15.

27. Killeen AA, Leung WC, Payne D, et al. Certification in molecular pathology in the United States (Training and Education Committee, The Association for Molecular Pathology). *J Mol Diagn*. 2002;4:181–184.

28. Griffey PA. Fundamentals of financial management. In: Harmening DM, ed. *Laboratory Management: Principles and Processes*. Upper Saddle River, NJ: Prentice-Hall; 2003:163–179.

29. American Medical Association. 2006 CPT. Current Pnocedural Terminology (Professional Edition). Pathology and Laboratory Medicine Guidelines. Chicago: Americian Medical Association; 2005.

30. Grody WW, Cutting GR, Klinger KW, Richards CS, Watson MS, Desnick RJ. Laboratory standards and guidelines for population-based cystic fibrosis screening. *Genet Med*. 2001;3:149–154.

31. Laboratory Accreditation Program—College of American Pathologists. Molecular Pathology checklist. Northfield, IL: College of American Pathologists; 2005.

32. Department of Health and Human Services, Centers for Disease Control and Prevention. Subpart Q—Inspection. *Fed Regist*. 1998;63:986–987.

33. Department of Health and Human Services. CLIA Program: approval of the Joint Commission on Accreditation of Healthcare Organizations as an accrediting organization. *Fed Regist*. 1995;60:130–132.

Chapter 12

From Research to Clinical Practice

Karen Snow-Bailey

Molecular pathology cannot be discussed without including the translational nature of the clinical practice. While the number of Food and Drug Administration (FDA)-cleared or FDA-approved molecular pathology in vitro diagnostic test kits and analyte-specific reagents is increasing, the development of commercial test kits and reagents does not keep pace with the clinically useful genomic information generated by basic, translational, and clinical research. In the genomic in vitro diagnostic testing arena, the molecular pathology laboratory stands at the interface between science and medicine. With existing molecular biology methods, the vast majority of genomic discoveries linking genomic sequences or variations to disease states or risk can be translated into clinical tests in the molecular pathology laboratory. The laboratory director and personnel must understand the regulations and standards that govern this translational process to ensure that the high quality of clinical practice is assured.

Regulations for Clinical Laboratories

Laboratory Accreditation

State and federal regulations stipulate that only laboratories certified under the Clinical Laboratory Improvement Amendments (CLIA) may perform testing when test results are released to a patient or healthcare provider and results are used for medical management.[1] Many US laboratories participate in the Laboratory Accreditation Program offered by the College of American Pathologists, which has CLIA deemed status. New York State also has CLIA deemed status due to the high stringency of the state standards. The New York Clinical Laboratory Evaluation Program monitors the quality of New York State laboratories and laboratories in other states that perform testing on samples from New York.

Accreditation agencies in other countries include Clinical Pathology Accreditation Ltd (CPA; United Kingdom), the National Association of Testing Authorities (NATA; Australia), International Accreditation New

Zealand (IANZ), the Dutch Accreditation Council (RvA; the Netherlands), and the European Molecular Genetics Quality Network (EMQN). Standards and checklists used for accreditation vary internationally but include CLIA, CAP checklists, and International Standards Organization (ISO) standards. Unfortunately, the lack of global standardization creates somewhat of a barrier to using offshore laboratories for clinical testing, because equivalency of accreditation status has not been determined. This is of particular relevance in testing for very rare disorders, for which only one or two clinical laboratories worldwide may be performing the testing.

Proficiency Testing

A requirement for laboratory accreditation is participation in an external proficiency testing program or external quality assurance (EQA) program, where one exists. The CAP offers surveys for numerous analytes (covering inherited disorders, infectious diseases, and somatic mutations). Programs also are provided by the EMQN, the United Kingdom External Quality Assurance System, the Human Genetics Society of Australasia (HGSA), and the Royal College of Pathologists of Australasia (RCPA). At an international level, the Organisation for Economic Cooperation and Development (OECD) has surveyed laboratories in member countries regarding quality assurance (QA) and proficiency testing practices.[2] If external proficiency testing is not available for a particular analyte or test, then interlaboratory sample exchange, retesting of previously analyzed samples, or both, are options to demonstrate proficiency. Recommendations have been made for expansion of proficiency testing programs and development of a wider range of QA materials.[3]

Personnel Certification

CLIA regulations outline minimum requirements for laboratory directors. Some states require certification of technologists working in clinical laboratories. Certification processes and options have been reviewed.[4]

Regulation of Assays and Reagents

The FDA regulates commercial kits for clinical testing. Additionally, reagents making up assays developed by individual laboratories are regulated by the FDA as analytespecific reagents (ASRs). This means that the reagents are manufactured under current good manufacturing practices (CGMP) and are subject to restrictions on distribution, use, and labeling.[5] Laboratories using FDA-approved kits, ASRs or laboratory-developed methods are required to validate the tests under CLIA regulations prior to clinical implementation.

Participation in Research Studies

Regulatory Standards

Title 45, Part 46 (Protection of Human Subjects) of the *US Code of Federal Regulations* describes the policy of the US Department of Health and Human Services for the protection of human research subjects. The document covers functions of the Internal Review Board (IRB) and general requirements for informed consent. The relationship between study participants and researchers is addressed, including complex issues related to participants' access to test results from their own specimen(s).[6] Genetic counselors can play a significant role in facilitating access to research studies and ensuring appropriate informed consent.[7] Recommendations for consent form design and content are available.[8,9] Clinical laboratories that participate in research studies should comply with the research regulations, including assuring IRB review and approval of the research protocols, informed consent, and proper protection of the research information.

Academic Interest

Development of a clinical test may stem from a primary research interest within the laboratory or may develop through collaborations with basic science investigators, clinical investigators, or clinicians with a focused medical practice requiring molecular testing. Data gathered during research can suggest that a test will have clinical application. Ongoing investigation using clinical samples under an IRB-approved protocol may then be used to determine the clinical sensitivity, clinical specificity, and clinical utility of the test.[10] Even after a test becomes offered as a clinical service, ongoing academic interest can be very valuable in making further test improvements or furthering the molecular understanding of the disease (e.g., adding methodologies to increase the clinical sensitivity, elucidating genotype-phenotype correlations to enhance result inter-

pretation, or identifying additional genetic loci or variants associated with the disorder).

Definition of a Clinical Test

For the consumer, a clinical test is a test used for patient management that is performed within the scope of practice of an accredited laboratory. For the laboratory, requirements are analytical and clinical validation of the test, with internal, peer, or regulatory review, or some combination of these, of the validation data, as required by regulation standards applicable to the specific laboratory, usually based on location. All aspects of the clinical test must be determined, including test conditions, controls, procedure manual, personnel training, and all other aspects of clinical testing, as described in chapter 11. Mechanisms and materials for pre- and postanalytical steps also must be implemented, including test information, instructions for specimen collection, result reporting, and billing.

Considerations in Introducing New Clinical Tests

Oversight of Molecular Tests

In 1995, the Task Force on Genetic Testing was convened by the National Institutes of Health–Department of Energy Working Group on Ethical, Legal, and Social Implications of Human Genome Research. The task force was charged to review genetic testing in the United States and to make recommendations where necessary to promote safe and effective testing practices.[11] As a result of the task force recommendations, the Secretary's Advisory Committee on Genetic Testing (SACGT) was formed to address issues associated with new genetic test development, including analytical and clinical validity, clinical utility, laboratory quality, and healthcare provider education. Functions of the SACGT have subsequently been assumed by the Secretary's Advisory Committee on Genetics, Health, and Society (SACGHS), whose charter is to explore, discuss, and make recommendations regarding various issues (e.g., medical, ethical, legal, and social issues) associated with the development and application of genetic technologies. The Office of Genomics and Disease Prevention (OGDP) at the Centers for Disease Control and Prevention (CDC) also plays an active role in genetic test development and monitoring as related to public health. Similar processes have been carried out, or are occurring, in other countries,[12] for example, by the Human Genetics Commission in the United Kingdom, the Institute for Prospective Technological Studies (IPTS) and the European Society of Human Genetics in Europe,[13] and through the Australian Health Ministers' Advisory Council (AHMAC).

Economic Considerations

The cost-effectiveness of genetic testing requires consideration of the prevalence of the disease (and associated genetic defects), burden of suffering, availability and efficacy of treatment, and cost and accuracy of genetic testing. As illustrative examples, a recent article evaluates cost-effectiveness of genetic tests for hereditary nonpolyposis colorectal cancer, familial breast cancer, and periodontal disease; CYP2C9 pharmacogenetic testing for warfarin therapy; and thiopurine S-methyltransferase for 6-mercaptopurine therapy.[14]

Medicare payments for clinical tests are determined by the Current Procedural Terminology (CPT) codes that apply to the specific test. Each CPT code has a monetary value. For many tests, the value of CPT codes is insufficient to cover the cost of performing the test.[15,16] SACGHS has developed recommendations to address the inadequacy of reimbursement for genetic testing.

Predicted Test Volume

Test volume will affect how frequently a test is performed and the batch size of each test run. Test costs should be calculated, incorporating fixed and variable costs accounting for the batch size of each test run, with adjustment for control costs. Tests run in small batches will be more costly than tests with high batch sizes, predominantly because the labor costs are distributed over fewer tests with smaller batch sizes. The test volume should be high enough for the laboratory to maintain competency in performing the test and interpreting the results.

Resource Requirements

Staffing resources are required for test development, implementation, and ongoing provision of new clinical tests. The adequacy of staffing and equipment for the additional testing must be assessed and business plans developed and implemented to obtain any additional resources required for the new testing. New reagents will be required, including control materials (e.g., from repositories such as Coriell Cell Repositories, American Type Culture Collection (ATCC), European Collection of Cell Cultures, and the National Institute of Standards and Technology). Recent research initiatives have been successful in developing additional QA materials for genetic testing.[17,18] Novel testing platforms and technologies are being introduced into the molecular marketplace at an astonishing rate. Unfortunately, there is no one-size-fits-all technology in molecular pathology practice. The nature of the genetic defect, predicted test numbers, and instrument, reagent, and royalty costs should be considered in determining the most appropriate method and instrument for each test.[19,20]

Intellectual Property

Genes, mutations, methods, and technologies may be associated with intellectual property rights and patents. Many academic organizations now have intellectual property offices that work with researchers to identify "inventions" that can be patented. An overview of the patent process, a "patent primer," has been developed by the American College of Medical Genetics (ACMG).[21,22] The Genetics and Molecular Medicine section of the American Medical Association Web site contains additional overview material and useful links.[22] Clinical laboratories wishing to implement a new test should be aware that patents may limit the utilization of specific inventions pertinent to that test. Indeed, the patents and licensing practices for genetic sequences associated with disease processes have a significant impact on molecular pathology laboratories and have recently caused concern, particularly when licenses are not broadly available for clinical practice.[23] In response to this concern, the ACMG has prepared an educational document for consideration in preparing licenses with guidelines that are compatible with wide access to affordable genetic testing.[24]

The Test Development Process

ACMG Standards and Guidelines for Clinical Genetics Laboratories describe three levels in the development of a diagnostic test: research and development, investigational studies, and accepted clinical test.[20] In the United States, CLIA regulations require clinical tests to have been validated by the testing laboratory. As outlined in the ACMG standards and guidelines, test validation requires attention to pretest components (e.g., sample and information collection), assay methodology, analytical validity, clinical validity, clinical utility, and ethical, legal, and social issues. Many of these aspects and additional items such as cost analysis and billing have been discussed.[25]

Analytical Validity

The development of assay protocols should utilize appropriately maintained and calibrated equipment, testing standards, quality controls, and defined interpretation criteria. For numerical results, reference ranges need to be determined and sources of assay variability need to be defined and quantified. Analytical validity requires assessment of the analytical sensitivity and analytical specificity. Although publications have addressed analytical validity of specific tests among cohorts of clinical laboratories, each testing laboratory must determine the analytical sensitivity and specificity of its own test. The test procedure must be documented, for example, by following guidelines established by the Clinical and Laboratory Standards Institute (CLSI; formerly NCCLS).[26] Other CLSI documents, available on the CLSI Web site (http://www.clsi.org/source/

custom/sortby.cfm?category-category) under the section heading "Molecular Methods", provide guidelines for the application of molecular methods for genetic diseases, infectious diseases, hematopathology, and fluorescence in situ hybridization (FISH).

Clinical Validity

Clinical validity is an assessment of the frequency with which the test identifies individuals who have the disorder or clinical phenotype identified by the test. Components of clinical validity are clinical sensitivity and clinical specificity. Data may be derived from the laboratory's own studies or by assessment of published data, or both.

Clinical Utility

Clinical utility incorporates the impact and usefulness of the test weighed against the cost of testing and any adverse health or psychosocial consequences. Factors to consider include available interventions following positive or negative test results, economic or psychosocial benefits or harms of testing, and implications of results for other family members.

Informational Materials and Reports

In addition to development of a written test procedure, the laboratory is required to provide information for the healthcare provider on specimen requirements and transportation, test requisition requirements including informed consent, test turnaround time, and other information relevant to the ordering and use of testing.

The report format and content need to be established. Reports should be interpretable by nongeneticist healthcare providers. Studies undertaken during recent years highlight some of the difficulties encountered by primary care physicians and other nongeneticists in correctly interpreting genetic risk information and in appreciating the limitations of genetic testing.[27,28] These studies are instructive for laboratory directors in pointing out the need to avoid jargon as much as possible and to consider the importance of the report format. Standards and guidelines, best practice guidelines, and checklists for reporting are available.[20,29,30] Disease-specific guidelines also are helpful in report formatting and content. For example, both the EMQN guidelines for Prader Willi-Angelman syndromes and for Friedreich ataxia[31] and the ACMG guidelines for cystic fibrosis and for fragile X syndrome[20] discuss key elements to include in the reports and provide suggestions for interpretive comments.

Mutation databases are invaluable resources in the interpretation of sequence alterations detected in many genes and disorders. However, such databases are not peer-reviewed or quality-controlled resources. Therefore, peer-reviewed publications for a particular mutation are essential for providing the most appropriate report interpretation. A challenging issue is interpretation of missense alterations when no previous data exist to substantiate the change as either a pathogenic mutation or a benign polymorphism. Methods to characterize variants, using BRCA1 mutation interpretation as a model, have been described.[32]

Considerations for molecular pathology reports for tests other than inherited disorders are available.[33] Discussions include consideration of creating "unified" reports, for example, incorporating molecular, flow cytometry, and surgical pathology into a single hematopathology report.

Special Considerations for Rare Disorders

Conferences held in 2004 and 2005 evaluated the status of testing for rare disorders and considered issues related to quality, availability, access, and resources for rare disease testing.[34] Several recommendations for promoting quality testing were made, and issues requiring further discussion were identified. Subsequently, the ACMG published Technical Standards and Guidelines for Molecular Genetic Testing for Ultra-Rare Disorders.[35] These guidelines acknowledge unique challenges associated with rare disorder testing that affect test validation (analytical and clinical), quality assurance, and result interpretation.

A number of clinical laboratories offer testing to confirm mutations identified in research laboratories. These services range from provision of testing for a limited number of disorders to custom mutation analysis for perhaps any rare disorder for which a research laboratory has identified a pathogenic mutation. Laboratories that offer this clinical confirmation can be located in the GeneTests directory available at www.genetests.org/servlet/ under the heading "Custom Molecular Genetic Testing."

Resources for Locating Testing Laboratories

Association for Molecular Pathology Test Directory

The Association for Molecular Pathology (AMP; see the AMP Test Directory, available at: http://www. amptestdirectory.org) maintains a directory of laboratories that provide molecular testing for infectious diseases, solid tumors, and hematopathology. The directory is searchable by various fields, including name of the disorder, molecular abnormality, disease agent, and laboratory location.

GeneTests

The GeneTests laboratory directory (http://www.genetests. org) includes international laboratories that perform testing for inherited disorders. Listed tests include molecular, biochemical, and FISH tests. Searchable fields include disease name, gene, clinical feature, OMIM number, and laboratory location. The GeneTests resource also includes GeneReviews, a clinic directory, and educational materials.

The European Directory of DNA Diagnostic Laboratories

The European Directory of DNA Diagnostic Laboratories (EDDNAL; http://www.eddnal.com) provides information on molecular testing services for heritable syndromes and disorders offered by laboratories throughout the European Union countries and Norway, Poland, and Switzerland. Searchable fields include disease name, OMIM number, and laboratory name or location.

Orphanet

The Orphanet Web site (http://www.orpha.net/) provides information on clinical- and research-based testing for rare diseases, as well as information on support groups and clinical trials. Search terms include disease name, OMIM number, clinical signs, and laboratory name or location.

GENDIA

GENDIA (for genetic diagnostics; http://www.gendia.net/) is an international network of more than 50 laboratories located in the United States, Europe, and Australia. Samples submitted for testing are sent to a single laboratory for distribution to the testing laboratories. Available tests can be located by disease or gene.

Summary

Our knowledge of the molecular pathology of inherited and infectious diseases and of numerous cancers has vastly increased over the past several years. Additionally, the practice of molecular pathology has been transformed by the availability of new technologies, testing platforms, and automation. Alongside the growth in knowledge and available technologies has been the introduction of numerous standards, guidelines, and regulations that are designed to ensure the provision of safe and accurate molecular tests in the clinical setting. These documents provide guidance to laboratories that are introducing new clinical tests. Ongoing challenges such as the limited availability of QA materials and proficiency testing programs are being actively addressed, as are the economic, ethical, legal, and social issues associated with molecular testing. The continued growth of molecular pathology practice holds great promise for the future practice of medicine.

References

1. Schwartz MK. Genetic testing and the clinical laboratory improvement amendments of 1988: present and future. *Clin Chem*. 1999;45: 739–745.
2. Organisation for Economic Co-operation and Development. Quality assurance and proficiency testing for molecular genetic testing. Summary results of a survey of 18 OECD countries. Available at: http://www.oecd.org/dataoecd/25/12/34779945.pdf.
3. Williams LO, Cole EC, Lubin IM, Iglesias NI, Jordan RL, Elliott LE. Quality assurance in human molecular genetics testing: status and recommendations. *Arch Pathol Lab Med*. 2003;127:1353–1358.
4. Killeen AA, Leung WC, Payne D, et al. Certification in molecular pathology in the United States (Training and Education Committee, The Association for Molecular Pathology). *J Mol Diagn*. 2002;4:181–184.
5. Gutman S. The role of Food and Drug Administration regulation of in vitro diagnostic devices—applications to genetics testing. *Clin Chem*. 1999;45:746–749.
6. American Society of Human Genetics Ad Hoc Committee on Consumer Issues. Genetic lay advocacy groups: significant others in the conduct of human genetics research. October 1999 (revised November 10, 2000 and October 18, 2001). Available at: http://genetics. faseb.org/genetics/ashg/pubs/policy/pol-46.pdf.
7. Markel DS, Yashar BM. The interface between the practice of medical genetics and human genetic research: what every genetic counselor needs to know. *J Genet Couns*. 2004;13:351–368.
8. The American Society of Human Genetics Statement on Informed Consent for Genetic Research. *Am J Hum Genet*. 1996;59:471–474.
9. Hull SC, Gooding H, Klein AP, Warshauer-Baker E, Metosky S, Wilfond BS. Genetic research involving human biological materials: a need to tailor current consent forms. *IRB*. 2004;26:1–7.
10. American College of Medical Genetics Standards and Guidelines for Clinical Genetics Laboratories. 2005 ed. Available at: http://www. acmg.net/Pages/ACMG_Activities/stds-2002/stdsmenu-n.htm.
11. Holtzman NA. Promoting safe and effective genetic tests in the United States: work of the task force on genetic testing. *Clin Chem*. 1999;45:732–738.
12. Cox SM, Faucett WA, Chen B, et al. International genetic testing. *Genet Med*. 2003;5:176–182.
13. Godard B, Kaariainen H, Kristoffersson U, Tranebjaerg L, Coviello D, Ayme S. Provision of genetic services in Europe: current practices and issues. *Eur J Hum Genet*. 2003;11(suppl 2):S13–S48.
14. Higashi MK, Veenstra DL. Managed care in the genomics era: assessing the cost effectiveness of genetic tests. *Am J Manag Care*. 2003;9:493–500.
15. Root CB. Medicare coding and reimbursement for clinical laboratory services. *Clin Chem*. 1998;44:1713–1727.
16. Logue LJ. Genetic testing coverage and reimbursement: a provider's dilemma. *Clin Leadersh Manag Rev*. 2003;17:346–350.
17. Bernacki SH, Stankovic AK, Williams LO, et al. Establishment of stably EBV-transformed cell lines from residual clinical blood samples for use in performance evaluation and quality assurance in molecular genetic testing. *J Mol Diagn*. 2003;5:227–230.
18. Jarvis M, Iyer RK, Williams LO, et al. A novel method for creating artificial mutant samples for performance evaluation and quality control in clinical molecular genetics. *J Mol Diagn*. 2005;7:247–251.
19. Amos J, Patnaik M. Commercial molecular diagnostics in the U.S.: The Human Genome Project to the clinical laboratory. *Hum Mutat*. 2002;19:324–333.
20. Fortina P, Surrey S, Kricka LJ. Molecular diagnostics: hurdles for clinical implementation. *Trends Mol Med*. 2002;8:264–266.
21. Murphy PD. American College of Medical Genetics Intellectual Property Subcommittee of the Committee on the Economics of Genetic Services. Patent Primer. October 2003. Available at: http://www.acmg.net.
22. American Medical Association. Gene patenting. Available at: http://www.ama-assn.org/ama/pub/category/2314.html. Updated December 10, 2004.

23. Cho MK, Illangasekare S, Weaver MA, Leonard DG, Merz JF. Effects of patents and licenses on the provision of clinical genetic testing services. *J Mol Diagn.* 2003;5:3–8.

24. Tait JF, Intellectual Property Subcommittee of the Economics Committee of the ACMG. Points to consider in preparing license agreements for patented genetic tests. November 2004. Available at: http://www.acmg.net.

25. Association for Molecular Pathology. Recommendations for in-house development and operation of molecular diagnostic tests [statement]. *Am J Clin Pathol.* 1999;111:449–463.

26. Clinical and Laboratory Standards Institute. Available at: http://www.clsi.org.

27. Giardiello FM, Brensinger JD, Petersen GM, et al. The use and interpretation of commercial APC gene testing for familial adenomatous polyposis. *N Engl J Med.* 1997;336:823–827.

28. Sandhaus LM, Singer ME, Dawson NV, Wiesner GL. Reporting BRCA test results to primary care physicians. *Genet Med.* 2001;3:327–334.

29. Clinical Molecular Genetics Society. Best Practice Guidelines. Available at: http://www.cmgs.org/BPG/Default.htm.

30. Swiss Society of Medical Genetics. Best Practice Guidelines. Available at: http://www.ssgm.ch/sections/Documents/Statements/publications.htm.

31. European Molecular Genetics Quality Network. Best Practice Guidelines. Available at: http://www.emqn.org/bpguidelines.php.

32. Judkins T, Hendrickson BC, Deffenbaugh AM, Scholl T. Single nucleotide polymorphisms in clinical genetic testing: the characterization of the clinical significance of genetic variants and their application in clinical research for BRCA1. *Mutat Res.* 2005;573:168–179.

33. Check W. Fleshing out molecular pathology reports [and related articles by Check W and Gulley M]. CAP Today. February 2004. Available at: http://www.cap.org.

34. Available at: https://www.phppo.cdc.gov/dls/genetics/RareDiseaseConf.aspx.

35. Maddalena A, Bale S, Das S, Grody W, Richards S, ACMG Laboratory Quality Assurance Committee. Technical standards and guidelines: molecular genetic testing for ultra-rare disorders. *Genet Med.* 2005;7:571–583.

Index

CPSIA information can be obtained
at www.ICGtesting.com
Printed in the USA
LVHW06s1712160918
590309LV00005B/635/P